THE END OF
THE ROAD

THE END OF THE ROAD

THE FESTINA AFFAIR AND THE TOUR THAT ALMOST WRECKED CYCLING

ALASDAIR FOTHERINGHAM

BLOOMSBURY

LONDON · OXFORD · NEW YORK · NEW DELHI · SYDNEY

BLOOMSBURY SPORT
Bloomsbury Publishing Plc
50 Bedford Square, London, WC1B 3DP, UK
29 Earlsfort Terrace, Dublin 2, Ireland

First published 2016

British Library Cataloguing-in-Publication Data
A catalogue record for this book is available from the British Library.

Library of Congress Cataloguing-in-Publication data has been applied for.

ISBN: PB: 978-1-4729-1304-3
ePub: 978-1-4729-1305-0

Typeset in Adobe Garamond Pro by Deanta Global Publishing Services,
Chennai, India

MIX
Paper from
responsible sources
FSC® C013604

This book is dedicated to the memory of my father, Alex, who managed to write himself a cameo role in my recollections of the 1998 Tour after he came over to Dublin to see the Tour prologue and first stage. A bookseller by trade, my father also made the most of his visit to do a little bookdealing – as he would always do whenever he travelled any further than the end of his garden. But what was much more surprising was when he also somehow managed to inveigle his way past Dublin Castle security (no small matter in 1998 at least, and without a press pass, too) and into Bruno Roussel's press conference, standing behind a wooden screen to listen. After listening to Roussel's dismally inadequate explanation concerning Willy Voet's absence, my father came striding out from his hiding place and uttered in a theatrical whisper to me what proved to be very prescient words: 'what on earth is going to happen now?'

A NOTE ON THE AUTHOR

Alasdair Fotheringham is a freelance journalist, and was the cycling correspondent for the *Independent* and the *Independent on Sunday* from 2001 to 2016. He has covered 24 Tours de France and 20 Tours of Spain, the Olympics in 2008 and 2012 and numerous other major bike races. He is also a regular contributor to *Cyclingnews* and *ProCycling*. His previous books are *The Eagle of Toledo*, a biography of Spain's first Tour de France winner Federico Martín Bahamontes, and *Reckless: The Life and Times of Luis Ocaña*.

Contents

CONTENTS

Prologue

As Good As It Gets?

Saturday, 11 July. Prologue: Dublin–Dublin, 5.6 km

He stared at the toilet bowl, flushing away his drugs into Dublin's sewers. This should have been a highlight of his Tour, his year – his career, even. Because no matter how hardened the professional bike rider, taking part in a Tour de France prologue cannot fail to produce a little gooseflesh, a dash of anticipation. Cheered on by crowds lining the whole route for most of the peloton as they ride round, soaking up the applause, a Grand Tour prologue is a pleasurable, inconsequential reminder that they have made it to the pinnacle of the sport. As one-time Festina pro Christophe Bassons once put it: 'Eight minutes and 46 seconds of elation.' It couldn't get much better than that.

But for Rolf Aldag, a much valued domestique or team worker in the Telekom team for defending Tour champion Jan Ullrich, in Dublin it couldn't get much worse. Paranoia had kicked in, nerves were frayed to breaking point. At the very beginning of the Tour, it must have felt like the end of the road. His abiding memories of the 1998 Tour's start have nothing to do with racing at all. They have been eclipsed by recollections of sitting staring at a flushing toilet bowl in his team hotel room, watching his banned drugs spin out of sight, if not out of mind, as fast as possible.

Aldag was panicking for one simple, devastating reason: the arrest of Willy Voet, a soigneur from arch-rivals Festina, a few days earlier on the Franco-Belgian border. En route to the Tour de France,

Voet's team car had been found to be packed with an arsenal of illegal drugs. Everything was there that a team could need for a three-week race: 86 vials of human growth hormone (HGH) in two different formats, 60 capsules of Epistosterone, 248 vials of physiological serum, eight syringes containing hepatitis A vaccine, two boxes of Hyperlypen tablets (to lower fat levels in the blood), four ampules of Synacthene (to increase corticoid hormone production), two vials of amphetamines. And, most importantly of all, 234 doses of the banned, undetectable blood booster EPO.

In comparison, Aldag had in his suitcase just EPO – at the time the peloton's drug of choice. Nor was Voet providing 'gear' for the Telekom team. However, given Voet's arrest, and the waves of fear that an unprecedented arrest of this kind induced in a peloton where a significant percentage were involved in illegal doping, Aldag could only see one course of action: 'Flush it and peel the label off and put it in a plastic bag and really jump on it, those ampoules, and don't just put them in the trash, because there might be a policeman or journalist watching. We were so sure there was somebody in the hotel building following us, cars out there following us, so we had to stamp it into small pieces and get rid of it in the toilet. There it goes, 300 euros.'

Aldag argues this was not due to a sudden crisis of conscience: he, and many riders in the peloton, were well past that stage. Rather, this action was born purely out of fear of the police and French prisons.

'People were really screwed in their heads. Everybody was so confused. We pretended to be shocked about Festina's soigneur, and then we realised we had got so lucky. It was like, "now what" [do we do with our own supply]?

'For me, I didn't have a lot. It was already crazy to take it in my suitcase, but nobody was really aware of how wrong it was at that stage. It was part of the deal. It was only when the Festina scandal broke that it was like: "OK, shit".'

Somehow, suddenly, it felt as if the ground had shifted underneath the riders, and nobody could predict the consequences. All the riders knew was – they were vulnerable. And so was the Tour de France, the pinnacle of their sport.

1

Unbeatable Jan?

When you build a house of cards it is inevitable that one day it will collapse, no matter how firm the foundation. But in Rolf Aldag's case, long before Willy Voet's arrest left him feeling as if his cycling world could cave in at any minute, the German had also formed part of Telekom's spectacular rise to power in his sport. Their ascendancy, as Aldag sees it, didn't start with Jan Ullrich winning a Tour or any other rider succeeding: rather, it started with his team's radical change in racing mentality, on a day it *didn't* win. And it was all thanks to a tall, quiet, balding Dane whose biggest claim to fame up until then was as a Tour general classification (GC) outsider: third in the 1995 race, but not a likely winner in anyone's book, least of all Telekom's.

'It was a stage in the Midi Libre, 1996,' Aldag, blessed with a crystal-clear recollection of such incidents, recalls. 'There was a big, big break with all the top names in it – Rominger, Indurain, strong guys like [1994 Tour leader] Flavio Vanzella … And Bjarne [Riis] suddenly drops back to us in the bunch and says, "we have to chase." And we're like, "hello, where have you been for the last five years? This Indurain guy, he's won the Tour a few times recently", and Bjarne just says again "we chase."

'So we did. We chased all day. And we caught them 15 kilometres from the line. And the question we answered to ourselves that day was, "if we can catch these guys, why would we ever panic in the Tour? Who can attack that we can't pull back?" It made us mentally so strong, that in the Tour there was "no panic". It's just a matter of time and resistance: we will catch them. That was the big change. Bjarne was the team captain. He guided people and influenced them. The rest of us were too similar.'

On a single day Telekom went from being the rudderless formation of previous years to a squad which suddenly gained the self-belief it needed to win the Tour twice in a row, in 1996 and 1997. In 1995, Telekom had raced the Tour as part of a joint squad with ZG Mobili, winning two stages with Zabel. Yet as only 'half a team' and no overall contender to boot, Telekom could hardly be described as a key factor in the race. But 12 months later, Telekom gained a real sense of upwardly mobile purpose: suddenly it felt like anything was possible.

The 1996 Tour victory with Riis, Aldag – now a top team director – argues 'was the nicest of our victories because we were completely underestimated. I remember they had interviewed Bjarne during the previous winter, and he said he wanted to win the Tour. And we [the rest of the Telekom team] were all sitting in a room nearby and killing ourselves laughing listening to him, saying to ourselves, "there's this guy [Miguel Indurain] who's just won the Tour five times, what's so different now?"'

But when it came to the racing in the Tour itself, the riders – inspired by Riis in the Midi Libre – had fought hard. 'We figured the only way to survive was to support each other. Brian Holm was so ill he looked like he'd been in a war, but we were all there for each other, we all felt so keen to do that.'

By 1998, with two straight Tour victories in the bag, and Ullrich second in 1996 and the winner in 1997, Telekom were clearly the squad to beat. An initially difficult power relationship between Riis and Ullrich in the 1997 Tour de France had been resolved, too – in favour of the German.

'On paper, 1998 should have been a lot easier than 1997, because in 1996 Riis and Ullrich were first and second. So in 1997 it was clear that Bjarne, as the defending champion, could ask for a protected role.'

However, given the title sponsors were German and it was a German team, 'everybody understood that a win with Jan Ullrich was going to be 20 times bigger than in 1996.' (Already, as a podium finisher in 1996, Ullrich was Germany's first top three Tour finisher since Kurt Stöpel in 1932.) Thus, when Ullrich won in 1997, after claiming a key stage to Andorra when he first donned the yellow jersey, fortunately for Telekom it was with Riis's blessing. 'Ullrich's second place in 1996 had been a huge surprise, but in 1997, the only reason he attacked to Andorra was because Bjarne told him to go. Otherwise, he was a loyal kid: if he'd raced in his own interests he could have won the Tour in 1996.'

Rather, Aldag argues, 'he did not think too much about different options and that made his life simpler. He didn't get super-stressed.' And after winning the time trial in St-Etienne, Ullrich was en route to Germany's first ever Tour de France victory. By 1998, with the Riis–Ullrich power struggle resolved, rather it was Ullrich's weight issues that had briefly worried the team. Riis wrote in his autobiography that he and Ullrich 'looked like they had just got up from the buffet table' at the start of the season. But by July the team doctor insisted Ullrich had the same weight as in 1997 – 73 kilos after going up to 87 during the off-season – and two and a half hours of testing at Freiburg had indicated he was in good shape.

In fact, there was more concern that Ullrich's chances of becoming the twelfth rider to win the Tour twice in a row were under threat in other ways. The opposition looked stronger than ever: Festina, led by French champion Richard Virenque, had an even more formidable line-up than usual after their signing of

Swiss powerhouse Alex Zülle, already a double Vuelta a España winner and second in the 1995 Tour de France. Marco Pantani, the Italian climber, had just taken an exceptionally impressive victory in the Giro d'Italia in May. The Spanish Banesto squad, jointly headed by former double World Champion Abraham Olano with his firebrand co-leader José María Jiménez, was another major threat. Telekom knew that they could not rule out Laurent Jalabert, ranked the world's number one as the Tour began by a massive margin – 2,937 points compared to his closest pursuer Alex Zülle, with 2,201 – and his ONCE squad either. Prior to Riis putting Miguel Indurain to the sword in the 1996 Tour de France, the Spanish team had been the only one serious to trouble the Spaniard in the Tour de France in five years, with their mass attack on the stage to Mende airfield in 1995.

Telekom might have looked powerful on the outside but, as Aldag points out, the team was a mishmash of different cultures and potential conflicts, some only recently resolved, like Riis v. Ullrich. It didn't help either that the two leaders for the Tour's number one team could not have been more different: there was the vastly experienced Riis, from a small agricultural town in the flatlands of central Denmark, and Ullrich, ten years younger, and born in former East Germany in the industrial city of Rostock.

There were other bizarre, more inbuilt, contradictions in Telekom. The squad itself was directed by two former top Belgian pros, Rudy Pevenage and Walter Godefroot, and they ensured the team's structure was identical to any other squad from their native Flanders, the region that was – and still is – one of cycling's powerhouses. But while the financing was mainly West German and the day-to-day dynamics Flemish, the team's training structure and racing mentality – in Ullrich's case – came, 100 per cent, from East Germany. And it did not matter that the Berlin Wall had fallen nearly a decade previously. 'Our training plans did not change for 15 years,' says Aldag, who joined Telekom the year after it started in 1992 and remained with it until he retired in 2006.

'The thing was [following the reunification] the power stayed in West Germany but the cycling knowledge came from the East.' The former GDR was also where the country's top sports schools were located – to this day pros like Tony Martin and even Rik Zabel, the young son of Erik, the Telekom sprinter on the 1998 Tour, have cut their teeth as riders in these centres – and where Peter Becker, Telekom's trainer, had done much of his work. The arrival of some top former East German pros like Olaf Ludwig and Uwe Raab in the squad in 1993 only reinforced that tendency, 'and Godefroot was happy to leave [the training strategies] all to others because he had no idea what they were talking about'. It was, he says, a question of 'copying and pasting East Germany plans … from 1993 to 1998 it was a Belgian team with an East German training system'. Only by 2002 or 2003, 'when Walter stepped back', did Telekom really change.

This ultra-conservative attitude to training and dislike of innovation or improvisation extended to their leader: in fact, as had been seen when Ullrich came within a whisker of losing the Tour in 1997 when he was isolated by Festina with a surprise attack in the Vosges, no one else suffered worse from that lack of initiative than Ullrich himself. This failure to handle critical situations proved crucial, too, in the outcome of the 1998 race. If Ullrich was the favourite for that year, and Telekom had come 'to win it no matter what', as Aldag puts it, his innate shyness, uncharismatic personality and unexciting riding style meant he was anything but a natural leader. Instead, that role remained with Riis, just as it had done since June 1996, and his prominent role was to prove crucial in the fate of the 1998 Tour, and not just in terms of the racing.

According to Aldag, 1998's real issue inside Telekom, prior to the Festina scandal, was the increased desire among the team to benefit personally from the wave of success. Zabel, for example, had won the green jersey in 1996 and 1997, as well as seven stages, but had no leadout man. 'Jan had to defend his title, Bjarne was the road captain, and the rest of us were simply there. But then with that success you feel like a star, so it's more, "what do I get out of this?"'

Aldag points to a stage win for Heppner early on in the 1998 Tour as representative of the team domestiques' craving for a slice of the glory, and the evident risks that went alongside a group mentality where 'we never thought anyone could beat us'. During seven years of Lance Armstrong's rule at the top he points out, only one of the American's team-mates, George Hincapie, took a stage win. The chinks in the Telekom armour were there in many other ways, too, such as a dearth of mountain support for Jan, certainly not to stage a counter-attack if a climber began to threaten the German hegemony. Udo Bölts was on the squad and had performed well in the mountains many times, but he was more of an all-rounder whose strongest point was climbing. Telekom lacked the riders, in Aldag's opinion, 'to put a team like Marco Pantani's' – by far the most dangerous mountain climber in the race – 'under pressure'.

Would the drain on drugs provoked by Voet's arrest have worried Ullrich's team? Only up to a point, given that EPO was generally taken by riders prior to a race. 'You got there and the level was high, what I did then was take something once in a while because then it would last for a certain amount of time.

'You had this cooling stuff there that you could put in your suitcase, so that would keep it cool for 24 hours; you can store it for another 48 hours without cooling and that brings you into the third day and after that you don't really need it.'

Besides, as Aldag pointed out, 'When we came back to the Continent, you could have always got something if you really needed it. There was no testing, so they can never prove it, they can't prove it's from my toilet, it was more "hey, we got lucky". We were just happy it's somebody else's problem.' However, as the affair mushroomed, that was unlikely to remain the case.

Drugs scandals like the one breaking at the start of the Tour de France were hardly new in cycling. But the intervention of the police, rather than the anti-doping authorities, the possible penal consequences for some of the protagonists, and above all the scale of the amount of doping products seized brought the Voet affair into a new, completely unknown dimension for the sport. As French newspaper *Le Journal du Dimanche* reported the weekend the scandal broke, 'Marie-George Buffet, the French Minister of Sport, warned that "the consequence of this affair for the 1998 Tour could be disastrous if the enquiry establishes a link between these products, their destination and a French team".' Given Voet worked for Festina, France's number one squad, and was en route to Ireland, that link was already clear in most of the peloton's and the public's minds. The riders' overarching fear, therefore, was that the link turned into a chain of doping allegations – and of yet more police raids that could drag them all down.

'As is natural, [riders would] pretend to be really shocked and pretend you're the cleanest team on the planet,' Aldag says. 'The only shock was like, "shit, now it all blows" ... police methods to question them, that was the real shock.'

Even worse, they could not blame the police in themselves, Aldag felt. 'My assumption was we all do the same shit, so if we get caught, it's a risk you take. And if you don't get caught, then you continue riding your bike because that's what we're here for.

'Ultimately, we'd done something wrong and the police had the right to do it. It's not like they put EPO in our suitcases, so if they find it, what else should they do? You have to expect it.

'Dublin was just one big chaos after Festina, that's what sticks in the memory,' Aldag recalls. 'Voet's arrest dragged everybody off course, there was no focus any more from that moment.'

The news of Voet's arrest had been passed on to Aldag from the usual source of gossip in the peloton at the time, the community of soigneurs. The team back-up staff were all working for different teams, but as Aldag puts it, 'they were all connected to each other', and, therefore the first to hear what had happened to one of their co-workers. The fact that they worked for all the teams meant that the impact of Voet's arrest was felt deeply, too, and the reaction was instantaneous: 'the feeling in the peloton was that everybody was just busy getting rid of the shit [drugs].'

The similarities between Telekom's system for acquiring doping products and the Festina case can only have reinforced the sense of urgency. As Aldag explains, up until the end of 1996 they too had channelled their products through a particular soigneur – in Telekom's case, Jeff D'Hont, who, like Voet, came from the cycling heartland of Flanders.

'D'Hont had a book where he wrote down what had to be used. Obviously he had other names in there, so that's why I'm pretty sure others used stuff as well. So to give an example, in 1996 or before, I'd go to his room, and he'd say we should do this and this. I'd say, "OK, if you think so". He writes it down, he marks a number behind it, and after two weeks he says, I get 365 German Marks from you, this is the list we used. He doesn't have a licence as a doctor, but is it interesting for me where he gets it? No. And do I really want to know about others? No, not really.

'That was the most extreme, because if you asked him he'd say, "it's for the breathing". And what is this? "it's for the power". So whatever, OK, it means everybody is in the dark.'

After D'Hont moved on to French team FDJ.fr. Aldag says he used a doctor employed by the University of Freiburg. 'They got into this more and more, but it wasn't that much of a different system. I paid it straight to one of the doctors in cash, so I had no idea ... Normal medication was delivered by the team, Vitamin C and B and iron, and that special stuff, in my case, I always paid to one single person in cash.' However, once the news broke that Voet had been arrested, Aldag regarded the 'special stuff' in his case as close to radioactive.

Mutual mistrust and extreme secrecy enshrouding doping in Telekom meant there was no group decision to ditch the drugs. In the case of Bjarne Riis, as the 1996 Tour winner and Aldag's team-mate puts it in his autobiography, the Dane opted to wait until the race's return to France to dispose of his EPO. Riis acted on the rumour – false, as it turned out – that the police would indeed be descending shortly on the Telekom hotel. 'I gathered together all my syringes of EPO and rushed into my hotel bedroom,' he wrote in *Riis: Stages of Light and Dark*. 'I squirted the lot down the toilet and then set about carefully removing any evidence that it had ever existed.'

As Aldag explains, inside Telekom most riders' doping operations were – in 1998 – one-man shows, even if they mostly used the same supplier. The reason was simple: the potential for blackmail. 'I never was a witness of anybody sticking a needle of EPO into their arm, it would be stupid to do. I know people may not want to accept this, but why would a team manager or director bring himself into that situation?' he argues. 'Next year we would have to negotiate a contact, and I could stay there and say, "hey, you remember Dublin when you prepared the EPO for me. You want to cut my salary? You want to fire me? That's going to be fine, but you're going down with me."'

Nor did riders in Telekom discuss their doping among themselves, 'because imagine your room-mate takes nothing, you'd look like a complete idiot. And then it's also like the next level could be "he's better because he takes more". All that crap, you could avoid it' – by staying silent. There was no doubt that doping was frequent, although there is clear evidence, too, that some key individuals did not participate. 'Everybody knew it existed, nobody talked about it clearly.' To illustrate his point, 'if there was an attack in the peloton and then [somebody would yell out] "hey, here we go, 10,000 units! [of EPO]", you wouldn't get people [commenting] "hey, what does he mean, 10,000 units?" It was just so widespread.'

The tension at Dublin only eased slightly thanks to Chris Boardman and a French team taking the opening prologue, and therefore the control of the race from an early stage. It was also, ironically, a win for one of the few riders from the 1998 Tour de France never to have any links to a doping scandal, and who won, Boardman now says, precisely because he did not think he could do so any longer in the context of an increasingly drug-riddled sport. As he puts it, 'I won because I didn't expect to win.'

By this late point in his career, 'Racing [time trials] had become so unpredictable, it was depressing, you could have the form of your life and you'd get battered,' he now explains. 'Climbers could go as fast as you in one race, and then the next minute it'd be like, "oh, I can win something."

'I won it because I didn't think I was going to win so I didn't overextend' – a term which means racing too hard, too soon, in an event, and not leaving enough energy for a last sector that was, in Dublin, to prove crucial.

As Boardman reveals, 'I won it on the last corner, actually, with 700 metres to go which then led into a drag up to the line. If you got the corner wrong, which most people did cos you couldn't see round it, you'd kill your speed, and then spend most of your energy on the drag re-accelerating. But if you got it right and saved something, then you could make up huge amounts in the last part,' which was what he did.

When the classification finally became clear, Boardman had managed to go flat-out for victory by a margin of four seconds.

Describing it as his best prologue win ever – he had also won in 1994 and 1997 – at the time Boardman admitted ruefully that he could remember every detail of all of them, but that he struggled to recall the dates of his children's birthdays. He had overcome any fears of risk-taking, he said, on the circuit's five tricky corners, still drying out from the afternoon's heavy showers, 'by persuading myself it wasn't raining.' There was a nice personal touch when he dedicated it to his wife, Sally, although the reality behind that gesture was, as now emerges, much bleaker than suspected at the time, given Boardman and his wife were in the midst of major marital difficulties. It had been a fine result, with the second-fastest average speed for a prologue in the history of the Tour at 54.19 kmh – behind his own record at Lille. Boardman had managed to clock the fastest time at the midway point, and while there was a gap of four seconds between himself and runner-up Abraham Olano, the next six finishers were within an arc of some four seconds. Ullrich, meanwhile, had finished sixth.

Aldag on the other hand was fielding very different questions – the first battery of those about doping. '[I was] not happy getting the questions, we used to get them once every three years: "are you doing it clean?" But then [in the 1998 Tour] you had those questions 15 times a day, a minute. It was the first time it was really like that.'

But in the 1998 Tour it was certainly not the last.

2

'And When Did You Last See Your Soigneur?'

Sunday, 12 July. Stage 1: Dublin–Dublin, 180.5 km

Under normal circumstances, Dublin Castle would have felt like an odd place for a press conference about a bike race. The metal detectors and rigorous inspection of journalists' computer bags every time they entered the Tour's main press room made the castle an uninviting place to work. But given the scale of difficulties entangling the Festina squad, suddenly the castle did seem the place for the beleaguered French team to give its first press conference about a certain missing soigneur. After all, weren't castles built to withstand sieges?

By the end of Sunday's first stage – won in fairly uneventful style by Tom Steels, the Belgian sprinter, with Chris Boardman retaining the overall lead – Festina's efforts to circle up the wagons, as the media onslaught grew ever heavier, were more like fire-fighting exercises than an all-out defence. Their main problem was that there were too many variables: Festina had no idea of how serious the situation could become. They did not even know whether Voet, having been arrested with so many drugs in his team car, had confessed that they were for the entire team.

It was verbal shadow-boxing territory and sports director Bruno Roussel certainly looked alone and visibly stressed out as he faced the phalanx of journalists. He cut a solitary figure, too, seated at a long, broad table in an echoing, wood-panelled dining hall. As the questions rained down on him – when had he last been in touch with Voet? Did he know of Voet's current whereabouts? – Roussel's vulnerability was palpable. It was not so much a case of 'And When Did You Last See Your Father?' as 'And When Did You Last See Your Soigneur?'

Sitting beneath an enormous photograph of Dublin Castle and a giant logo of the Tour de France, Roussel's answers about Festina's missing soigneur seemed deliberately evasive. He clumsily stuck to one key line of defence. It was essentially the same answer he had given to race director Jean-Marie Leblanc, and Jean-Claude Killy, the head of ASO, the Tour's organisers, when he met them at seven o'clock on the morning of the prologue in order to avoid prying journalists. Roussel had no idea, he told ASO and the press, where his team soigneur Willy Voet was; all he knew was that a soigneur was missing. He even said that there had been some sort of confusion over the identity of the missing masseur, that he had thought at one point it could have been Michel Gros, the team's second sports director.

Roussel confirmed, though, that Festina's team *service course* in Lyon had been raided by police (twice, by that point), that 'we mustn't throw suspicion on riders who have always behaved properly, thinking that all their results are due to doping'. It was, he said, inconceivable that the team be excluded, or pull out itself, from the race.

Fed up with so much evident ducking and diving, Jean-Yves Donor, the long-standing cycling correspondent for *Le Figaro*, asked Roussel point-blank whether it might be better to tell the truth. Roussel slowly answered: 'What truth? I just want to get back to France.'

The truth was that Festina, at the time of the 1998 Tour, was ranked number one team in the world. But like a circus elephant perilously perched on a tiny ball, a significant degree of the squad's success pivoted on one dangerously tiny axis: Willy Voet and his access, via logistics manager Joel Chabiron and suppliers in Portugal, to a steady flow of banned drugs. As a result and as Roussel knew perfectly well, ever since 6.35 on the Wednesday morning, when Voet had been arrested 200 yards into France, Festina risked being at the centre of what the *Guardian* had already described as 'cycling's greatest ever doping scandal'. On the other side of the Irish Sea they were hardly more sympathetic: 'Tour de Farce,' snarled that weekend's edition of the now-defunct Dublin-based *Sunday Tribune*.

Since the Wednesday afternoon, when he had received a call from Festina's Michel Gros in Meyzieu, the Festina team HQ, Roussel knew exactly where Voet was, too: in custody in Lille. Gros had informed him that the French police had paid a lengthy visit to Meyzieu, seizing more medical products. Another search was then carried out two days later.

By Saturday, Voet had already been placed under formal investigation (an intermediary step in French law prior to charges being made) by the judge Patrick Keil in Lille, close to where he had been arrested, for 'the importation of banned products and the illicit transport of banned products'. Roussel had already informed his leader, Virenque, of Voet's arrest. His reponse, Roussel claimed, was brutally self-centred: 'and how am I going to perform without my products?'

Roussel had then gone on to inform the Festina staff and squad, staying at a hotel some 50 kilometres south of Dublin, that Voet was in the hands of the authorities. Then, when the riders headed for the team presentation in Dublin on Friday, he urged them to ignore any questions about Voet's non-appearance.

'That afternoon, the nightmare started,' Roussel recounts in his autobiography. 'At the other end of my phone, Sylvie Voet was in a right state.'

'Willy's in prison, Bruno. Don't let him go down, eh?'

By that point, too, on the Friday evening Roussel had attended a reception in Phoenix Park to commemorate the Tour's departure, where he had met, for the first time, the French Minister for Youth and Sport, Marie-George Buffet. Buffet had greeted Roussel with a smile, but she already knew, he says, of Voet's arrest.

'Before the Tour started, I remember I asked Bruno if he knew where Willy Voet was,' comments Jean Montois, AFP's long-standing cycling correspondent, who broke the news of the Belgian's arrest to the Tour management on Friday afternoon while they were watching the teams' presentation ceremony in central Dublin. 'He insisted he had no idea, but only after a long silence. I could see him hesitating.'

As for the top Festina Tour riders, Roussel argues that their principal concern was 'how to face up to this sudden crisis'. But in some cases they were not so worried about the team's survival; rather, they were concerned about breaks in the supply line of their banned drugs. Less than a week after Voet's arrest, Roussel says, 'a new source' for the drugs had been found and a fresh possible supply route established. But the team's fate, in any case, still remained intrinsically linked to their old one.

At that point, Festina was not just ranked professional cycling's top team: in France it was bordering on 'national treasure' status. Among French fans in particular and the public in general, Richard Virenque-mania was at its height in his homeland and the squad was rubbing shoulders with the French political establishment, even hobnobbing with President Jacques Chirac and his wife, Bernadette.

A month before the 1998 Tour, for example, Jean-Marie Leblanc had called Roussel to ask if any of his riders could visit the Corrèze region, which the Tour was visiting on stage seven. The request had come from an adviser of Mme Chirac, at the time one of the Corrèze department's leading authorities. Mme Chirac wanted to do a special pre-stage TV report in order to highlight both its tourist attractions and her own involvement in the area. Roussel was so enthusiastic about the project that he brought not just one rider, but the whole Tour de France line-up, the Festina team bus and the mechanics' truck. The TV feature closed with a debate between Roussel, Jean-Marie Leblanc – 'praising him for his professionalism,' Leblanc recalls – and Mme Chirac.

Given the ensuing developments in the Tour, the feature was quietly dropped from stage seven's coverage. However, the reportage (to this day still not broadcast) remains a good indicator of how Festina was moving in some of the highest circles of France's social and political elite.

It didn't matter, apparently, that Festina was actually a foreign team. A watch-making company from Andorra, Festina had taken over as the main sponsors of a medium-sized Spanish squad, Zahor, in 1989, briefly using the brand name Lotus, one of their lines of watches. Then, when it merged with the Dutch squad PDM in 1993, the renamed Festina team continued to be registered in the principality of Andorra, and Miguel Moreno, one of Spain's top directors, stayed on the team books but was joined by Jan Giesbers, the former PDM boss. Thanks to the merger, Eric Rijckaert, the Flemish doctor who was to become a key figure in the Festina scandal, also came on board.

Key elements from a French team, RMO, further swelled the ranks of Festina after RMO's initial plan of renewed financial backing from a mysterious Arab prince to avoid folding collapsed in dramatic style. The 'prince' first wheedled a spectacular sum of money from the previous RMO management that he claimed he needed to release £5 million from his Swiss bank account to fund the squad in its provisional new 1993 format. Then he disappeared without a trace. It later emerged the so-called prince was an international conman.

RMO's riders and management now had to look fast and hard for an alternative employer, with Voet, Virenque and Roussel, as well as long-standing 1992 Tour leader Pascal Lino all joining Festina. It was not an ideal choice: after the three-way merger, Festina was an ungainly squad, with 50 riders on its books, of whom only some 35 actually raced. Furthermore, each former part of the squad – PDM, the old core of Festina riders and the RMO group – initially formed their own cliques.

Lack of management leadership did not help matters. 'Jan Giesbers directed the team but without much authority,' Virenque claimed in his second autobiography. 'We practically didn't see him, at the start of the season we had no bikes, no equipment.' Finally, following a scandal in May 1993 where Festina riders were accused of selling their services to the Banesto team during the Giro d'Italia – won by Banesto's Miguel Indurain – Giesbers was shown the door and Roussel found himself running the team.

Voet, though, would have been familiar to most of the Festina riders regardless of their background. Even if he was largely unknown to the general public, he was a long-standing figure in cycling's backstage world. Born in July 1945 in Belgium, Voet had a brief, unsuccessful amateur career before working briefly as a bus driver then returning to cycling as a soigneur in 1975. Prior to Festina he had worked in nine other teams, mostly Belgian, Dutch or French, where he forged a reputation as a Mr Fixit.

'He sorted out everybody,' Roussel commented, '… toothpaste, a missing spectacle lens, a little something wrong with your knee or your heart. He always found the right word or the right thing. His organisational skills were not poor, either. So good that the Willy I knew at RMO, whether it was taking musettes to the feed station or carrying suitcases, became the doctor's right hand at the races.' Such was Voet's dedication and attention to detail that when, as ever, at hand for the riders' breakfast, he would even bring them a missing spoon to save them another trip to the buffet table.

Anybody who reads Voet's *Breaking the Chain*, his slim autobiography published following his arrest and 16 days in prison, will realise that Voet was not just good at logistics. He was a home-grown expert both in doping products and in avoiding getting caught using them. For page after page in his book Voet interweaves the stories of his arrest, subsequent detention and police statements on the inner machinations of doping at Festina with a series of anecdotes centring on banned drug use in cycling. He also relates, in sometimes vivid detail, the procedures employed by different generations of riders for dodging positive dope tests. These ranged from sodium drips hung from picture hooks in hotel rooms for lowering hematocrit levels prior to dope testing, to condoms of untainted urine used by riders to provide non-doped samples during the testing itself. The condom would be inserted into the anus – 'handy for warming it up and giving it extra authenticity' he points out with almost gleeful practicality – with a tube coming out of one end then curving round the perineum. Most commissaires, Voet claims, had never noticed the difference between human 'plumbing' and the artificial kind used during tests, until one rider unwisely boasted about its effectiveness to someone connected to the anti-doping authorities, after which that particular method was consigned to the unofficial history books.

Voet was also both witness to and participant in the changing fashions and trends in the types of drug used – banned or otherwise – in the sport. As a soigneur he gave his first intravenous injection to 1968 Tour winner Jan Janssens, with 'stuff to help recovery'. Then he 'went through the full spectrum. Amphetamines injected into the arm or the stomach, corticoids, steroids, anabolic agents, even testosterone. Daily rituals, nothing out of the ordinary.' Amphetamines became less popular because they later were detected in doping tests, 'but until the start of the 1980s, drug tests were as sophisticated as a gasworks ...

'No one thought of it as fraud, cheating or dangerous,' he writes, although he does cite cases of top riders, like France's Charly Mottet at RMO, refusing to have anything to do with them. Another, in Festina, was Christophe Bassons, who was later hounded out of the sport over his refusal to maintain the *omertà* surrounding banned drug use. However, it is hard to avoid the impression that the Bassons, Boardmans and Mottets of this world were the exception that proved the rule. Or, as Voet puts it: 'Drug taking is to top-level sport what batons are to a troupe of cheerleaders: you rarely find one without the other.'

Voet was also – as was the case for many of those involved in maintaining the cheating that for decades permeated parts of cycling – a very keen fan of the sport. It may seem impossible to square Voet's cynical observation of how some results were obtained, acquired through insider knowledge, with his love of the sport, but such a contradiction was very much the norm within some sectors of the professional cycling world in its pre-1998, pre-Armstrong format. Every year, for example, Voet would drive his family to the French national championships. He describes in his autobiography how in 1997 he dined with the Festina riders the evening before the race, ordered champagne because it was his birthday, nipped upstairs to their rooms to inject a dose of cortisone into the buttocks of five Festina riders, came back down and drank some more champagne, watched the race the following day then drove home – his wife in the family car, he with a team vehicle. All in a day's work, in other words. At Festina, he wrote, he 'lived out his passion for cycling'.

For all that his father was a top amateur rider and then a trainer of the French junior team, Bruno Roussel himself was rather less conventional – and as one top insider comments, 'that meant he wasn't liked'. First a coach then a director, Roussel's first team as a manager was the US Creteil amateur squad based outside Paris. He then moved into the professional world with the Swiss squad Helvetia in 1990 before heading RMO – where he was to come across both Voet and Virenque – in 1991.

Roussel had the ability to micro-manage and a love of logistics; with 25 riders on the team's books, years later he could still recall the exact flight schedules of individual riders. But he was also an innovator. Festina were the first team to organise riders' reconnaissances of Tour mountain stages and time trial stages prior to July, for example. Their attention to detail even embraced the hotels they would use in the race so they could check out which rooms were the least noisy – 'overlooking a park rather than an airfield' – and could therefore be sure to maximise riders' recuperation.

Years before Team Sky made 'controlling the controllables' one of their key catchphrases in their drive to spearhead the modernisation of the sport, then, Roussel was doing the same thing, only he described it as 'minimising what was left to chance'. Equally, rather than leaving it up to the last minute or creating a 'long list' in mid-May, as teams even now are wont to do, Roussel would choose the nine Tour riders the winter before.

His crucial decision in 1993 was to act on Voet's advice and talk to Rijckaert about Festina's lack of results during the early Classics campaign and the lack of understanding between the different 'clans' – the Festina, the RMO and the PDM cliques – in the squad. Rijckaert's proposal was, as Roussel puts it, to modernise Festina's doping, and run it as an organised team operation. His argument is that given professional cycling 'has become medicalisation on a grand scale ... pills in the morning, injections in the evening, drips to speed up the recovery process', it is best to keep it 'under medical control ... to limit the excess'. After three days' reflection, Roussel agreed, and Rijckaert began producing personalised doping plans. As Daniel Delegove, the judge overseeing the Festina trial in 2000, wrote: 'he was the instigator, the conceiver, the director and the organiser of the system in place in Festina.'

But there were, Roussel says, limits designed to protect riders' health. Hematocrit levels, an indirect indication of EPO use, were only allowed up to 54 per cent, six points lower than some notorious cases in cycling and only four points above the 50 per cent barrier later introduced by the UCI.

However, these limits, along with his hands-off policy for the running of the doping programme, were also a means for Roussel to maintain a distance from the chemicals powering the Festina machine. It is noticeable that for the first 60 pages of his autobiography, for all its suggestive title, *Tour de Vices*, there is not one mention of the team's banned drug use. Then, when he does refer to doping, a word he uses for doping products and their use – *soins* 'care' – initially makes no reference to its illegality. Roussel kept his head in the sand in other ways, too. On the team bus purchased from the almost equally nefarious PDM team, for example, a false TV screen was used to hide a hugely sophisticated piece of equipment – price €30,000 – used to measure the riders' different blood values, among them hematocrit. However, Roussel did not, unlike Voet and Rijckaert, have a key. Similarly, when the two Belgians discussed the doping programmes on the squad, they would do so in Flemish, a language Roussel did not speak.

Can we label this purely and simply as an exercise in self-deception? Perhaps. Perhaps it was also a way of ensuring that, as Aldag said happened in Telekom, there was less chance of Roussel's finding himself blackmailed by unscrupulous riders. But, finally, it was an indication how compartmentalised doping had become in the sport and how straightforward that made it for figures like Roussel to operate on different levels. With so many barriers in place, it was easier for Roussel to keep the fact he was overseeing a highly elaborate and systematic programme of cheating almost entirely separate from his everyday thought processes.

The sense that this was not really cheating was reinforced by the widespread belief that, as Voet says, 'everybody had the same weapons', and that the playing field was somehow more level because everybody cheated to the same degree. This theory, which still has a number of exponents in cycling, has several large holes in it, and it's worth a brief digression to explain what they are. Firstly, and simply, not everybody did cheat to the same degree and some did not cheat at all. Secondly, the argument ignores the fact that different riders have different reactions to drugs, banned or otherwise, even assuming the drugs used were exactly the same type. And they were not, neither from one rider to another nor from one year to another. The effects of these differing circumstances were never so noticeable, either, as in the 1990s in cycling, when, as Voet himself put it, 'The difference was that the old drugs helped a rider to maximise his own potential. The new drugs transformed the rider.'

Michele Ferrari saw things differently, stating in July 1996, 'If a doping technique becomes widespread, then the level of the riders goes back to what it was. A donkey remains a donkey and a champion remains a champion. It's just that both are charging uselessly and risking their health for the same results they would have had anyway.' This kind of generalisation implies doping techniques have the same effects on all riders. But they did not – and do not – have the same effects, just as legal performance-enhancing activities, like altitude training, cannot affect riders the same way. What Ferrari's comments show is not just an invitation to self-deception, they also subtly edge people who are already doping towards a series of questions: if I'm cheating anyway, what products out there would break the stalemate with the other dopers, do me less damage, and where can I get them? Ferrari would, as it emerged, be only too happy to provide answers.

In Roussel's case, just like in Telekom, this nether-world of doping was only occasionally visible above the surface of the team's everyday existence. Not that that mattered too much either way; it was all seen as part of the deal. 'After four years there came a point,' Roussel writes, 'that we did not distinguish the good from the bad, the authorised from the forbidden.'

Yet this hidden world and the success it brought with it was, even before the 1998 Tour, threatening to overwhelm Roussel's control of the squad. As Virenque's popularity continued to rise in France, in part thanks to his steadily improving performances, his ego grew correspondingly larger, and he became less willing to listen to Roussel. For example, Roussel's attempts to reduce the number of interviews Virenque gave – far more than his rivals and considerably reducing his recovery time – failed miserably. At the same, time, the riders closest to Virenque – Pascal Hervé, the reigning World Champion Laurent Brochard, Didier Rous and Christophe Moreau – often left Roussel in no doubt where their loyalties lay, too.

'We were a little blinded by Virenque's aura. His stardom. The enthusiasm there was around him,' Brochard said in an interview in 2014. 'We benefited from that, too.'

'He wasn't just an individualist attracted by TV cameras. I think he was always [if a team-mate won] very happy. Even if it wasn't him, it was his team.'

It reached the point in the 1997 Tour, Roussel recounts, that not only Virenque but his entire clique of riders – nicknamed 'The Barons' – ignored the management. On one stage in the Alps, to Morzine, Roussel specifically ordered the squad not to work chasing down breaks. But when Roussel drove alongside the bunch, it was to find Festina, spearheaded by Brochard and Hervé, leading the charge behind a harmless lone attacker – Laurent Jalabert, by then no longer a threat – on Virenque's orders.

The division between Virenque and Roussel grew even wider when news broke in the third week of the 1997 Tour that Festina had signed double Vuelta winner Alex Zülle as their new co-leader for 1998. Virenque, sensing that he might be sidelined, was furious, but there was no denying that, compared to the Frenchman, Zülle had a better chance of winning the Tour. Festina, whose salary for their new star was the equivalent of €1.6 million a season – making Zülle the best paid rider in the peloton – certainly thought so.

Virenque's strategic ineptness at winning Grand Tours of any kind had become painfully clear in the third week of the 1997 race, when he and Festina had Ullrich up against the ropes in one stage through the Vosges. After shaking off the German – who was suffering from a bad stomach – early on, Virenque and three team-mates found themselves in a group of favourites ahead of Ullrich and with 80 km left to race. Telekom, meanwhile, were scattered to the four winds, with only one rider, Udo Bölts, left with Ullrich.

Under the circumstances, Virenque could, with some deft negotiation and working alliances with the other top names in the front group – Olano, Pantani among them – have gained a huge margin on the German. Instead, he failed to convince the other riders and, with Roussel stuck in race traffic behind and unable to act as negotiator, the front move fizzled out. Yet for all Roussel's frustration afterwards, who was Roussel to risk attacking the goose that laid the golden eggs?

'I think I can claim, without boasting, that due to what I have achieved in my sport, I am the incarnation of its top values: courage, overcoming one's natural limits, the refusal to admit defeat in any battle. This chivalric spirit pleases me, it chimes with the strong feelings I have about riding a bike.'

So writes Richard Virenque in his 2002 autobiography. Despite finally confessing to doping, two years after the 1998

Tour, Virenque himself clearly still felt his nicknames of Richard Lionheart or Sir Richard remained untainted.

This was self-delusion on a grand scale. To a significant part of the French public after the 1998 Tour Virenque had become little more than a caricature of himself. This went right down to a sketch of *Les Guignoles*, France's equivalent of *Spitting Image*, where with his new, post-1998, team Virenque was incapable of eating – preferring to stick the fork into his arm, saying that 'in Festina, these only had one tine'. (His new team end up giving him a bib, which proves pointless since he then attempts to inject himself with a bottle of water.) There was one of Virenque's alleged comments when denying he did not dope, *'à l'insu de mon plein gré'* (willingly but not knowingly), which has, as Wikipedia puts it so adroitly, 'passed into French popular culture as a sign of hypocritical denial'.

Virenque's fall from grace was a heavy one, particularly for a figure who was so venerated. It is worth recalling, given all the media fallout of the 1998 race, that in *L'Equipe*'s history of the Tour, 1997's race carries the headline 'Virenque, the semi-god'.

'If Raymond Poulidor' – the most popular French rider of the 1960s and 1970s – 'was popular for his earthly wisdom, Virenque is a star on tour,' the article insists. 'We identified with the former, we are carried away by the second. The first is a friendly uncle, the second the boyfriend or son-in-law who excites us ... who turns us on.'

This was no exaggeration. By 1997, Virenque – courageous, passionate, headstrong and magnetic, with his little-boy-lost curls and swarthy looks provoked widespread physical attraction and motherly feelings in France. So popular was he with the French public that he comfortably outstripped previous, far more successful local idols of the sport.

His impetuous attacking style in the mountains, the long lone breaks, the constant facial expressions every time a TV camera came near him as he was riding along – all were part of the

Virenque show, all part of his appeal. His fans crammed the mountainsides, too, wearing the polka-dot jersey of the Tour's King of the Mountains – for which Virenque holds the all-time record number of titles – and waving red-dotted posters with a hundred different varieties of the *Allez Richard* versions. Deafening chants of *Ree-chard, Ree-chard* as fans surrounded the team bus for day after day were equally inescapable (and increasingly irritating and tedious for Tour journalists), while his tactical blunders were generously overlooked in most quarters. In 1997, Ullrich's final victory margin of 9′ 9″ over Virenque had made it clear who was the head of the Tour. But there could be no doubt either who, for the French at least, was the Tour's heart.

Virenque's idyll with the Tour had begun in 1992, his first ever Tour, on stage two. The 'happiest day of my life', as he was to call it, came after an attack across the Pyrenees – that year tackled exceptionally early in the race – that culminated with Spain's Javier Murguialday and Virenque reaching the finish line in Pau together. Murguialday took the stage, Virenque the green of points jersey holder, the race lead and the King of the Mountains jersey. The yellow jersey was only his for one day, before Pascal Lino, his RMO and future Festina team-mate, took over as race leader at Bordeaux; the green jersey remained in his possession as far as Nogent-sur-Oise in the north, the polka-dot jersey a little longer. Having lost the overall and points lead and their corresponding jerseys, which race protocol dictated were to be given priority when a rider simultaneously topped different classifications, 'I finally wore the King of the Mountains for the first time between Roubaix and Brussels,' Virenque recounted. 'It was the start of a long love affair.' He finished a notable second in that classification, behind the equally fiery climber Claudio Chiappucci.

Virenque claims that he rode his first two years as a pro completely clean, something he states was both unremarkable and yet indicates, he argues, his natural talent for racing, the wholly natural basis for his all-out attacks. But his argument to explain why he had to take drugs from his third year onwards is well worn: 'Before 1998, if you didn't do EPO to fight your fatigue, you had to stop riding your bike. You couldn't compete with the rest.'

Yet further down the same paragraph in which this statement appears, he is equally adamant that EPO only had a certain effect: 'the victories I have seized were done on energy and courage, that doesn't change anything.' He is at pains to emphasise the doctor's insistence on the controlled use of banned drugs, claiming that the maximum hematocrit level permitted in Festina, for example, was 50 per cent – four points lower than at least one other Festina insider recollects – and that he himself asked the UCI for it to be dropped to 47 per cent. But there is no getting away from the fact that Virenque – who claims even now that he was a scapegoat, that he and his team were unjustly singled out in a world plagued with cheating – systematically and willingly doped for one season after another. Equally, from one year to the next, Virenque's popularity rose in France. His victories might be few and far between in the Tour. There was one at Luz Ardiden in 1994 after a 110-km breakaway, 40 of them alone, and bursting into tears as he crossed the line. And another came at Cauterets in 1995, where he celebrated unaware that fellow-rider Fabio Casartelli had lost his life earlier in the day on the same stage, and a third at Courchevel in 1997, where it looked suspiciously as if Ullrich had let Virenque win. But each time they broadened his fan base further and further.

Why was he so popular? In 1993, France was in need of a cycling hero, following the retirement of Laurent Fignon, the double Tour winner, in 1992, and the self-imposed exile of Laurent Jalabert to Spain and the ONCE squad, where Jalabert grew increasingly isolated from his compatriots. Virenque's fighting talk might have been clichéd, but it was what every cycling fan, particularly after years of relatively uneventful domination by a time trialling 'machine' like Miguel Indurain – and fears that Ullrich might be equally predictable – liked to hear. And not just in France, either. This was the era when *Cycle Sport*, at the time the UK's only publication focusing on mainland European-based professional cycling, dedicated an entire issue to the 'death of the climber'. Virenque, at least, seemed the embodiment of the kind of rider who, apparently dead and buried, could break out of his coffin and go and haunt a few time triallists.

'In the mountains there is a fairground atmosphere, a feeling of euphoria and joy,' Virenque claimed in 1995, explaining his liking for the big climbs. 'The real mountains are what I like, where the roads are black with people, where they just move apart enough to let you through. It makes your spine tingle. The backdrop you have on the cols in the Tour is fabulous. You have the feeling that you are going onstage, that you are the star of some great show.'

At the same time, Virenque's willingness to perform for the cameras played wonderfully for French TV, and chimed, too, with the increasingly television-oriented nature of the Tour. Last but not least, Virenque's team played along with him, realising that in terms of publicity, if not in actual results, Virenque was a winner all the way. 'We knew Richard's limits. We played the game of trying to get the yellow jersey, but winning it, that would have been a miracle,' Brochard says now. At the time, though, Brochard would never have admitted it.

Yet if strategy and time trialling were never his strong points – it is notable that Virenque, in his 13-year career, had no stage race wins whatsoever – that didn't matter. The 30,000 fans who turned out in the tiny market town of Lisieux for a post-Tour criterium in 1997, headlined by Virenque, were not concerned. Nor were the crowds that were so desperate to get close to the Festina team bus in the final week of the 1997 Tour that the vehicle itself needed a police escort.

At 28, in 1998, Virenque was at the height of his powers. He knew that when racing in the Route du Sud that year that he could afford to reject a team hotel as too uncomfortable. He opted instead to take the entire squad back to the previous night's lodging, despite it costing a reported 20,000 French francs. There were even reports that he allegedly asked a helicopter pilot for a French television station to bring his machine as close as possible in time trials so he could benefit – in theory – from the lower wind resistance caused by the helicopter blades. Just as in the story of the emperor's new clothes, nobody tried, or dared, to put Virenque right.

Riding at the Dauphiné Libéré, his last major preparation race, Virenque was in good shape. He had taken a mountain-top stage win, at Megève, and finished sixth overall – slightly out of the frame, perhaps, but the best placed of all the Tour favourites by a long shot. (Ullrich was at the Tour de Suisse, Pantani resting up after the Giro.) So it was all but inevitable that on the Friday before the Tour de France, *L'Equipe* dedicated four pages to him and the three other top Festina riders: Brochard, Dufaux and Zülle. (All of them bar Zülle, curiously enough, had dyed grey hair, not, as one might have thought, an ironic comment on their post-Voet arrest worries but simply a nod to fashion.) *France-Soir*, meanwhile, had a headline that might have raised eyebrows in other circumstances – 'Sont-ils dopés?' – but it turned out *France-Soir* was referring to the ongoing World Cup and its football players. The paper reassured its readers – 'not to worry, of the 240 [anti-doping] tests in the first 60 games, none were positive'.

The same was already not true of one Festina rider on the Tour: Christophe Moreau. Moreau had returned a positive 'A' test for anabolic steroids in the Critérium International in March. But he was still waiting for the results of the 'B' test before a sanction could be applied.

As an example of the prevalence of a more relaxed attitude to doping at the time, reactions to the Moreau positive could hardly be bettered. Rather than keep their rider off the Tour, when the news broke of his positive nearly three months after the race, in June, Roussel argued that his rider had been given the drug 'by somebody outside the team' and left it at that. 'Christophe has been abused, his honesty has not been questioned,' Roussel claimed to *Le Parisien*, blaming the positive on someone who 'was not part of the medical staff but who formed part of the entourage'. He had instructed his rider, he said, 'to continue racing in the Dauphiné Libéré', where Moreau had just taken second in the prologue, 'so he could do an anti-doping test and demonstrate his innocence. It's the best way of showing that he's not a cheater.' Asked whether his Tour de France berth in the Festina line-up was in doubt, Roussel argued, 'why should I keep him off the Tour on top of the punishment he's already going to receive?'

But Moreau's positive remained, too, the first major slip-up of this kind inside the doping 'system' established by Roussel, Rijckaert and Voet, and hinted that the team's doping cauldron was beginning to boil at least a little more fiercely. Certainly, as Virenque's ambitions grew ever stronger, the internal competition to race alongside him (and the rewards, too) was greater. The pressure resulted in riders feeling determined to perform at higher and higher levels.

As a result, the Festina system was beginning to crack at the edges. As Bassons reports in his book *A Clean Break*, 'Left to their own devices, these ingenues took reckless risks. The increasing number of those involved in the whole doping process also led to overdoses or to links with characters of a dubious nature, which resulted in riders getting worse rather than better.' Even as early as 1997, Bassons records that 'there were signs of revolt within the ranks ... throughout the 1990s, our Belgian doctor had built up his reputation through his knowledge of EPO. His star was fading thanks to the arrival of a new range of pharmaceuticals that he viewed with scepticism.' By 1998, for example, some Festina riders – it is not clear who – were already bypassing Rijckaert to consult doctors in Italy. The notorious Dr Michele Ferrari was among their number, while Voet says Dufaux told him he was visiting another in Switzerland. (Virenque had paid a visit to Michele Ferrari as early as 1996 – although he did not return, given, as Voet puts it, 'it was very expensive and teaming up with Ferrari was like putting a saucepan up your backside: it was immediately very obvious what you were doing'). Even so Ferrari's popularity was such that Rijckaert acquired the nickname Dr Punto – the far less powerful brand of car, although made by the same manufacturer.

Equally, Virenque was willing to go outside Rijckaert's system in order to increase his own chances. In the 1997 Tour, in preparation for the St-Etienne time trial, despite Roussel's and Voet's opposition the Frenchman insisted on obtaining a phial of an unknown substance from a Spanish soigneur, not on his team. Not knowing that the substance had in fact been switched by Voet for a harmless placebo, Virenque punched well above his weight in the time trial, first losing three minutes to race leader Ullrich but then holding the German's back wheel all the way to the line.

Not only that, but Rijckaert himself was in trouble, as early as that spring. His name had already come to light during a police investigation in Ghent, Belgium, into a local chemist, a neighbour of Rijckaert, suspected of attempting to defraud the Belgian social security. The chemist recognised during a police interrogation that Rijckaert had bought EPO from him.

By 1998, according to Bassons, Rijckaert had been 'evicted' from the team – and then brought back in. As a result of the Ghent investigation, Roussel had 'ordered his staff to destroy everything in the archives that contained a reference to his name. The outlaw had been removed from the team's technical staff. He had disappeared from the new edition of the team presentation brochure. Overtaken in terms of science, he had become dangerous from a legal standpoint. The management were looking for a replacement and other, more efficient and discreet dopers, had been approached.'

However, given the Moreau positive, and the increasingly tumultuous system, Roussel panicked and, having all but shown Rijckaert the door, late in the spring of 1998, the Belgian was reinstated again as the team's top medic. 'Roussel put in an emergency call to Rijckaert,' Bassons recounts, 'who had to control this dangerous and appalling mess in the big races.' Voet's pre-Tour visit to Rijckaert, then, would probably never have happened had it not been for an attempt to bring the Festina doping 'programme' back under control. As Bassons puts it, 'Paradoxically, this reorganisation and the centralisation of products in the hands of specific people would eventually result in the downfall of those behind this system.'

Festina, then, might have been the number one team in the world, but even before the customs officials just inside France waved Voet and his EPO-packed car to a halt on the Wednesday morning before the Tour, the squad was already sailing in perilous waters. In fact Festina, like the Tour itself, was an accident waiting to happen.

3

Le Tour en Irlande: Red Wine, Guinness – and EPO

Monday, 13 July. Stage 2:
Enniscorthy–Cork, 205.5 km

While the Tour de France faced mounting problems about its credibility thanks to the mushrooming Festina scandal, the race's first visit to Ireland also provided some potent reminders, even in a football World Cup year, of how the Tour de France had become the biggest annual sporting event on the planet.

From the streets of Dublin to the ferry port at Cork where the Tour set sail for France, the size of the crowds lining the roads on all the Irish stages was vivid testament to the public interest the Tour had provoked. France and Ireland had often been political allies in the past, and certainly France's sporting event received the warmest of welcomes, too: the tricolour flags – both red, white and blue and green, orange and white – were out in force, and an unlikely but apparently drinkable mixture of red wine and Guinness flowed in the roadside picnics. Ever since it had first begun outside French borders in Amsterdam in 1954, and as 2014's three-day visit to Yorkshire, Cambridgeshire and London confirmed again, the Tour's popularity has always tended to soar when it heads abroad. Ireland in 1998, its first and to date only visit to the Republic, was no exception.

'I was already a fan but even if Irish cycling was at a low ebb in the 1990s after the Kelly and Roche years and there was no Irish rider in the race, it was still quite a big deal. I remember a lot of people on the roadsides, even if they didn't know much about the sport,' comments Ireland's Barry Ryan, now a cycling journalist.

As a teenage fan, Ryan was present on the Tour as a spectator both in the Dublin prologue and again on the roadside at Midleton, where he says, 'I remember there was a sprint there sponsored by Stena Line' – the company which shipped back the Tour's 1,500 vehicles that night from Cork to Brittany – 'and the crowds were very big. People came out to see the spectacle and it had been very well publicised. You could call it a typical foreign *Grand Départ*.

'It wasn't too long after the Nissan Classic [Ireland's top race of the 1990s] had finished, people were still pretty nostalgic for the Kelly and Roche years. The press wasn't entirely welcoming, though. The *Sunday Tribune* had run an article detailing doping problems in cycling the week before and I think one paper had the line "people should draw their curtains when the Tour goes past". A week later that was kind of proved right!'

Cycling, too, had made it onto the mainstream Irish TV channels, although it wasn't always given priority. Part of Friday's presentation and Saturday's prologue were shown live, as was Monday's stage 2, but Sunday was quietly dropped in favour of the Munster hurling final between Clare and Waterford in the town of Thurles. Ryan says that the fallout from the doping scandal had not really filtered into the public's collective consciousness by that weekend. 'You've got to remember it was pre-internet time, so the news of it was very slow-burning. It would have been on Irish radio the night before the Tour began, because I remember my mother telling me she'd heard a soigneur had been caught with drugs in his car, but I didn't have much detail about that beyond the radio report.

'It was only when the Tour went back to France that the details were really fleshed out. People would have been aware of it, but whether they paid much attention to it is another story. Apart from that one *Tribune* journalist maybe, I certainly don't know of people not going to the race because of it. We never thought it was going to come to anything. As a cycling fan you assumed it would peter out like other cycling doping stories had.'

So that day Ryan, his parents and his sister drove to Midleton, some 30 km from his home town and went to enjoy the race like any other fans. 'With hindsight it was maybe not the best place. There were very big crowds and car parks set up on the edge of town. A lot of people had congregated there from a very long time before, right from the morning, to see the race.'

News quickly reached them, too, of what was going wrong in the race – on Monday's stage 3, disaster had befallen the British leader of the Tour, Chris Boardman. For a second time in four years, Boardman had crashed in the first half of the Tour and was forced to abandon. In terms of injuries, this was nothing like as bad as 1995 when he skidded out on a fast downhill corner at Saint-Brieuc in the prologue and broke several bones. But the Briton had still fallen heavily, lost consciousness for several minutes and been evacuated to Cork, ahead of the peloton, in an ambulance – out of the race once more.

'We'd already heard he was out and saw the ambulance coming through,' Ryan recalls, 'although I can't recall whether we knew that Boardman was in it or not. A guy in my class at school was standing near where Boardman crashed, and snatched his bidon. I refused to believe him until he came in to school with a Coke bidon with *CB* written on it in marker.'

The crash, around 50 km from the finish, happened just as the bunch was beginning to speed up for a hot spot sprint, just before the somewhat dilapidated coastal port of Youghal. As daylong headwinds gave way to coastal sidewinds, further raising the tension in the bunch, the Briton, lying 20th or so in the lined-out peloton, hit the deck. The GAN pro went spinning across the tarmac and only came to a halt when his head slammed to the ground, and was clearly in a state where he could go no further.

Clutching the hand of his sports director, Roger Legeay, as he was stretchered into the waiting ambulance, Boardman's speedy trip past the peloton to Cork University Hospital meant, as one paper drily put it, 'He was to be first into Ireland's second city, but not in the way he would have wanted.' Instead, the Wirral man became the first yellow jersey wearer since the ill-fated Luis Ocaña in the 1971 Tour de France to crash so heavily that he could not continue.

Boardman, who had a large gash on his left cheek, his right arm in a sling and cuts and bruises all over his body, said in a press conference the next day he recollected nothing of the crash. But with time, he now says he has been able to reconstruct events.

'It was so simple. We'd just gone up a big drag as I remember, it was windy, I was following [team-mate] Eros Poli up to the front. I was coming up on his wheel as he was slowing and he just went round a cats-eye, our wheels overlapped and he took out my wheel. It wasn't his fault, he was just changing direction, it was a combination of the momentum. But when you overlap, you just go straight down. I came down next to a dry stone wall, people thought I'd hit it, but in fact I hadn't.

'It's the only time I've ever been unconscious, it's like blinking and suddenly you're looking at the roof of an ambulance. It felt like a minute, but it was like, "Christ, was I in a bike race? Christ, I wasn't in the Tour? Christ, I wasn't leading?" Wiggle toes, that's OK. There's that whole reconnect with reality cos it was quite something, my face was burning because the side of my face got ripped and had to be sewn back together.'

Back in the 1998 Tour post-crash press conference, he had displayed his usual wry humour. His worst injury was to his left wrist, he said, pointing out, 'Have you ever tried eating Cornflakes with your right hand when you are left-handed?'

In reality, though, Boardman was feeling anything but humourous inside, and it had nothing to do with bike racing or the Tour's steadily worsening crisis. As he now says, his dedication to his wife Sally at the prologue victory had come as he was trying – and at that point, failing – to save his marriage.

'We were having marital issues, she'd had enough of me putting myself first. Then in that last couple of years I had been miserable, too, and was still putting myself first, and Sally had mentally left by then. She'd had enough.

'I realised that she'd gone, because even when I went to hospital in Cork, she was with friends still in Dublin, I think, and she stayed there. It was a massive stock-taking moment for me, and there was where I decided I had to stop my career and save my marriage. I couldn't say, "oh, I'll be more considerate and I'll return to the path," because I'd already been saying that for years. So I had no credibility any more.

'It took quite a few months. I was very lucky, but it was very good for me, because it was a proper perspective check. So I wasn't paying attention to cycling exploding in the background; I went home and I was quite relieved to be out of the Tour. I wasn't bothered, although I realise that was not what I should have been feeling. But I had health issues developing as well. I left and forgot about cycling or watching it for months and just focused on my marriage,' which he did, indeed, manage to salvage.

Meanwhile back at the Tour, Boardman's accident had come on a day where narrow roads, big crowds and fraught nerves made for a tough day for the peloton. But another crash, this time involving spectators, was far more serious, when an 11-year-old girl, Laura Sewell, and her mother were struck a glancing blow by a rider, Federico de Beni. The mother was uninjured despite landing heavily in a ditch, but the girl suffered severe head and neck injuries and remained unconscious for more than a week, before eventually recovering. De Beni was traumatised by the news of her injuries and abandoned, saying he could not stop thinking about the accident, shortly after the Tour returned to France. He rode a few more races that season but then retired from racing, aged just 25.

As for the rest of the riders, after a comparatively staid first mass-start stage, barring a late crash for top sprinter Mario Cipollini, Boardman was not the only one to have a difficult time of it on the Tour's third and final day in Ireland. Pantani, Virenque and Ullrich, the top three finishers from the 1997 race, were all dropped in the crosswinds on the run-in to Cork and forced to work hard to regain contact. 'Pantani rode an appalling prologue in Dublin and now has the look of a man who wishes he was on the beach at his home near Rimini,' the *Guardian* claimed.

There was another big pile-up, eight kilometres from the finish, with Virenque, Laurent Jalabert and Laurent Brochard all coming a cropper. None, though, were injured, and they could continue to the finish, where, thanks to the strong headwind, the peloton arrived an hour late. Then, on the big western approach road to Cork, the Carrigrohane Straight, Czech sprinter and national champion Ján Svorada took the victory in what was a somewhat anti-climactic finale to a dramatic stage, while Zabel, having shaved seconds off Boardman's lead, was automatically crowned the new leader. The post-stage question as to whether Boardman would still be wearing the *maillot jaune* had he stayed upright might have been annoying for some riders with overly large egos, but Zabel, even though he had never led the Tour before, took it well. 'I wish Boardman well, but even without his crash,' he said, 'I am sure I would still have got the jersey.'

As for Festina, Roussel and his team continued to tell themselves and their sponsors that they had the situation under control. This collective self-delusion was surely helped by the fact that, by Sunday, the only brush with the organisation's system of fines and suspensions for misdemeanours to that point had occurred when Brochard was forced to pay all of 50 Swiss francs for wearing white shorts to match his World Champion's jersey. A day later the entire squad were forced to hand over a similar sum for having their race numbers printed on their jerseys – both in terms of their budget and the credibility with the fans and what was to come later, very small drops in an ocean.

The Tour itself, though, was facing increasing numbers of questions about the absence of Voet. 'Let's calm down,' Jean-Marie Leblanc commented during the long Irish weekend. 'It's a doping case, but it doesn't involve a rider, it's not connected with this race, it's hundreds of kilometres from here.' That distance between Voet in Lille and Leblanc in Dublin was obviously unplanned by the Tour when it came to Ireland, but hardly inconvenient when it came to conserving the Tour's image. There were some other questions circulating, with a few people still scratching their heads as to why the Tour was in Ireland at all. After all, the prologue was the most distant from French soil in the race's history – albeit closely followed by the Berlin *Grand Départ* in 1987. But one of the reasons became very evident as early as Monday morning.

While the Tour made an early start en route south and west towards Cork – its final stop-off point for the Irish stages – France was waking up to a huge collective hangover after beating Brazil in the World Cup final. The Tour had already started a full week later than usual, in order not to overlap excessively with the World Cup. Then, when it was proposed to ASO that it could make its first ever start in Ireland, a nation not expected to make it into the final, the idea was warmly accepted.

From ASO's point of view, Ireland represented part of the increasing internationalisation of the Tour as a commercial as well as a sporting product. For example, speculation in Ireland over future *Grand Départs* a long way outside France like the one planned – and quietly dropped, post-1998 – in Dresden in 2006 were increasingly par for the course. Even in the increasing furore over Festina, the rumour of a start in Guadaloupe in the West Indies, too, still persisted. The Tour was equally important as a vehicle for boosting cycling in Ireland, its aim being to leave a better legacy than the freshly tarmacked – and therefore more bike-worthy – 400 km of roads over which the Irish Tour route ran. (Boardman insisted, in his post-crash press conference, that the roads were in great shape.) During the build-up to Dublin, there was much speculation about the possibility, for example, of a bid to host the World Championships in the west of Ireland in 2003. Sky's Philip Deignan, from Letterkenny in Donegal, still recollects how he was inspired to become a racer by watching the race in Dublin. Much of this optimism concerning Irish cycling was blighted by the Festina affair, as Stephen Roche once said. 'It [the Dublin start] didn't produce the spin-offs it might have. That said, cycling fans in Ireland really appreciated being able to see the sport on their own doorstep and logistically it was faultless.'

So much for the future. As for the past, the Tour's connections with Ireland at that time were much more significant than those of the UK. Stephen Roche's Tour de France win in 1987, a first for Ireland and 25 years before Bradley Wiggins rode into Paris in yellow and took Britain's first victory, was the unquestionable high point. But if 1987 was Roche's year, with wins in the Giro, Tour and World Championships, Sean Kelly's multiple stage wins and points-jersey triumphs in the Tour, as well as his huge number of

Classics wins and Vuelta a España victory, produced a much more consistent, if less obvious, interest in the sport that rumbled on for well over a decade. The appreciation was mutual: Jean-Marie Leblanc once revealed that it had been a wish of Jacques Goddet, the previous Tour director, that the race could have been designed so that Sean Kelly could have tried to win it, saying 'he greatly admired Kelly, but the route was too mountainous for him'.

The opportunity to take the race to Carrick-on-Suir, Kelly's home town, was not the key reason why the Tour was present in Ireland. But it did represent a golden opportunity to pay homage to the great Irishman. Carrick-on-Suir, redubbed by media as Carrick-on-Tour for the race, responded equally well to the honour, organising special seminars, literary evenings and amateur bike races for the week-long build-up. There was even a timed race to Clonmel, the next town on the Suir, with a prize of a car as a reward for anyone who could beat the record set by – who else? – Kelly himself. At the same time, and of equal importance, following a neutralised ride through Dublin, the Tour's first stage got underway in Roche's home town of Dundrum, the riders passing by a sculpture commemorating his achievements on two wheels. Finally on the Friday, hours before the Festina earthquake hit the Tour, Leblanc and other Tour organisers honoured their promise to lay a wreath at the grave of Shay Elliot, Ireland's first Tour de France leader (for three days) back in 1963 and the country's pioneer in professional European-based cycling, in the churchyard at Kilmacanogue. Leblanc recalled to one newspaper that he had once met Elliot at a race in the Pas-de-Calais region when he was an amateur and had asked him for his autograph. The Irishman's friendliness to the young Frenchman helped nurture Leblanc's fondness for English-speaking riders, and his development into a lifelong Anglophone. It was perhaps not so surprising, therefore, that the Tour – under Leblanc's direction since 1989 – spent two days in England in 1994, or that he lent a sympathatic ear to the Irish bid for the *Grand Départ* in 1998.

That *le Tour en Irlande* was organised by Alain Rushton, local organiser for *le Tour en Angleterre* in 1994, and by Pat McQuaid – president of the Irish Cycling Federation and later to head the UCI – gave additional credence to the bid. The actual bill was footed by the Irish government, to the tune of two million Irish pounds with Bertie Ahern, the then PM, presenting the first yellow jersey in Dublin. (Media claims that up to 35 million Irish pounds would be netted by the Irish economy in return for the outlay allayed most worries about the cost.)

Logistically, the crucial piece of the jigsaw when it came to taking the Tour to Ireland was the support from the transport company Stena, who provided three giant ferries to ship the race back to France on the Monday night. (One of their more visible rewards, as Barry Ryan points out, included hot spot sprint banners bearing the company's name in Ireland.) There were some notable hiccups in the visit: complaints from the locals over the Tour's initial plan to avoid Sean Kelly Square in Carrick-on-Suir because it was too dangerous, a threatened Gardai strike – the so-called blue flu as it involved calling in sick en masse – and a very public row between Roche and the local organisers, that had begun as far back as April, over his role in the Tour's visit. But ultimately as the 'Jostle stone', a local landmark, was removed at Carrick to allow the Tour through, the Gardai failed to go on strike and Roche continued to appear for interviews – for the British press, at the utterly improbable location of a Dublin greyhound stadium – these sorted themselves out. Without the Festina scandal, there is little doubt *le Tour en Irlande* would have been as resounding a success as *le Tour en Angleterre* had been in 1994, and would be again in 2007 and 2014.

But the arrest of Voet meant the cracks in the Tour had widened to a degree so painful that it was all but impossible to ignore by the time the race left Ireland. As the *New York Times* veteran cycling reporter Sam Abt pointed out in an article at the time, 'in the publicity buildup for the Tour, no Irishman seems to have been forgotten except for Paul Kimmage. His name appears nowhere except in the *Sunday Independent*, the Irish newspaper for which he writes' – *Rough Ride*, the first book to deal head-on with drugs in cycling in any language – 'which has just been reissued eight years after it scandalized many in the world of professional bike racing'. This was despite *Rough Ride* selling 15,000 copies by 1998, and winning the William Hill Sports Book of the Year in 1990.

'My perception at the time was that we were victims of a corrupt system,' Kimmage said in an interview before news broke late on the Friday about the Festina scandal, and before also identifying EPO, the new drug of choice after amphetamines and steroids, as 'a very bad change'.

'This attitude of sweeping it under the carpet, the law of silence, has done a lot of damage to the sport,' Kimmage said. 'I think they're paying for it now.'

Drug scandals or no drugs scandals, during its three-day sojourn in Ireland the Tour de France had towered, albeit briefly, above almost all other social events, sporting or otherwise. But within cycling the Tour has never done anything else. Dwarfing the other events in racing as it does, every incident on the Tour is magnified, every error has the potential to ruin a rider's career, every triumph the ability to give a rider a lasting legacy.

The death of a Spanish rider, José Luis Viejo, in the late autumn of 2014, illustrates this. Viejo took one standout triumph in his career, a minor transition stage of the Tour in 1976. That would not be so remarkable except that the time gap between Viejo when he crossed the line and the rest of the field was a record-breaking 22′ 50″. When he died in November 2014 that record still stood, and Viejo, his name honoured in his local town, had obituaries in every major Spanish daily. The victory in a nine-year career may have been his only top win, but because it happened in the Tour it was enough to earn him a place in cycling's history books. As such, the Tour has always been innately conservative in nature. It is not just the intrinsic logistic difficulty of getting such a large institution to change its format. Such aversion to change is also because – and this is true of any sporting event – it would have made it harder for the Tour to remain a historic point of reference, for achievements ranging from Viejo's stage win to Anquetil, Hinault, Merckx and Indurain winning it five times outright to be contrasted to more contemporary performances.

In an interview in 1996 with the magazine *Cycle Sport*, Jean-Marie Leblanc described some of the priorities he faced as a director of the Tour de France, which included its role as cycling's benchmark. But it was also, he said, a cultural and social reference point for France as a nation.

Speaking on a personal level, he explained, 'The Tour is a *fête*, part of France's national heritage. You have to say *bonjour* to the old lady with her little dog and to the child who comes up to you to say "Monsieur Leblanc, bravo."' That social role went hand in hand with the Tour route's constant nodding towards events or new infrastructure which had modernised France's image, as well as recognising landmark achievements in France, Leblanc said. As examples, he cited the Tour using one of the first trains to travel through the Channel Tunnel, prior to its opening to the public, in July 1994. Then there was the time the Tour paid homage to another gigantic achievement in the world of transport by crossing the recently opened Pont de Normandie in 1995. As a way of linking the competition with the bridge itself, the slight rise to its centre was classified as a minor climb in the King of the Mountains competition.

The Tour was also a reflection and idealisation of French social values, Leblanc revealed. For example, if faced with multiple bids from localities for the same stage start, 'the Tour would try to prioritise visits to towns with high unemployment, because if a mayor is trying to boost morale with a Tour visit, I like that. It's our social role.' Another simple point illustrates the Tour's position in France's collective consciousness. Unlike the other two Grand Tours, the Giro d'Italia, which almost always finishes in Milan, and the Vuelta a España, which used to finish in the Basque Country and recently ended in Galicia, the Tour de France has never finished anywhere except Paris, and to celebrate its 2003 centenary it started in the French capital as well as ending there, just as it had done 100 years before.

Leblanc's role as director of an event which was so much a part of France's social fabric and which was at the same time a major international event was a complex one. His trying to combine different responsibilities and obligations was as evident, too, in the Tour's battle against doping, pre-1998, as it was in other areas. 'When I became head of the Tour I thought – and I don't think I was mistaken – that the Tour was too hard,' Leblanc said in his 1996 interview.

'There were too many summit finishes and too many mountains at a time when we wanted to fight drugs. You can't fight drugs and put in more and more mountains, more and more sprints, more and more classifications, more of everything.' But another ingredient in the Tour's recipe for success is implicit in what he says, too: there was the constant demand, and pressure on him, for a more spectacular race.

This determination to resist excessive focus on *spectacle* dovetailed with another favourite bugbear of Leblanc's, the need to reduce what he called *gigantisme* – the tendency for a creeping but steady increase in the Tour community's size – and manageability.

'I reduced the summit finishes a bit, the sprints, the jerseys [classifications] ... the need each year is to find a balance, but the levers we can pull are not that numerous. You can't take out the mountains or the time trials, it's always a bit more or a bit less.'

Such a softly-softly approach on the part of the Tour later led to a broad-based criticism, with the considerable benefit of hindsight, that in the early 1990s, the organisers had not done enough to fight doping. But beneath the apparently placid waters of one Miguel Indurain Tour de France win after another, their 'anti-doping' pedalling was perhaps not as furious as it could have been. But that is not to say that that pedalling did not exist. It is also possible to argue, as Leblanc does, that the anti-doping struggle was not the Tour's direct responsibility, but that of the authorities running the sport. However, what is undeniable is that, regarding doping, cycling was getting increasingly out of its depth: and regardless of what precise measures each separate institution in cycling should have taken, the *combined* efforts of all the authorities and organisations were insufficient.

By the time Jean-Marie Leblanc fully retired from the Tour de France directorship in 2007, he had been present on 32 editions of the race. He had seen the race from several perspectives, having experienced the Tour as a fan in his teens, then as a racer, albeit as a domestique and for only a couple of years before retiring in the early 1970s, then for over a decade as a journalist for French newspapers *La Voix du Nord*, the specialist magazine *Vélo* and the semi-official publication *L'Equipe*.

Present in the Tour's management since October 1988, Leblanc was therefore well aware of how the Tour, given the importance of the race and its visiting all the different continental *départements* – minus Corsica – was woven into France's collective consciousness. In the introduction to his autobiography, *Le Tour de ma Vie*, he quotes a French President of the Republic as saying that the race 'presents France to the entire world'. This might sound a shade exaggerated, but it's symptomatic of the density of the Tour's relationship with France, and how important, therefore, it was when the Tour hit its huge crisis in 1998. The Tour's identification with France beyond the merely geographical was partly due to its 100 year history, and partly because the only times it had stopped were when the country itself was in crisis.

Such was the case, for example, in the Second World War. As Jacques Goddet, its long-standing director, said in 1999, the year before he died, 'The occupying authorities and the Vichy regime wanted the Tour to take place at any price to make the world believe that France was a normal, happy place. I refused, in spite of the fact that, in a time of shortages, any resources we needed – food, petrol, vehicles – would be made available. I saved the Tour from being sullied, and that was important for its postwar future.'

Yet by the end of the 1980s, with the arrival of Leblanc, the Tour was definitively outgrowing its French roots and western European-oriented outlook. Greg LeMond had already become the first non-European Tour winner, teams from Colombia and the United States taking part in the Tour were no longer viewed as unusual purely on the basis of their nationality, riders from the former Soviet bloc were featuring more and more strongly. The Tour's image was also moving with the times: Leblanc recollects worrying in his first year of directing the race that switching the Tour's official transport sponsor from French Peugeot cars to an Italian make, FIAT, could go down badly with the public. By the time he retired, he said, he would have had no such scruples about looking for a non-national backer from any part of the world.

Dynamic, articulate, and, as his autobiography suggests, passionately attached to the Tour de France, Leblanc was a charismatic and combative director – all of which was to stand him in good stead in the Tour of 1998. He was also far less patrician than Goddet, which was perhaps crucial in the across-the-board negotiations in 1998 that were sometimes needed to keep the Tour from sinking completely.

Leblanc sometimes refuses to discuss doping in interviews – perhaps understandable given, as he also writes in his autobiography, 'from the moment I arrived in the Tour, right up to my exit in January 2007, one word, one evil, one obsession marked this long period: doping'. He is, he said, heartily sick of the subject.

Does that mean he has something to hide? As a rider, the question of doping came up, he claims, but only intermittently. Large hints had been dropped to him before a difficult criterium that he would be better off 'preparing'. Then he caught sight of a small handful of pills, that turned out to be amphetamines, taken by top pro Désiré Letort in a French national championships – and which duly saw Letort both win the Championships and test positive. But Leblanc himself never had any problems with the anti-doping authorities, and if the number of anti-doping tests during his five-year career was risibly small (less than half a dozen), they all came back negative. His career, in any case, was never in the higher echelons of the sport, its high points a second place in the Four Days of Dunkirk, a win in a stage of the Tour of Portugal and two completed Tours de France.

Rather than his career, Leblanc claims his first eye-opener to the existence of doping was when Francesco Moser took the Hour Record in 1984 – although it should be underlined that Moser's activities were not illegal at the time and blood doping only began to be banned in 1985. As for the point when it all but sunk his morale, that came after reading Jesús Manzano's revelations of mass doping in the Kelme squad, principally concerning the same, by then illegal, practice used by Moser – blood transfusions – in March 2004.

'I wondered,' he writes, 'what the point was of staying at my post in the face of such practices, which make the human organism a common-or-garden tool for experiments by mad doctors.' He did not resign, however, battling through that summer's 2004 Cofidis affair, the revelations in *L'Equipe* of potential positive tests for Lance Armstrong in 2005, the Landis positive for testosterone and the massive Spanish anti-doping investigation, Operación Puerto, in 2006, and finally retiring just before the publication in 2007, by former soigneur Jef D'Hont, of a book outlining the doping practices in Telekom.

Doping became an increasingly major concern for him in the mid-1990s. By that point, EPO use had become far more generalised, as Rijckaert's advice to Roussel about making doping more systematic in Festina makes clear, and the evidence is inescapable.

'We now know exactly what was the significance of the Gewiss taking all top three places in a breakaway in the Flèche Wallonne in 1994,' Leblanc repeated on several occasions, the significance being the team medic, Michele Ferrari, was one of the most notorious doping doctors of the last 25 years. (That year, Ferrari's comment in an interview about EPO being as safe to take as orange juice if correctly used is still a chilling one.) Leblanc has cited numerous other examples of suspect racers in that era, ranging from Claudio Chiappucci, winner of the Tour's most famous breakaway on the stage to Sestriere in 1992, to Ivan Gotti and Evgeni Berzin, winners of three Giros d'Italia between them.

There is no indication, either, that by 1998 Leblanc was any part of a major, across-the-board campaign to wipe out banned drugs – or that he would have got significant support had he been doing so. The small amount of official information sharing, for example, between the Minister of Sport and Jean-Marie Leblanc would suggest that. By Thursday lunchtime Marie-George Buffet had been informed, via contacts in Lille and Paris, that Voet had been arrested. By the evening she had reportedly received two faxes containing information about the drugs that had been seized. However, Leblanc did not discover for himself that Voet was in prison until he was informed by a journalist late on Friday afternoon. Buffet's reaction when he told her about Voet? 'I know.'

But it would be equally inaccurate to say that the Tour's director had not ventured down the anti-doping warpath at all. In his autobiography, by way of indicating his increasing interest in it, he cites a meeting of one of cycling's top authorities, the Professional Cycling League, in 1996 between race organisers, riders, teams and federation officials. After one official had alerted the meeting to rumours of EPO circulating even at junior level, a collective letter was sent to the French authorities and the UCI's president, Hein Verbruggen, pleading for more concerted action – 'to press on the accelerator,' as Leblanc puts it – in the fight against doping.

The communiqué issued after the meeting said that the letter had asked the international federations, the IOC and the state authorities in general to modify legislation so that, among other requests, blood samples could be tested. It also called for increased research against other substances such as corticoids and testosterone, and a single legal protocol that could be applied to speed up anti-doping justice.

While the French authorities responded by warning of potential human rights issues involved with blood testing and the need for a thorough scientific basis, the UCI indicated that their anti-doping commission was planning new measures to combat banned drugs. Among these was the establishing of tests for a maximum permitted hematocrit level: although nominally a health protection plan and put into place in March 1997, it was widely seen as an indirect way of limiting the use of EPO.

By the summer of 1998, a second new line in the sand had been drawn: the embryonic form of the biological passport was set up. Coming into effect in 1999, the testing four times a year of key physiological values and accumulated 'normal' readings for athletes would, it was hoped, indicate off-the-wall readings of doping. However, it was only approved by the UCI in June 1998; at the time it was seen, to quote the UCI, 'as a preventative measure, not an anti-doping one', and would take years to function fully. Even now, the passport's validity is subject to debate.

Leblanc recounts, too, that he made a last-minute trip to see Hein Verbruggen at the Dutchman's second home in the west of Ireland, days before the Tour started, with the use of EPO amongst the subjects for discussion. Leblanc's concern had been renewed, he said, after Yvon Sanquer, a French director of the tiny Mutuelle de Seine-et-Marne squad, had 'forcibly expressed a warning' about the drug's use in the peloton during a meeting at the French Nationals – the same race where Willy Voet had injected corticoids into the French Festina riders. Verbruggen's response, Leblanc claimed, was that EPO would not be detected for another three or four years.

That was not the case. But even if, speaking hypothetically, Voet had not been arrested and the tumult and drama that was to rip the Tour apart never happened, the chances are that, given the speeding up in the intensity and effects of doping during that decade, the underlying problems would surely have emerged elsewhere, if not with such force. In hindsight, the 1998 Tour would simply have risked being branded as equally dope-ridden as the rest of the races in that era. Boardman's abandon even before the Tour reached home shores meant it was lacking one of its few undisputed moral compasses in terms of the anti-doping struggle. But in terms of the Tour's credibility, Boardman's exit was irrelevant. Well before it set sail from Cork, like the *Titanic* when it left the same Irish port 75 years earlier, cycling was already heading for its own iceberg.

4

From Aspirins to Vacuum Cleaners: The Life of a Young 1990s Professional

Tuesday, 14 July. Stage 3: Roscoff–Lorient, 169 km

As the Tour returned to France by ferry and plane, in an attempt to lighten the tension black jokes abounded. 'We reckoned that the fish in the Irish Sea were all going to grow wings because of the amount of gear being dumped overboard,' one top journalist recalls. On the riders' Monday evening flight back over the English Channel, meanwhile, the craic was all about Cork being the *Titanic*'s last port of call. There were other half-serious stories doing the rounds of the ferry's bars that night: that teams had hired unmarked vehicles in Cork and Dublin that were now transporting their arsenals of doping products in other, less closely watched, ferries; that the hire cars' tyres were jammed full of drugs; that some teams had reverted to their tactics of the 1996 Giro d'Italia after its own foreign *Grand Départ*, in Athens. When they had discovered that Italian customs would be awaiting the car ferries in Bari on their return to Italy, the story went that the teams sent unmarked vehicles through the former Yugoslav republics. Jammed, of course, with drugs. There were smirking comments, too, that some riders' WAGs were now engaged in another race – the one to book up hotel rooms as close as possible to the Tour to ensure that their partners could dope up in peace.

The line at which the truth ended and the alcohol-fuelled imagination of the Tour's journalists kicked in was rapidly becoming blurred. But did it really require alcohol for that? With the underbelly of the racing scene exposed so clearly by Voet's arrest, the sport was now acting in an area where its usual parameters had been broken. It could not be said that the wall of silence surrounding drugs, professional cycling's inner certainty that it was somehow immune to French legislation, which had begun to outlaw doping in the mid-1960s, had begun to falter. But it was certain that a large chunk of the wall had suddenly broken away, and at the Tour, cycling's flagship event, too. The question was, firstly, what would happen to the Tour when it returned to its usual arena of French roads and mountains; and, secondly, if Voet talked, how much would that *omertà* crumble?

The overnight return to France, at the small Breton port of Roscoff, also witnessed the race's re-encounter with the World Cup, which outside Ireland had overshadowed the Tour completely – and on that Monday in the Tour's mother country, even more so. France's 3-0 defeat of Brazil in the final the night before left the country's sports fans nursing a collective hangover.

The news in *Le Parisien* the following Tuesday morning was not easy even for teetotal cycling fans to digest, though. According to the newspaper, Voet had now confessed that the drugs he was carrying were not for his personal use, as had been his initial line of defence. Instead, he had revealed that they were for the team as a whole, and he had been acting under orders from team management.

Some fans in Brittany, French cycling's heartland and Roussel's home region, were not in the least pleased at the way their Tour *fête* had been ruined by the news, and were determined, instead, to put the blame firmly on the media. They hammered on the roof of *L'Equipe*'s car and spat at its windows as it struggled to make its way through the narrow Roscoff streets in the midst of a gigantic traffic jam to the start line. This was quite possibly the first time the media, rather than the riders or – as would have perhaps been more just – the entire structure of professional cycling during that period, were to be singled out for blame for 'ruining' the sport.

As it happened, neither the police nor the customs were waiting for the teams when the riders and staff reached their hotels late on Monday night, or when their team vehicles crawled off the ferries and into the Roscoff traffic jam early on Tuesday morning. However, Roussel had an unpleasant surprise when he opened the curtains of his hotel room in Brittany and saw, as he told his lawyer over the phone, '40 journalists looking at me'. But Roussel was by no means prepared to quit, not even when Jean-Marie Leblanc reportedly appealed to him directly at the start that day to take Festina out of the race.

Instead, according to *Un Cyclone Nommé Dopage*, published the year after the Tour, Roussel continued categorically to deny there were any problems, telling journalists he 'did not understand anything' and he needed 'to know more. I understand people are going to ask questions, it's not going to be easy.' His riders also batted away the questions: 'it does not concern me and doesn't interest me,' said Brochard. 'All I know is my conscience is clean.' 'I'm not a policeman or an investigating judge, so I don't have any access to that [Voet] dossier,' added Hervé, a touch smugly. Moreau even claimed, somewhat hypocritically since he had tested positive that March, that he could not be using those products of Voet's because 'we have anti-doping tests on the races. So we've got nothing to worry about.'

Virenque meanwhile – his hair still dyed grey – was busy at what he did best: milking his popularity. While Roussel and company were handling the press, Virenque was glad-handing local dignitaries as he was presented with a giant red onion by Roscoff Town Hall, presumably one of the town's highest civic honours. (One paper wondered if this was to help Virenque in 'producing the Gazza-style tears which have endeared him to every Frenchwoman'.)

Jean-Marie Leblanc dropped increasingly strong hints, though, that Virenque might be shedding more than onion-induced tears in the near future, when he indicated that Festina's expulsion might only be a question of time. 'I am waiting to receive something official either from the police or the Ministry of Justice saying that, yes, Festina have done something seriously bad, which will allow me to make a decision and take some measures,' Leblanc said. 'Right now all I have is newspaper reports.'

Rumours spread rapidly that the first team cars on the Tour were being inspected by French police in the evening, allegedly Telekom and two minor squads, TVM and Polti. The story, if true, would have seriously harmed the Tour with two of their former winners in the German squad's line-up – but it turned out to be the first of many false trails. However, Roussel's statements, Leblanc's hints and the stories of possible investigations within the Tour itself meant the doping chickens were coming to roost much closer to home. This was no longer just an enquiry into the Festina team soigneur, hundreds of kilometres from the race. Suddenly it was a sports scandal the Tour itself would have to face on its own doorstep. As Jean-Marie Leblanc, showing his journalistic past, said in Roscoff: 'we're no longer on the sports pages, we're in the news section.'

At the same time, rather than involving one squad the Roscoff rumours about Polti and Telekom, even if inaccurate, were the first indication that the French police were now searching for new angles outside Festina themselves. In other words, just as

Rolf Aldag had feared, everybody was under threat – not just Richard Virenque and company.

Joerg Jaksche, a second-year pro with Polti racing his first ever Tour de France and first Grand Tour, has very clear memories of – of all things – the squad's vacuum cleaner on that year's race. After all, following Willy Voet's arrest, that was where the German and his team-mates in the small Italian squad, Polti, decided to hide their drugs.

Between sips of coffee at a McDonald's in a small town in central Austria, Jaksche recalls an experience that could, given it is nearly eight years since he left the world of cycling and that he has studied for a Business MA, be taken from a former life on another planet.

'They cut out the plastic, made a second "floor", put some ice in it and then covered it with aluminium paper to keep it cold. It was actually like a fridge, really cold,' he says about the vacuum cleaner-cum-doping container. Asked if there was enough room, Jaksche said, 'there was not so much, little vials and so on'.

The procedure, he said, never varied: 'Everyone was carrying their own stuff. It was always the same, we would all meet up in the bus or in our camper van after the race for a coffee. And then one of our soigneurs would open the vacuum cleaner and everyone would grab their stuff, destroy their syringes and then get out.

'The system is not that different from that described by Tyler Hamilton' – the rider who would later help lift the lid on doping in US Postal, the American squad. 'It's just that there one person would bring the stuff.'

Albeit a rider with a minor team, the German's concerns were identical to those of the big hitters in the Tour that year. Jaksche says that he did talk to other teams about their path of action in the same situation. He claims one French team 'kept theirs [drugs] until a certain moment … then decided to bury it in the ground somewhere. I have that from [name supplied].' Others like Saeco and Cofidis, Jaksche claims, 'hid them on vehicles that were part of the publicity caravan'.

In fact, Cofidis rider Philippe Gaumont, who died in 2013, gave a different version in his autobiography of what he and other team-mates did. On 18 July, the day of the Tour's first long time trial, Gaumont recalled that he and other members of the Cofidis squad were told by the management that they should hide their drugs 'because "otherwise we'd be in the shit"'. Some were duly passed on elsewhere; a lot of them, he reveals, were 'taken out into a wood and all the vials were broken: cortisone, caffeine.

'Nobody went to the bottom of the problem, or asked about the future of cycling. We were just told, "looking at what's happening, we're stopping everything, at least for the moment". And the only worry in the group was to find out where we could hide our EPO without being worried about doping in danger.'

In any case, Jaksche had heard, too, that other teams kept their banned drugs, 'because otherwise it would be like an admission of your doping, because what would you do if the team broke down [stopped performing so well] in the middle of the race? You had to continue in order to tell the story that you're successful.'

Jaksche feels that 'a majority' of the teams continued using doping products like EPO. 'My impression was that the Italian teams kept it, too. I certainly don't buy this idea of people getting rid of it and never doping again. Of our team, of nine riders nine people kept it. So why should other teams be different?'

He had no sudden feelings of guilt, Jaksche says, brought on by the surreal way Polti hid their Tour de France stash of banned drugs, no sense of another line being crossed – perhaps another bleak indication of how widespread doping was in comparison with the current era of cyclng.

'You could always have cut it out, always have said, "there's another option in my life". But the presumption was you wanted to stay in cycling, and then there was no other option.'

At the 1998 Tour, having opted to keep their doping supply in the vacuum cleaner, Jaksche says for Polti it was 'back to business as usual. We had our shots every night. But then in the last week we threw it all away because they said it was senseless by then to carry it.

'It was just the same, they said, "do it but don't get caught".'

Yet for all the collective cheating, doping was invariably a lonely existence. Jaksche's parents, he said, 'thought for sure their son couldn't do it. That's why they were happy when I went to Telekom [in 1999] too, and moved to Freiburg; they thought "ah, it's German, it's better, you don't cheat". Which was,' he adds wryly, 'wrong'.

In the 1998 Tour his team, Polti, were one of the smallest in the race. Their leader, Luc Leblanc, a former World Champion with a fourth and a sixth place in the Tour to his name, was the only cyclist of note, but his career was going downhill and he would retire at the end of the year despite being only 32. And if the Telekoms and Festinas of the cycling world could ill afford to lose their focus, Jaksche says that collectively a squad like his were 'too worried' to perform properly.

This was despite the fact that, from the doping point of view, Polti were so minor he believes they were not a priority for the French police: 'the amount of drugs we had was so small, we mostly flew under the radar.' The team lorry was, he says, 'searched once', as was one of the team cars late in the race. But although the gendarmes stood outside their team hotel one night, investigating another squad, nobody looked in the Polti bus, still less in the vacuum cleaner.

Jaksche also argues the squad's financial outlay on illegal drugs was much smaller than what would have been needed to buy the amount seized in Voet's car for Festina. But at the same time, he points out, given the most a squad like Polti could hope for was a stage win, the police raids made it far less likely to happen – because the riders were so worried about the consequences of being caught.

'A cyclist's life was so "into drugs" at that time, starting from 1992 to 1998, EPO was so widespread, they had so many concerns they lost their – not their ambition, but their concentration on the race. Probably they had the stuff at home. Imagine – I don't say that he had – Luc Leblanc with a fridge in the basement: it's difficult, you're three weeks away from home, you don't know what the police have got, you cannot talk on the phone because you would think our phones were tapped – at least I certainly did.' Jaksche says he found himself in that predicament a little later in his career, 'when T-Mobile riders' homes were being raided because of a legal problem and I was, like, "it could also happen to me". Then you are worried – and I think that was the situation [for other riders in 1998].'

Telekom's way of responding to the extra strain was perhaps noticeable in their willingness to let a break, albeit one containing a domestique like Jens Heppner, move away as soon as the Tour returned to France, on the short, hilly trek south from Roscoff to Lorient. Nine riders, including Festina's Hervé – both the *coureur régional* of the break, Xavier Jan, and Hervé were given extra loud cheers by the crowds on the roadsides, the latter in sympathy with his team's predicament – went clear and on an ultra-fast stage, run off at an average speed of 47.472 kmh with a tailwind spinning them along. Then, in the finale into Lorient, Heppner and Bo Hamburger sheared away, with the German taking the stage – a sign, Aldag says, of increasing restlessness among the Telekom rank and file – and the main bunch coming in a minute down, led in by Jaksche's team-mate Fabrizio Guidi. But the day's prizes were well out of reach by that point. Hervé snaffled provisional top spot in the King of the Mountains ranking while he or another member of Festina continued to troop up on to the podium every morning as leaders of the Tour's team classification. Just as they had done since Dublin. Yet beneath the surface the pressure was beginning to tell, and badly. 'The strain is doing my head in, I don't want to be here any more,' Neil Stephens said after the stage. 'I saw a crash and almost steered into it, so I could go home.'

Even so, despite the increasing concerns about the police raids, which were to get more and more serious as the race continued, Jaksche said on one level he was curiously happy. The race might be disintegrating but at the same time he was a Tour rookie, on the inside of the event that was the pinnacle of the sport. 'I was always concerned but I was really happy to race the Tour. It was my first Tour, it's this mixture, you have these huge impressions, the way you race, the spectators and everything, and I was able to distinguish these two things, I said, OK this is big-time shit, but I enjoyed racing. Because I loved what I did. So I was tired and happy when the Tour was over for me, but I still enjoyed it, the scenery, the impression, it was still beautiful.'

His ability to separate the racing from the doping was so well developed, even in just 18 months as a pro, that he turned in some very solid rides for a second-year racer. 'I was never sick of things in the 1998, I wanted to continue. I was good at [stage 11's summit finish] Plateau de Beille, I got there with [top racers Daniele] Nardello and Riis, and I had a good day in the Alps where [Polti leader] Leblanc told me not to wait for him on the climbs and I got into the second group. I was feeling happy, I enjoyed that.'

Evidently, the compartmentalisation that sports directors like Roussel clearly developed about doping was also present among the riders. Jaksche, too, kept his day-to-day racing 'mind' barriered off from the systematic cheating, the 'very negative side', as he calls it, that went on in the hotel rooms every evening. It was, he said, very hard to sleep at night. 'Yes, I was very nervous, thinking what do you do if you go to prison, stuff like that.'

He agrees that the 1998 Tour, then, did not act as stern advice to him of the wisdom of giving up. Instead it marked a point where Jaksche's ability to separate the enjoyable part of being a racer and the tougher times – the doping at the heart of the sport – became an absolute necessity. That July he developed an impermeable mental barrier between the two. If not, he argues, in his case he would have had to leave the sport. 'There were two different things, there was racing and the illegal side of things. I accepted it as part of the job, it was my way to handle it, I had to. I was able to cut those two things apart, otherwise you couldn't survive.'

But it only worked up to a point: 'on the bike you were happy, even though I suppose you could have been arrested. But it was more when you were back at the hotel, or in the room where the stress started.' Sources of information, with no internet and few mobiles around, were limited to the manager, Gianluigi Stanga, 'telling us rumours'. Inside the peloton, he says, the shouting and joking around with doping that had always been present dried up completely 'and afterwards also. Personally I never talked about it, until …' – and he laughs softly, given that he lifted the lid in dramatically thorough fashion on drug taking in the peloton a few years back – 'I talked about it. But this stuff – "ahhh, the Spanish"' – a favourite topic of doping conversations given their reputation, at the time, for taking a soft line on banned drugs – 'or "I took 100,000 units [of EPO]", I never did that.'

Jaksche's presence on the Tour was not as a last-minute stand-in, as could well have been the case for a young rider. Rather, he had been told by Stanga in March that he wanted Jaksche to be 'the revelation [stand-out new rider] in the Tour de France'. This, in fact, had been the team's plan since over a year before and which, ironically, had meant Jaksche had stayed doping free for a large part of that time. 'The main reason was because of the 1997 season, where I did Paris–Nice clean and I got over the Ventoux with all the top names' – he finished 19th and the first Polti rider home on that particular stage, a remarkable result for a first-year pro. 'One team-mate had done that race and he was "prepared" and I dropped him clean.'

'So I had this meeting after the race and Stanga came up to me and said, "*cosa hai preso?*" [what did you take?] And I had no fucking idea what he was talking about.' Jaksche's only drug, he said, was an aspirin, 'just because it was the first stage where it was hot, and in the German national amateur team we'd had a good [health] education, so whenever it was hot, we'd take an aspirin just in case you'd get a fever. So I told Stanga that I'd had an aspirin and he just looked at me and said to others, "I don't trust this guy." And Stanga came in the room the next day with a centrifuge and he said, "OK, we're going to test you [for your hematocrit]."'

Far from being fuelled up with EPO, Jaksche's hematocrit turned out to be 39 per cent, and Stanga, he said, was delighted. 'Partly because he realised I wasn't lying to him', and partly, presumably, because he realised that Jaksche was an unsullied talent, who could, if correctly 'treated', go far. (This had been the reason he had been signed in the first place, 'because Germans weren't like the Italian amateur scene at the time, where they were doping even worse than the amateurs, so I wasn't burned out'.)

At the 1997 Paris–Nice, then, Stanga was so pleased with Jaksche having looked at the centrifuge results that on the spot, 'He said he was going to give me a five-year contract – which didn't happen, but still this was the way of thinking at the time. And after I took EPO and then got third in a stage in the Tour de Suisse that summer ahead of top riders like Francesco Casagrande, he told me that I shouldn't take anything for the rest of the year' – the idea being to make sure Jaksche's organism could be exploited to the maximum in the next, when, as Jaksche puts it, 'he said he would "put me on the [doping] programme" – just in time for the 1998 Tour'.

As Jaksche recalls, the doping system in place at Polti worked as it did in many Belgian teams at the time, where the doctor would be the brains of the operation, but would leave the practical (and legally incriminating) aspects to the soigneurs. 'The doctors knew everything and they are the most intelligent people on the team. They are also the most frightened because they could lose their titles [right to practice], so they don't touch anything. They just tell the soigneur' – whom Jaksche describes bluntly as 'the poor guys who work for €1,300 a month, travelling for 300 days a year, and they have only this so they can be put under pressure [to collaborate in the doping process] by the team manager' – 'and the soigneur tells you'.

Even if some soigneurs, like Voet and D'Hont, had been around the block so many times they had considerable medical knowledge, Jaksche says that in all his teams – and he was in six – 'the doses were decided by the doctors'. For example, regarding EPO they would prescribe 'every day 1,000 units', with criminal activity becoming so tediously normal that Jaksche says, 'it was a bit like taking an aspirin. It wasn't generally very sophisticated, just in a few ways, like you'd need to make five separate calculations to be sure you had the right dosage.' After that, it was into the routine of 'every day, 1,000 units, then if your values were going up like crazy, you'd stop it'.

There was, unlike in Telekom, no secrecy about it whatsoever, with other riders having 'the stuff shipped in before each race. For example, at the Tour of the Basque Country in April a top rider got a package from a Belgian doctor as if it was the most normal thing in the world.' This helped reinforce the routine nature of it all, Jaksche recounts: 'I started to be the same, I was like, "oh, everyone is doing it, the police cannot do anything because it is my earnings." You easily get into that mentality and then suddenly it was like ... it was not a real thing.'

And so his own countdown for the Tour, in terms of doping, began: 'in my personal experience, you started at least ten or 15 days before [with EPO], doing 1,000 units every day, then you start controlling it [your hematocrit level] and maintaining it with 1,000 [units] every three days. So if you have 40 hematocrit, you would do it for longer, if it's 48, then much less.'

By the time he reached Dublin, though, his sense of anticipation was as great as any sportsperson's – clean or otherwise – would be when on the point of starting the biggest event in their discipline for the first time, and appreciating how much more spectacular the Tour was than anything else previously experienced. 'We'd have races in Nurnberg around the castle, with a lot of spectators, but that was like, say, at the Tour de Suisse. But at the Tour de France, it was just enormous, the whole city of Dublin was closed down, it was good.'

Jaksche had a mission of working for Polti team leader Luc Leblanc: 'with me, he was always OK. Many people have problems working for the team leader and they are speculating on what they can do for themselves. But the Tour was so overwhelming for me, I said I would ride for him as much as I could and then whatever happens, happens. Whatever they told me to do, I did it.'

This came at a price, though – a doping price. Each rider's physiology could vary radically and Jaksche's hematocrit average was about 43 to 44 per cent, meaning that in his case he had to continue injecting throughout the Tour. 'If you did too much one time, then your values go up too high.' That was an issue that a person with a different series of blood values, perhaps using a different type of EPO and with different reactions to the drug, would not have to face. But Jaksche was not alone; apart from EPO, other substances he used or saw being removed from the vacuum cleaner included human growth hormone and 'maybe testosterone patches, two or three things ...'

However, Jaksche knew that this time round the arrest of Voet had shifted the goalposts radically. 'I heard about it from Luc Leblanc. We were sitting at dinner and he was talking to [Casino sprinter Stéphane] Barthe.' Barthe, as Jaksche recalls, had had an offer from Festina the previous year, and 'he was like "Oh shit."' In turn, 'Luc just went "phewww" and we all looked at him.'

A long discussion ensued between all the team members, over 'what we should do with the stuff'. Again unlike Telekom, 'Nobody flushed it down the toilet … Our conclusion was, if the French police are going to raid the aeroplane bringing the peloton back to France, then the whole Tour is over, and our question was, "would the police want that?"'

'So we thought we'd risk it. But the whole situation was very stressful and then at the end we threw it away in the last week.' Jaksche points out that the normal attitude of team management was 'always the same … they tell you officially "don't do this" [doping] and they hope you want to continue. They don't want to be incriminated, but if you are performing badly then the team is bad, the sponsor is bad [unhappy], it's just a chain.'

On this occasion, rather than keep his head buried in the sand and ignore the doping, Stanga 'decided directly, where do we hide it', Jaksche recounts. With the police – for the first time ever in cycling – potentially making raids on the Tour itself, rather than the occasional customs search of vehicles, there was too much to lose. Riders and management, traditionally two very separate parts of a team, were beginning to establish who the common enemy was: the police, and – probably for the first time in the history of cycling – the press.

5

From Vegetable Basket to Victories: Behind the Scenes with Festina

Wednesday, 15 July. Stage 4:
Plouay–Cholet, 252 km

Thursday, 16 July. Stage 5:
Cholet–Châteauroux, 228.5 km

For Bruno Roussel, getting taken into police custody must have come as something of a relief. For just over a week, as the impact of Willy Voet's arrest and the discovery of the team's stash of drugs reverberated ever more loudly at the Tour, the pressure on the Festina team manager had steadily, and unbearably, mounted.

Exhaustion was setting in on all fronts. By his own admission Roussel had slept for a little less than three hours on the Friday night before the Tour started, given he was up talking to his lawyers, who had hotfooted it over to Ireland, until 4 a.m. Subsequent photographs of him from the first week show Roussel's increasingly weary and worried face, brought on by the constant tension.

Then, in one single moment, the lying was over. Roussel had been on the telephone to his lawyer in the car, steering with one hand as he was directed off the course with other Tour de France vehicles round the side of the finishing straight at Cholet. Business as usual, in fact: normally other directors would park their cars by their team bus and then wait for their riders, having crossed the line, to pick their way through the heavy Tour traffic to their waiting vehicles. On this occasion, the waiting was the other way round: the blue-clad figures at Cholet's finish were on the lookout for Roussel.

'Ever since I had got off the plane in Brittany, I had been expecting, at every moment, to be approached by a plain-clothes police inspector,' Roussel later commented – and presumably not just because, ever since Dublin, he had been publicly demanding an opportunity to talk to the police about the case. His lawyer, Thibault de Montbrial, wished him luck and they ended the call, then Roussel was asked to drive away from the race, behind the police vehicles. At Cholet police station he was formally placed under arrest. At the same time, Roussel learned that the Festina team doctor, Erik Rijckaert, had also been detained and was in an adjacent cell.

Roussel probably did not recall it at the time, but, bizarrely, Cholet had been the town where the Festina 'system' of organised doping had started its first lease of life five years earlier. According to Voet, it was in Cholet that Festina had had their Tour de France riders tested for their normal hematocrit levels prior to the 1993 race – as a precaution before the team initiated them into its first ever systematic, team-run administration of EPO. As the 1993 Tour's *Grand Départ* in the Vendée came ever closer, the riders had grown increasingly concerned about the non-arrival of the batch of EPO they were due to use. Voet recalls that Roussel 'called Spain, then put down the receiver and reassured us: "it's coming in tomorrow by plane"'.

Fast-forward five years and, the day after Roussel's arrest, a lengthy police interrogation concerning that half-decade of EPO use by Festina's top riders began. Initially the director attempted to cover up his team's tracks, and he held out for nearly 24 hours. But at around 5 p.m. on Friday, 16 July, when Roussel was informed that Rijckaert had confessed to the doping system and he was shown both Voet's and Rijckaert's statements, he too decided to stop lying.

Like Voet and Rijckaert, Roussel pulled no punches when he began his confession. He said that around 1 per cent of the team's total annual budget – some €40,000 euros – was used as a 'war chest' to buy drugs like EPO and HGH. The money was siphoned off the top riders' bonuses for their best results (with those riders' agreement), while Voet added that cash from the start money paid by criterium organisers to Virenque and his fellow 'barons' was also used.

Just like Jef D'Hont in Telekom in the mid-1990s, Voet wrote down the drugs used – in code – in notebooks to keep tabs and to ensure the correct money was paid at the end of each year by each rider. In keeping with their unofficial place in cycling's virtual 'black museum' of doping, the notebooks can be seen in the central photo section of his autobiography, page after page of semi-coded graphs, revealing to those in the know exactly how a top team could dope its way to the highest level of the sport.

According to the three individuals' statements – although Rijckaert later retracted his – not all riders took part in the system, but the upper echelons of the Festina hierarchy, such as Zülle, Virenque and the Frenchman's most loyal lieutenants were all involved. However, Rijckaert partly contradicted another of Roussel's central claims – that the system in place was for the benefit of their health – by pointing out that those who did participate were willing to act as guinea pigs when the team tested the effects of insulin-like growth factor 1. IGF1 is a hormone which was reported as having very dangerous side effects. Even though it was not clear if this had any effect on performance, in keeping with the 'total war' philosophy that seems to have predominated in the second half of 1990s cycling, the team added this to their lists of medicines, just in case.

When the USADA report into Lance Armstrong and US Postal's use of banned drugs for the Grand Tours was made public, their cheating was regularly described as 'the most sophisticated organised doping program in the world'. Yet, intriguingly, no matter how polished an operation the purchase and use of banned drugs had become in the years after the 1998 Tour, the Festina management's statements are a reminder of how little one of the most disturbing facets of organised doping in cycling had changed: how the process of using banned drugs could inveigle its way into the most inoffensive activities and areas of the protagonists' lives – and then hide behind them.

Looking back, an example of this – described by Tyler Hamilton in his book *The Secret Race: Inside the Hidden World of the Tour de France* – is how riders on the Postal team bus disposed of used syringes. They were screwed up and crushed into empty Coca-Cola cans then taken out of the bus by soigneurs, who mingled with the crowds waiting outside for the riders and dropped them in rubbish bins at a discreet distance from the bus. The mixture of what appears to be an act of good citizenship – 'please be sure to dispose of your rubbish correctly' as the anti-littering campaign catchphrase goes – and the sinister is a jarring one. But so, too, is the way one Tour rider comments that drugs would be shipped in to his team-mates in the late 1990s: what could be more natural than a wife and baby visiting a partner on the race, he said, as long as you overlooked the vials of EPO taped to the inside of the baby's nappies?

Go back a little further and, in the case of the doping material used by Festina in the 1998 Tour, and found in Voet's car, there were some equally surreal moments when everyday domestic life was juxtaposed with hard-core drug use. The Belgian had explained to police in Lille, for example – where Rijckaert and Roussel would be taken on Friday, 17 July – that he had stored the doping material for Festina's Tour in the family fridge, more specifically in the vegetable basket. 'This had not gone down too well with my wife,' he writes in his autobiography, 'but not so much because she had no idea where to put the carrots, but because she doubted that the stuff was harmless.' Whether Voet's wife knew that it would be part of the 'fuel' used by Festina as they battled to remain the number one cycling team in the world is another story altogether. Whatever the case, the 'domestic' element of the Festina doping organisation, as revealed by Voet, is a reminder of how unsophisticated and grassroots a sport cycling had somehow, at one level, managed to remain. Despite all the scientific, technological and doping innovations of the 1990s, banned drug use for the number one cycling team came down to this: an amiable looking, bespectacled, balding, middle-aged man, driving halfway round Europe in the family car (without a licence) and hoping his wife won't get annoyed with him because of the 'other products' in among the vegetables in the kitchen.

Adding to the sense of unthreatening, almost mundane routine for such illicit activity, Voet would later tell how the drugs in his car had been handed over to him a week earlier by Joel Chabiron, the team's logistics manager, in the anonymous surroundings of a chain restaurant car park situated near Merignac airport in Bordeaux. As Voet recalls in his typical matter-of-fact style, Chabiron had purchased the drugs in Portugal and transported them as far as Bordeaux. The two had parked – 'bumper to bumper' with the briefest of nods to the clandestine nature of the deal – outside the restaurant, the material had been transferred and Voet then headed for home. All business as usual, both in terms of trying to win the biggest bike races on earth and what all too often truly lay behind that.

A few days later, the unlikely but vital link between all the drama and hype of professional cycling (in Festina, culminating with Virenque's rock-star status in France) and Willy Voet's fridge resurfaced. With the drugs now removed from the vegetable basket and placed in large boxes and ice-filled flasks in the car boot, Voet was on the road again – first stop the team headquarters in Lyon to pick up a team vehicle. From there he travelled to Evry, in the Paris suburbs, where he collected an official Tour de France car at the race organisation's base. And from there he proceeded to Rijckaert's home in Ghent, to collect ten boxes of glass drips – unavailable commercially in France, but which Rijckaert had in abundance at his surgery. At that point, on the Wednesday before the Tour, all that was left prior to meeting the rest of the Festina staff was, on paper, a quick spin across the plains of western Flanders and northern France. Instead, the police intervened.

Voet himself was on drugs when he was stopped: he was under the influence of the infamous *pot belge*, a combination of substances injected in doses of 10 to 20 millilitres. Used occasionally by riders, *pot belge* was, Voet later discovered (he had no idea at the time) a mixture of amphetamines, caffeine, heroin, painkillers and, sometimes, corticosteroids. He was using it, on this occasion, to stay awake after a short night and very early start.

Not only that, Voet had another vial of *pot belge* in his car, destined for Festina's Laurent Dufaux, as part payment for a Yorkshire terrier puppy Voet had bought from the rider as a Christmas present for his daughter. Voet had, in turn, received one of the two *pots belges* from a former pro he had run into at the Flèche Wallonne Classic, in exchange for some Festina team clothing Voet had 'borrowed' from the bus.

It hardly seems surprising that cycling was somewhat complacent about drug use at the time, given that Voet says when the customs officials waved him to a halt that Wednesday morning it was the first time he had been stopped in 30 years. For months, too, he had been driving without a licence – having lost it the previous winter for speeding. Nobody had noticed.

Voet knew that at the time police raids on teams were as rare as hen's teeth. Rather, any battles against drugs were left to their respective sports federations and national anti-doping bodies. One exception to the rule had been when a medium-sized Dutch squad, TVM, had had EPO seized from a soigneur's car in March at Reims – a case which was to play a major role in the 1998 Tour.

There had been the attempt by Italian customs at Brindisi to stop teams on their return from Athens in 1996, but after the teams diverted their vehicles through former Yugoslavia it was cancelled. Probably the biggest case of a police raid prior to a drugs seizure had been in 1997, during the Giro d'Italia, when the prestigious MG-Technogym squad's hotel in Cavalese was visited at 3.30 a.m. by Italy's NAS – the equivalent of the British police's Drug Squad. Twenty vials of anabolic steroids, three of HGH and a bag of syringes were discovered in a soigneur's room. The sports director, Giancarlo Ferretti, allegedly claimed the drugs were for his own health – to improve his sexual performance, he said – but that did not convince MG-Technogym, who pulled the plug on their sponsorship at the end of the season. Ferretti, though, continued, with another small squad – Riso Scotti. The case itself, as Barry Ryan has pointed out, petered out.

However, the previous occasion the police had appeared at the Tour had been as far back as 1967, when they searched the British team's hotel following the death of Tom Simpson. As for French customs, their previous big swoop had been in 1959, when they seized amphetamines allegedly due for 1958 Tour winner Charly Gaul. Hardly a track record, then, to cause cycling's underworld any sleepless nights, but also one which explains why the arrest of successive Festina management figures caused such shock waves both in and outside the sport.

Voet's police statement, though, is not entirely convincing. Having to make a huge detour from his Paris–Calais route to pick up glass drips, particularly for a team with such a huge budget as Festina's, does not really ring true. There are conflicting accounts from his family over when he actually left their home in Veynes, one member saying it was as early as Monday. Then witness accounts of what Voet was carrying at that point – a bag for personal items plus the drugs in several boxes, or just the bag – vary radically.

Police statements do not clarify, either, why Voet was willing to risk the British and Irish customs with such a huge quantity of drugs, when the race was set to return to France in less than a week. Last but not least, Voet's decision to come off the main Ghent–Lille highway to use an A-road which, as it happened, was one of the favourite rat runs for local drugs dealers, also adds to the mystery.

Voet offers no explanation as to why the police swooped on him at all, either in his statement or in his book, although it does not appear to have been a random check, given – he says – that the police told him, 'we would have picked you up in Calais if we hadn't stopped you on the border'. But what sparked the tip-off? At the time Roussel was convinced that the raid was politically motivated, given that Virenque supported Jacques Chirac, the Tour de France was regarded as a conservative institution and France had a left-wing government. In addition, there could be no doubt that the Festina case reinforced the need for new, tougher anti-doping legislation, being shepherded through parliament at the time by the communist Marie-George Buffet, France's Minister for Youth and Sport. Yet this does not completely make sense either, given that the TVM case in March would have been ideal political propaganda, but in fact barely registered in the French media and had been all but dropped by the French police at the time. Rather, the TVM enquiry only sparked back into life thanks to the Festina case.

Other arguments seem even more offbeat. There were claims that the dispute was due to a complaint made by a chemist's assistant in Veynes, Voet's adopted home town, to the police. One top French journalist who reported on the Tour for over two decades said the tip-off was due to a conflict between different Masonic lodges. Miguel Rodriguez, boss of Andorra, argued on the evening of Roussel's arrest – this was an idea which underpinned much of the Spanish teams' subsequent actions in the Tour – that 'at times it has occurred to me that a significant part of this situation could be due to chauvinism.'

The most consistently coherent argument, though, is probably the one a long-standing French cycling insider supports. Roussel was deeply unpopular with his colleagues, many of whom were jealous of Festina's rapid metamorphosis from a wildly disorganised, ungainly squad of 1993 into the number one team in the world. The most likely explanation, he said, was that a fellow director had, at some point prior to July 1998, made an anonymous phone call to the police – who were, as we have seen, already quietly investigating top cycling teams as early as March that year, and not just TVM.

The race itself, albeit completely overshadowed by the events of the evening after the stage, continued, with Jeroen Blijlevens taking the bunch sprint into Cholet and Australian Stuart O'Grady becoming his country's first wearer of the yellow jersey since Phil Anderson 16 years before. Regaining the jersey for Boardman's GAN team had not been straightforward for O'Grady, a winner of the PruTour of Britain in May, after he came within three seconds of taking the jersey the day before, at Lorient. O'Grady was able to snatch a six-second advantage when he won the first intermediate sprint of the day, at Plumelec, which made him 'yellow jersey on the road'. The Australian then increased his advantage over defending race leader Hamburger with another first place in the day's second sprint a little further on.

The tide seemed to be flowing in his favour, but the 24-year-old from Adelaide subsequently came a cropper in a major pile-up two kilometres from the finish line. However, although when he rolled battered and bruised across the finish line he was behind the main pack of sprinters, neither Hamburger nor George Hincapie, also in contention for yellow, were ahead of him. O'Grady had made it into yellow but given the events around the Tour some newspapers barely mentioned it.

At the same time, the Tour continued to fulfil its familiar role as an opportunity for the teams' sponsors to wine and dine leading clients. Telekom, for example, flew 20 business executives out to western France for a 'day at the races', where they were duly entertained, and chaperoned by a former top Portuguese pro, Acácio da Silva. Whether da Silva plied them with insider accounts of life on the road, given the increasingly grisly stories circulating in the press, we shall never know.

The morning after Roussel's arrest, at the stage start three of the nine Festina riders held a press conference, which, despite the pouring rain, was attended by most of the Tour's media. Their mood coupled defiance with self-righteous indignation, with Virenque, flanked by Brochard and Dufaux, insisting that even with Roussel and Rijckaert out of the picture the show would go on.

'This has got its good side,' Brochard claimed. 'The public is more on our side than ever before.' 'Festina is the best answer to this, but we are all family men and we are being treated like delinquents,' added Dufaux. 'Our consciences are clear and we have faith in French justice,' Virenque insisted, 'we have come to win and we will do our job as professionals.' Media reports stated that he claimed, absurdly, that Roussel's arrest had not been such: 'he had asked to be interviewed and they came to collect him.' Virenque then attempted to make a resounding conclusion, saying, '*Vive le Tour de France et le vélo*'. Given the controversy surrounding him and his team, this merely sounded cheesy, even by Virenque's standards.

Virenque's press conference came too early to deal with the main news of the day, which was that Roussel had been provisionally suspended by the UCI and his director's licence withdrawn. The scapegoat, it seemed, had been found and a replacement Festina manager, Miguel Moreno, flown in from Spain. 'We judge the facts are sufficiently serious to do this,' Martin Bruin, the UCI's head commissaire on the Tour that year, told reporters. The silver-haired Dutchman said he had received a fax from Cuba, where the UCI's top figures were holding their annual congress in conjunction with the Junior Track Worlds, authorising him to suspend Roussel. 'Priority has to be given to the interests of the majority.'

Together with Festina, the remainder of the peloton continued to race onwards, with O'Grady retaining the yellow jersey and Mario Cipollini finally doing justice to his unofficial title as the world's fastest sprinter and winning his first Tour stage of the race.

While the stage was unremittingly dull – a 228-km run from Cholet to Châteauroux with no classified climbs, with the main feature of the day (a break by Aart Vierhouten, Fabio Roscioli and Thierry Gouvenou) reeled in thanks to GAN's hard work prior to a bunch sprint – a constant series of crashes which had marred the Tour since stage one in Dublin continued apace. O'Grady fell early on again, and although Cipollini avoided the by now predictable pile-up in the finishing straight, his compatriot Silvio Martinello hit the deck hard and broke his pelvis. As for stage two winner and green jersey holder Ján Svorada, the Czech was relegated to last in his finishing group for the part he played in causing the *chute*.

If Festina were in the eye of the storm, for the peloton in general the broadsides of doping accusations being fired off in the media left them feeling only marginally less exposed. Thursday's headline in *France-Soir* of '*Ils sont tous dopés*' was a fine example.

'I'm being cautious,' Dr Gérald Grémion, the chief medic at Lausanne hospital told the newspaper, which was perhaps debatable considering he went on to say, 'I'm going to say 99 per cent of all professional riders are doping, the ones who do the Tour de France as much as the rest of them.

'In total, around four to five hundred pros destroy their health by taking doping products.' He cited the case of Mauro Gianetti, the former Classics star and World Championships silver medallist, who had taken PFC – a drug which was said to be on the point of overtaking EPO as the peloton's drug of choice – 'who had suffered a serious kidney and liver failure. He could have died.'

Meanwhile, the French police were reported to have widened their net, to Big Mat, Lotto and US Postal – in Postal's case to check whether the team's import licences for their bikes were in order, as was the case. Big Mat's riders, meanwhile, had the contents of their suitcases checked by customs officers. Nothing illegal was discovered.

The heightening of the pressure, though, and the beginning of raids on riders who were not from Festina, increased the tension even more in the peloton. 'The riders are fed up and with all of this stuff going on, it is very difficult to get them to concentrate on the race,' one unnamed team director told Spanish sports daily *MARCA*.

'We feel a bit intimidated,' Fernando Escartín, one of the top Spanish riders, added, while insisting his Kelme team was free of all potential scandal. 'The worst thing about this is the damage it is doing to the sport.'

MARCA also claimed that 'with the Festina director out of the scene, things are slowly coming back to normal'. It could not have been more wrong.

6

The End of the Road

Friday, 17 July. Stage 6:
La Châtre–Brive-la-Gaillarde, 204.5 km

Saturday, 18 July. Stage 7:
Meyrignac-l'Eglise–Corrèze, 58 km

It could have been a normal Tour de France stage. After all, Mario Cipollini had notched up a second triumph in two days, despite falling so often since leaving Dublin he was contending with eight different injuries.

'I could have won four or five times without those crashes,' Cipollini said with his usual bravado. But perhaps that is unkind, given his hindsight might have benefited from one of the more exotic figures in the 1998 Tour, an Italian fortune-teller named Diamantena, whom Cipollini swore brought him luck and who was to be seen wandering the corridors of the team hotel along with the rest of Cipollini's back-up staff. Whether she could foresee the storm about to engulf the Tour is another matter.

Certainly *MARCA* claimed in their Tour reports that day that normality was returning to the race. Their reasoning was that early on the morning of Friday, 17 July, Rijckaert, Voet and Roussel may have all been charged with supplying drugs at sporting events, but Festina, despite rumours to the contrary, remained part of the Tour.

But by 8.30 that evening, the sense of a seismic shift in the Tour's future was too hard to ignore. It was common knowledge in the media that Roussel had been taken by police vehicle to Lille, and had finally found himself in the same location as his soigneur, albeit in a separate cell. But what nobody expected was the bombshell his lawyer subsequently dropped from the steps of the Lille courtroom. This came in the form of a statement on a single sheet of paper, written on top of a police office A4 ringbinder folder. Far from *MARCA*'s business as usual, that single statement would send the Tour de France reeling in a completely different direction.

Roussel's lawyer admitted that his client had, finally, revealed Festina's dark doping heart to the French police in full. As he put it, 'Bruno Roussel has explained to the inquiry the conditions under which a co-ordinated supply of doping products was made available to the riders, organised by the team management, the doctors, the *soigneurs* and the riders themselves. The aim was to maximise performance under strict medical control, in order to avoid the riders obtaining drugs for themselves in circumstances which might have been seriously damaging for their health, as may have been the case in the past.'

The Tour de France and all multi-day races in cycling are defined, in many ways, by their predictability: there is a stage start, a finish, someone wins, someone leads the race. But this statement, a full-blown admission that the Tour's leading French team, the world's number one ranked team and some of the top contenders, had cheated the system, flung the race, and professional cycling, into uncharted waters. That it was a body blow of enormous consequences to the credibility of cycling was undoubted. But how big a body blow? And with what longer term effect? Nothing could be ruled out, because if doping stories had been part and parcel of the Tour since its inception, this one dwarfed any of them.

Rumours, sometimes strong ones, had implicated a few squads in the past. But a legal statement providing direct, unquestionable evidence that doping took place on such a large scale, and above all, that it had been *team-organised* rather than by lone individuals made it something that could not be explained away as 'bad apples in the barrel'. The soigneur could no longer be dismissed by Leblanc as a distant, isolated problem in Belgium. The only certainty was Leblanc had promised he would make an announcement that evening.

Inside the giant, white canvas pavilion that acted as the Tour's press room that evening, the journalists sat waiting in rows at long wooden tables. Paranoia within the Tour was beginning to become the norm, though, with some journalists agreeing to pre-arranged signals to go outside to exchange information they did not wish to share with the rest of the press corps. Reporters involved stood outside the tent, attempting to explain what they had heard to journalists less familiar with French – but who were desperate that their equally linguistically challenged rivals did not get the same story.

A hitherto unexpected factor for the journalists set in: hunger. While some English-speaking correspondents had already headed for their hotel and a restaurant, the most junior of those who remained – in this case, me – was sent out in search of sandwiches for the rest. The only place open that I could find willing to sell me some food at that time of night turned out, of all things, to be a brothel, which only helped add to the sense of unreality already surrounding the Tour.

At 10.45, Leblanc strode up to the little wooden table at the front of the pavilion to make the announcement that, as Jeremy Whittle would write in his book *Yellow Fever*, made this 'The Night Which Changed Everything'.

'*Messieurs*, it's late, you have a difficult job, we do too sometimes, because the information which we have received in this Tour de France about the Festina affair comes solely from the press,' Leblanc said first of all. 'These are sometimes rumours, contradictions or interpretations.

'A week ago, in Ireland, we said that it would be necessary to wait for the evidence to be confirmed to take an official decision about the Festina affair. Afterwards, the UCI has decided to withdraw the licence from Bruno Roussel.

'This evening, in Brive, from 6 p.m. onwards after the finish we have received, also from the press, information coming from Lille. Similarly, M. Thibault de Montbrial, Bruno Roussel's lawyer, has made a statement in the press during the day' – which Leblanc duly reread in full, before continuing.

'And it has seemed terrible to us, the organisers of the Tour de France, organisers of the biggest cycling competition in the world, because it constituted no more nor less than a confession. A confession that doping took place in the Festina team and even that it was organised.

'That has seemed sufficiently serious for us – and when I say us, I talk about the Tour de France organisation, but also the sports authorities present here at my side in the shape of the chief UCI commissaire on the race, M. Martin Bruin – to base our action on article 29 of the Tour's regulations which says, and I quote: "the race management reserve the right to exclude from the Tour all riders or members of the course who have infringed the general principles of the race".

'This is why, after having learned about the general elements of information coming from the Lille tribunal and having deliberated for some considerable time, we have taken the decision to exclude Festina from the race, from this day forward. It's been a difficult decision, because we have thought a great deal about the riders, but it is a decision which we feel is essential and we hope is healthy for the Tour de France and for cycling, and which, we hope, will also put an end to this unhealthy atmosphere which has pervaded the race ever since the start in Dublin.'

His announcement – sitting next to Bruin, the same official who had confirmed Roussel's expulsion – constituted a sea change the like of which the race had never known. Ever since its inception, the Tour had either indirectly tolerated doping, as it did in its earliest years, or since the 1950s, had, as was logical, left it to the appropriate authorities to deal with. Leblanc's statement marked the point where, for the first time ever, rather than leave matters to the UCI, or the police, or the riders' and teams' own consciences, the Tour itself opted to act directly against dopers.

The effect, according to *Un Cyclone Nommé Dopage*, was nothing less than apocalyptic. *'C'est une bombe nucléaire qui explose sur la planète vélo!'* But as the mushroom cloud of Festina's expulsion erupted, the instant effect was not uproar or chaos, and certainly not applause, just the usual buzz among journalists as any standard press conference draws to a close. The reason? Probably that the implications were almost too much to take in at one sitting: in one fell swoop, the top team in the world and two of the key favourites had been ejected from cyclng's biggest race for systematic doping. Just a few days after France's football team had seemed to place the country on top of the sporting world, the image of its biggest national sports event was left looking seriously battered. The Tour organisers had had to take this action, so they said, because it was unavoidable. Whether they could have interpreted their rule book differently or not, Festina's expulsion was an attempt to stop the rot – or what had become visible rot, at any rate – with amputation of the most radical kind.

No questions were taken as Leblanc left the room. One was offered – would the President of France, as promised, be present at the race? – but this was ignored. Then silence fell, before the European newspaper correspondents, realising they were running up against the latest possible deadline, began typing furiously. The tumult grew in intensity when it was realised that communications were soon to be cut off, given the Tour's telephone operators' announcement that they would be closing down the fax lines – at that time the only means of communication for most reporters – in their adjacent pavilion by midnight at the latest.

At 11.30 p.m., the floodlights started to go out as the Tour's ground staff began rolling up operations in order to begin moving all the race finish infrastructure to the next stage town. Chaos ensued as journalists first raced to finish their copy and then to send it; rushing from one giant tent to another, from light to pitch darkness, they found themselves tripping over cables and guy ropes and barging into each other. And as the lights went out and the curtain came down on an event that had been suddenly pitched, after 95 years of existence, into a whole new, unknown, dimension, such scenes of stumbling, blind confusion could not have been more appropriate.

As chance would have it, Leblanc had been due to spend that evening and overnight at a palatial residence belonging to M. and Mme Chirac in the Corrèze region, and Leblanc said later he was immensely appreciative that, despite his very late arrival, France's first couple had kept open their invitation that he stay with them. 'They had even thought to be sure my suitcase was taken there from the race,' Leblanc recounted. Despite the lateness of the hour, the Tour director was even able to have some supper, with his glass of wine being steadily refilled by M. Chirac himself as he recounted the day's tumultuous events. As a gesture of support from the French political establishment, albeit of the wholly unofficial variety, for his course of action, Leblanc could hardly have failed to appreciate it. From inside the Tour, too, came some key backing – that of former director Jacques Goddet, present on the race to receive an honorary award and also at the Chiracs'. Instead of getting an award, he gave Leblanc an unofficial one: a huge hug and his insistence, 'Congratulations, you have saved the Tour.'

Many of the press, meanwhile, were on an all-night stakeout at the Festina hotel, an immense 14th-century chateau named Castel Novel. (Belgian manager Patrick Lefevere, whose Mapei team happened to be there at the same time, said later it was the nicest hotel the Tour organisation had allocated to his squad in 15 years – but that the Festina affair had rather cast a pall on proceedings.) Truth be told, apart from the sound of journalists crashing through bushes in the chateau's darkened grounds and others using their car bonnets to ostentatiously hammer out articles on their laptops that could far more easily have been written inside their vehicles, there was little to see or hear. Certainly none of the Festina team were available for comment, the only access to the main part of the chateau being over a small white bridge, guarded rather zealously by a white-suited member of the hotel staff. By midnight, the only member of the Festina management to be found was Michel Gros, sitting in the hotel exterior dining room, swigging beer and allegedly stating, 'they're blood doctors, not sports doctors'. At least, as *Un Cyclone Nommé Dopage* pointed out, he was embarrassed enough not to mention the name Rijckaert.

Gros and Virenque had both been contacted by Roussel's lawyer, shortly after he made the statement about his client's admission to the press, and Virenque, for one, was determined to continue regardless of the team's exclusion. This was partly because he had been told by his own lawyer, Bertrand Lavelot, that he and the rest of the team could go on, unless he was suspended by the French Federation of Cycling – under whose legal auspices the Tour was run. The team with Miguel Moreno now at its head, had decided that despite the expulsion they, too, would continue racing. A good night's sleep for everybody was therefore in order, the next day being the first time trial of the race.

Earlier in 1998, Hillary Clinton was taken on a guided tour of the region of the Corrèze, to show America's First Lady what was meant by *la France profonde*. This was the area where, in theory, she could best be exposed to timeless French rural life – verdant meadows, fields of sunflowers and the clack of dominos as ruddy-faced *paysans* whiled away endless afternoons with glasses of cassis in the village square.

On paper at least, a start village like the tiny Merignac-l'Eglise – population, at the time, just 53 – and the finish at the charming country town of Corrèze were the ideal setting for the Tour de France's first major challenge for the overall contenders, too. The Tour has always considered itself to be a vehicle for displaying France's attractions to foreign and domestic tourists. With over an hour on the bike for each of the main contenders, alone against the backdrop of lowing cattle and cheering country folk – certain, somewhere along the course, to encounter tractors forming letters reading '*Vive le Tour*' in a recently mown hayfield – this was meant to be all sleepy rural tranquillity and sporting excellence. Instead, however, Corrèze became the backdrop to the Tour's biggest crisis in decades as Virenque and his team-mates made a daylong attempt to convince the organisers that Festina constituted an indispensable part of the race.

With the first team vehicles due to arrive at 10.30 at the stage start, Miguel Moreno ordered the squad's mechanics to load up the bikes two hours early. This process was interrupted, however, by the arrival, by helicopter, of Jean-Marie Leblanc's right-hand man, Jean-François Pescheux, with a notification of Festina's expulsion from the race.

Virenque, for one, was still adamant that he would continue and he rang Leblanc to tell him he and the riders intended to race the time trial regardless. 'In that case you will not be timed,' Leblanc responded, ironically, considering the fact that the Festina company remained, despite the expulsion of their team, the race's official timekeeper. Virenque remained unmoved and for several hours deadlock ensued.

Rumours that the organisers would finally let Festina ride the course without being timed, though, were firmly denied, but they persisted until very late in the day. The situation was tense, but the organisers had one vital factor in their favour: the format of the stage. With riders leaving the start area individually at two- or three-minute intervals, it made it far more difficult for a collective protest against Festina's expulsion to take place than if it had been a mass-start stage.

This was more likely than may be imagined. Far from simply treating them as cheats who deserved to be expelled, since the Tour returned to France popular support for the Festina riders had been steadily increasing. Posters and banners in favour of the soon-to-be absent Virenque and his team-mates were dotted along the time trial route: 'Free Festina', 'We Want Festina' and 'No Tour Without Festina'.

Moreno then sent logistics manager Joel Chabiron to the start to try to convince Leblanc either to let the Festina riders back in or to race the time trial as a 'last farewell' to their fans before quitting. Leblanc's response was a flat 'no', at which Chabiron stormed out of the start area. By early afternoon, three of the nine riders – Neil Stephens, Armin Meier and Alex Zülle – had already opted to leave the race. But another call from Virenque, informing Leblanc the remainder were en route for the start and ready to go, saw the two agree to a most unlikely rendezvous to try to settle their differences once and for all: the backroom of a *bar-tabac* named Chez Gillou. Possibly Leblanc had realised that the location had its advantages. Chez Gillou was conveniently close to the finish at Gare-de-Corrèze, given that it was a long way from the start and therefore reduced the chance of Virenque storming out and trying to ride again regardless.

'What happened, happened, it was like I was there for nothing,' Gilberte 'Gillou' Boulegue, the eponymous owner of the bar, told French television reporters a few years after that bizarre encounter between the Festina riders and the Tour boss. 'I certainly didn't tell them they could use it, I wasn't expecting them.' Nor were the customers, who, myself included, had gone in there to stock up on cigarettes.

In what was a perfectly normal French roadside bar – green PMU flashing neon sign, formica tables and chairs, telly blaring sports in one upper corner and metal-topped bar – I had just completed my purchase when I got a front-row view of Virenque and five other tracksuited Festina riders plus Leblanc walking full-tilt across the bar room and into the back corridor. I tried to follow them but by the time they got to the door of the backroom where the meeting was to be held, a Tour de France official had waved me and most of the reporters back. 'Too full', he insisted, which was, as it happened, blatantly untrue.

The meeting lasted no more than a quarter of an hour. There were some raised voices, but when Leblanc emerged he was adamant there had been no change: 'If they insist on racing, their times won't be taken and it will be a charade. They are out of the race, period,' he said over his shoulder as he hurried away. He had, though, handed over the key document of the day: a formal notification of their exclusion from the race. This time, the Festina riders admitted defeat. While negotiating with Leblanc, they had tried, unsuccessfully, to get the French Federation to back their case, contacting, via their lawyer, its president Daniel Baal as he flew in that morning to Charles de Gaulle airport from the

Junior Track Worlds in Cuba. But the Federation sat on its hands and refused to provide any support. With a third of the team – Stephens, Zülle and Meier – already heading for home, Festina's French contingent realised their Tour was over.

Fifteen minutes after Leblanc's departure, the Festina riders began to depart with their spokesman, once again, Virenque. 'We've been ordered out; OK, let the Tour continue without us,' he said. 'It has to continue because it's such a great, popular event. We asked to continue because there are no charges, no witnesses against us. They said no. This is very difficult personally and professionally for the riders. We'll continue as a team and ride the Vuelta in September,' he added. Unsurprisingly, he also denied, yet again, taking banned substances. Other reports say that Virenque even attempted to claim that Festina themselves had decided to quit. If so, nobody was fooled.

'We'll be at the start of the Tour de France next year and we'll come to win. Vive le Tour de France 1998,' Virenque concluded. Then, as those outside Chez Gillou cheered and applauded, his voice cracked and the tears flowed. That was just about the only predictable element of the entire day.

And what of the other Tour riders? 'We all lied through our teeth about how we were the cleanest team in the world while being thankful it wasn't us that had been expelled' is Aldag's succinct analysis of how the defending champion's squad saw Festina's departure. Asked if – sneakingly – he and the Telekom riders might be glad to see the back of Virenque and company given that it was one major rival out of the game, Aldag laughs appreciatively at the idea, but denies it. Yet looking at the race purely in sporting terms, the German seems more ambivalent.

'We were so much caught up with it ourselves, we certainly didn't have that feeling of "lucky me". We should have been happy that they, our biggest competitors, went home. For sure we weren't sorry for them, either, with them there was really no connection at all. But they were clearly our number one enemy. With other teams, sometimes you'd say, "let's drop the rest and then fight each other". With Festina, we were fighting right from the start.'

While remaining silent about their own guilt, or lack of it, the bulk of the remainder of the peloton refused to support the Tour's action either. They pointed out that the standard methods for suspending a rider had not been observed. 'Guilt by association and innuendo isn't the way to go,' Bobby Julich told the *New York Times*. 'These guys haven't been proven guilty. It's bad for them and worse for the sport.' 'You can make assumptions where these products were going, but these riders did not fail drugs tests,' added US Postal rider Marty Jemison. As well as a sense of their own vulnerability, there was also a noticeable underlying sense of fear. 'The Mapei team is stunned,' Freddy Viaene, a Belgian masseur with the squad, told the *NYT*. 'It's like a hammer is coming down on everybody and the riders say, "Who's next to be accused?"'

The most intriguing comment made to the *NYT* came from none other than Tyler Hamilton. The man from Marblehead, Massachusetts, had punched well above his weight in the time trial – despite US Postal having emptied an estimated $25,000 dollars' worth of doping material down the toilet in a reaction to Voet's arrest – by posting the second-best time. 'The scandal's a shame; it's terrible for the sport of cycling,' Hamilton told the newspaper. 'But maybe this is going to open some eyes and change things.'

Somehow, that day in Corrèze, even without the usual 'top-up', Hamilton had ridden the time trial of his life, with a hematocrit of just 44 per cent, an indication both of his underlying, non-artificially enhanced strength as a racer and that – although he does not state this clearly – there was a big enough margin up to the legal hematocrit limit of 50 per cent to allow for considerable room for artificially induced 'improvement'.

'It felt weirdly good,' Hamilton wrote in *The Secret Race* after hearing of Voet's arrest and the ensuing mass panic and disposal of drugs, 'knowing that it'd be a level playing field, that we'd all be riding the rest of the Tour *paniagua* – Spanish-based slang for "bread and water", i.e. clean.' Hamilton says he believed this even though he'd already made it plain he was still possibly riding under the beneficial effect of some drugs. Not only that, he had heard, he later said, a few rumours that some 1998 Tour riders were resorting to Plan B, like Polti, and using very risky systems to keep their drugs in place. For him to insist he and the peloton were now racing *paniagua* is, therefore, a bit like the alcoholic who insists he has cut down on his drinking when he goes from drinking two bottles of whisky a day to one.

There is a similar sinister ambiguity to Hamilton's suggestion to the *NYT* that he would prefer cycling to be a cleaner sport, given that, according to the US Postal doctor Pedro Celaya, the time trial had provided Hamilton with the most compelling evidence to date about how far he could go in the sport. After that, it did not matter that two days later, Hamilton was dropped, suffering from heat exhaustion and, after telling his team-mates not to stay with him in support, rode 40 km to the finish alone. His defining performance as a Tour contender of the future had come two days earlier. Yet the heat exhaustion, which saw Hamilton lose 20 minutes, had indicated he had his limits. When it came to improving from one strong time trial ride into a winning performance at three weeks, the Postal doctor's delighted repetition of Hamilton's hematocrit level – 44, when the permitted level was 50 – when he greeted the rider after the finish strongly suggests how he was planning on increasing it artificially.

Cyrille Guimard, who won seven Tours as a team manager between 1976 and 1984, was probably one of the few voices to make it clear Festina were not alone in banned drugs use. 'You cannot deny a quantity of other riders are doing the same thing, that is certain,' Guimard said. 'The riders are victims of the doctors and the sponsors who pay the doctors.'

As for Philippe Gaumont and Cofidis, he wrote in his autobiography, *Prisonnier du dopage*, it was no coincidence the day after Festina were expelled that his team received instructions to stop using banned drugs 'at least for the moment'. That order was immediately by-passed, but, as he put it, the seeming sense of invulnerability that surrounded French cycling – 'we weren't subject to the same laws as the rest' – was finally broken. 'We finally realized that we were witnessing something really serious. As for the expulsion of Festina, everybody had a different opinion. There were those who asked why them and why not the whole peloton given we nearly all operated in the same way. And there were those who laughed. Festina riders had the reputation of being arrogant and some people were happy to see them go.' However, he insists, too, that all those riders were also immensely talented, and they continued to net top results after their expulsion.

But perhaps Gaumont's most perceptive comment of all is that 'at no point did the peloton show any sign of solidarity. Me no more than anybody else. A boat was sinking right next to us and nobody extended their hand to try and stop it. We were simply happy that it wasn't us, we just thought about our position and the money there was coming through for it. The salary and the family were way more important than the terrible injustice taking place in front of us. The Festina team were leaving, with their heads lowered, but who, in the peloton, was taking less drugs than they were?'

That Jan Ullrich had opened up his campaign for a second straight win was, in fact, all but ignored. And his stage win was powerful enough to all but constitute a knockout blow. True, the closest rival was Hamilton, whose 70-second time loss over such a long-distance time trial was comparatively small. But the closest pre-race rivals were Laurent Jalabert, 1′ 24″ down, and Abraham Olano, 2′ 13″ back. Neither the Frenchman nor the former World Road Race Champion were anywhere near as strong climbers as Ullrich.

Jaksche's team leader, Luc Leblanc, was the closest of the top mountain men, and he lost nearly three minutes. As for Pantani, a loss of 4′ 21″ pushed the little Italian to beyond the five-minute limit overall, which meant he could be all but ruled out. Futhermore, two of Ullrich's top rivals, Zülle and Virenque, were no longer part of the race.

Ullrich might not have won the Tour – events both off and on the bike were way too unpredictable for that – but the German had both fulfilled his number one status and looked to be well on course for a second straight win. As timid as ever, Ullrich said he was surprised to have taken the jersey so early, but that it 'shows the work has paid off'. This and other bland clichés made up his press conference, where – and this is yet another indication of how much cycling, and its reporting, have changed since 1998 – he was barely asked about the Festina affair. However, given the Tour's ongoing credibility crisis, his comments were barely remarked upon either way.

Equally, the Tour's most crucial stage to date provided a clear reminder of the cycling establishment's creaking attempts to fan flames in the anti-doping struggle, as the UCI opted to carry out surprise checks of riders' hematocrit levels that morning. Fifty-three riders were checked, but none failed the tests – the first carried out since the race had left Dublin. Among them was Hamilton, who, despite witnessing the Tour's drastic effort to clean up the sport, nonetheless complained to the *NYT* that they had been awakened at 6 a.m. by the UCI's inspectors. Considering the measures taken against Festina, that hardly spoke volumes for riders' commitment to the anti-doping struggle.

'Although the use of illegal drugs has long been suspected in the professional pack, the thousands of drug checks carried out every season convict fewer than a dozen riders. A major question has been whether the rumors are unfounded or whether the doctor that most teams employ is far ahead of the drug inspectors,' the *NYT* solemnly observed.

There was continuing proof, though, that they were not that far ahead of the police. Even as the Festina team were finally accepting their fate, other difficulties for the Tour were beginning to creep into view. That morning *Le Parisien* had revealed that, on 4 March in Reims, a TVM team vehicle with 104 doses of EPO – bought in Spain – had been intercepted. One major team might have been expelled, but another, albeit much smaller, was now immediately being brought into the spotlight. That it should emerge just as the Festina affair had reached fever pitch was a coincidence, by all accounts – given the Reims authorities had been planning an enquiry at the Tour de France since 10 June. But it was one which would undoubtably help maintain the tension in the race, and shape the Tour in the two weeks left until it reached Paris.

As for the race organisers, Leblanc reportedly told *L'Equipe* journalist Philippe Brunel, 'in a few days, thousands of spectators will applaud their heroes as if nothing at all had happened. I don't say that's right, I just say that's how it is.'

With their fight now over, the Festina team that remained at the Castel Novel for a second night opted to move into a different mode: that of *après-Tour*. Several of them – Virenque, Hervé, Rous, Moreau and Brochard – 'celebrated' their early exit from the Tour by dancing the night away at a disco in Brive-la-Gaillarde. For one, Christophe Moreau, whose positive doping test had been one of the earliest leaks to spring in the Festina system, a second night of partying on 19 July included his initiation, as he later declared to police, into what he supposed were the joys of Ecstasy. 'In a discotheque where' – he added as if this somehow made all the difference – 'they also played techno music, I was contacted by a young man of 25 who sold me a white pill, smaller than an aspirin, telling me that would allow me to forget my problems, for the sum of 100 francs … it's the first time I took what I think was Ecstasy. Effectively, I danced all night.'

But one element of Festina, in any case, remained inside the race. The publicity vehicles, not to mention the Tour's timing system – a sponsorship deal estimated to be worth five million francs a year until 2003 – stayed firmly in place, where they remained until 2015. 'Festina and cycling,' the logo ran on the team's website, 'a story that never stops.' On the evening of 18 July 1998, though, it was not at all clear what kind of future anybody had: Festina the team, the Tour de France and cycling in general.

7

The UCI and Anti-Doping: From Cuba to India (via France)

Sunday, 19 July. Stage 8:
Brive-la-Gaillarde–Montauban, 190.5 km

Monday, 20 July. Stage 9:
Montauban–Pau, 210 km

Two days after 'Roi' Richard Virenque and his band of not-so-merry Festina barons had admitted defeat outside the Chez Gillou *bar-tabac*, and on the same morning that Christophe Moreau had walked bleary-eyed out of a disco in Brive-la-Gaillarde after taking his first ever dose of Ecstasy, the head of professional cycling's governing body, president Hein Verbruggen of the UCI, finally arrived at the Tour de France.

Verbruggen's single visit to cycling's deeply troubled flagship event that July was to be very brief. Presumably he must have thought he had more important things to do. From 15 to 19 July, he had been overseeing the UCI Congress and Junior World Track Championships in Cuba – where, incidentally, a certain Bradley Wiggins had just become Britain's first ever junior individual pursuit gold medallist. And shortly after visiting the Tour, Verbruggen then headed off to a family holiday in India.

Verbruggen's comments to the press were – as was so often the case at the time regarding anti-doping – snappy, but singularly failed to address the underlying issue. Verbruggen supported the ejection of Festina from the Tour, something he was in any case constrained to do given the UCI commissaires on the race had already backed the Tour's organisers. But he then denied that banned drugs was a generalised problem in cycling, saying, 'if 99 per cent of the peloton were doping, I would resign'.

Given the bunch's drug of choice at the time was EPO, which was in any case undetectable, that kind of comment sounded good, but lacked any real substance. Verbruggen's failure to be present at the Tour and his preference for the balmier climes of the Caribbean and India spoke volumes about the UCI's hands-off attitude to professional cycling's greatest ever credibility crisis. As Aldag puts it, 'do you go on holiday to India while your house is burning down?' Regrettably, it was a rhetorical question.

But why was EPO so popular, particularly when blood transfusions offered similar effects and, while banned in 1986, were equally impossible to detect? In a lengthy essay for the website *Cyclingnews* on the history of blood doping, Feargal McKay says that 'as early as 1988 bodies were beginning to pile up on mortuary slabs as athletes in several sports began to experiment with EPO and die in their sleep … On a simple cost/benefit comparison EPO trounced transfusions, made them redundant. Though expensive in the early years EPO's price quickly fell. But even above the cost, EPO was logistically less complicated than transfusions, vials of EPO could be transported in ice-packed thermos flasks.

'There was simply no reason to engage in the hassle of expensive transfusions. Until, that is, tests for EPO' – the drug was banned by the IOC in 1990 – 'came along in 2000/2001. At which stage transfusions – which were still undetectable – once more became part of the doping armoury.'

It would be a mistake to regard the 1980s, for example, as an era in which doping was any less dangerous. Brains could be addled by speed just as easily as any other drug. 'I can name you riders who were addicted to amphetamines when they were pros, and who are convinced they are still, even now, racing the last lap of a Six Day [track] race,' Aldag says. 'So don't tell me EPO was any worse.'

But what is different is that EPO use was so intense and that its effects were so broadly felt. As David Walsh put it in *The Times* in 2003, 'What happened in the Nineties was that the drugs improved and became too damned good.'

To give a rough figure: retroactive testing carried out in 2004 indicated that 44 out of 60 urine samples from the 1998 Tour contained EPO. This is only approximate: the passing of time and allegations that the chain of custody might have been broken means the validity of the testing has been questioned. It might be possible, of course, that some of these tests, given they were anonymous, were for the same rider. However, it should also be remembered that the testing continued after riders like Aldag and Riis had poured their own doses of the drug down the toilet. Deprived of their 'top-up doses', by the end of week two at the latest its presence in the body, if not its effects, should have been wearing off.

The French Senate report on drug use in the 1998 Tour, published in 2013, is equally damning: it claims that subsequent tests showed that 18 different riders of the 189 starters that year took EPO and a further 12 were under suspicion. Up to one in six of the total may not sound that many until it is remembered that the retroactive tests were only for EPO and testing at the time was limited to three to five riders a stage, including those in Ireland.

Anti-doping records show, too, that no Festina rider was ever tested – and eight of them later confessed to doping. Records indicated the total number of Tour urine samples sent to the testing lab at Châtenay-Malabry, France's main anti-doping facility, on the Tour that year came to a paltry 108 – a figure also confirmed in an article for *L'Equipe* by former Tour boss Jacques Goddet in July 1999. If further indication of how vulnerable the Tour was to potential damage from banned drugs scandals was needed, for all that 1998 is remembered as the year when the Tour nearly collapsed, not one rider actually tested positive. 'All 108 tests were negative,' as Goddet writes, 'and what did we find in the team cars?'

Exactly why Verbruggen and the UCI failed to be more proactive in the Tour's most difficult moment in its history is something that has reverberated through the sport since 1998. Indeed, the question of what was going on, or, rather, *not* going on, in the UCI in the 1990s which may have meant doping could flourish so effectively is one many cycling fans still ask themselves today. It has been partly answered by the recent Cycling Independent Reform Commission (CIRC) report, which has reviewed the UCI's attitude to and actions against doping throughout the era of Armstrong's Tour de France victories. But, regrettably, the CIRC's investigative brief only extended as far back as 1 January 1998. Not early enough, then, to look in detail at the initial roots of the issue that led to the near-fatal breakdown of the sport in the 1998 Tour de France.

It's worth noting that the UCI rarely, during the 1998 Tour or in the years immediately afterwards, conclusively admitted its failure, or even its partial failure, to combat the doping issue. Instead, someone else tended to be blamed. This is clearly illustrated in 2001, well after it had had time to reflect on the recent past, when the UCI published a lengthy booklet entitled *40 ans de lutte anti-dopage*, a history of its anti-doping struggle. This simultaneously seeks to present the UCI at the forefront of the fight against banned drugs, to firmly reject accusations that it could have been at all lax in that question and to wriggle out of the failure to anticipate the Festina crisis – only mentioned in passing – in time.

Focusing mainly on the ten years from 1991 to 2001, the booklet starts off by stiffly reprimanding 'the insinuations that the UCI waited until the 1990s to start fighting against doping'. As far back as 1967, it recalls, it published 'An Appeal against Doping' in a popular cycling magazine, urging governments to help them and claiming that 'this plague can be exterminated'. Such an appeal, it claimed, was made 'despite knowing that it [the UCI] could not overcome a phenomenon that overcame the federation's resources and the sport of cycling'. It pointed out, for example, that at the time the UCI only had five full-time employees.

Yet these declarations of good intent are followed by the cheerful admission that between 1900 and 1950 the UCI had 'only occasionally' battled doping. After all, it insists, doping 'shocked nobody'. A high degree of self-deception here is palpable: can it really be possible that when Tour de France stars Henri and Francis Pélissier told reporter Albert Londres in 1924, for example, that their toenails had dropped off and they were 'drained from diarrhoea' as a result of drug taking, this was greeted with total equanimity by the newspaper's readers?

There is a similar underlying ambivalence in the booklet's insistence that riders taking cognac and amphetamines were 'all part of the same [doping] folklore of *other* times' (my italics). This suggests that these substances had long been abandoned by riders, when in fact in 1967 the death of Tom Simpson on the Mont Ventoux during the Tour was ascribed partly to amphetamines and, very possibly, dehydration from alcohol. Equally, the explanation as to why the UCI had begun its anti-doping struggle in 1955 more seriously hardly gets it extra brownie points. The UCI's Damascene moment, it insists, came 'after discovering a soigneur had been actively participating in encouraging systematic doping in his team in 1955 ... doping had become a problem and we had to fight'. Doping, it seems, was not a problem before; it was only when it was organised that they realised something had to be done about it. Considering the UCI only drew up a list of specific regulations governing soigneurs in 1994, for nearly half a century its reaction to this discovery that its sport contained dodgy members of that profession was non-existent.

Even if further descriptions of doping by the mid-1960s as 'relatively new and little-known' can be seen as stretching the truth, other parts of the document ring flagrantly false, such as the claim that the UCI spent around 10 per cent of its budget on anti-doping. That might – just – have been true when the booklet was published in 2001, yet it seems very unlikely given that when Hein Verbruggen was confronted by a French court just a year earlier he did not contest the judge's accusation that they spent just 1 per cent of their budget, £180,000 out of £25 million, on anti-doping. A further requirement that teams annually donate £1,600 to finance blood testing, in the context of a team like Festina with a budget of four million pounds, was, as the judge put it, 'ridiculous'. At points like this, the booklet comes dangerously close to mere propaganda. It opens itself to accusations, too, that the UCI's refusal to highlight its lack of financial firepower at the times when it was clearly a handicap – in the 1960s and 1970s – is a way of ducking awkward questions about why it did not spend more of its budget on anti-doping as it grew richer, in the 1980s and 1990s.

Some definite progress is highlighted in the booklet, too, such as the UCI's creation of an anti-doping committee, the first in the world by any federation, on 31 January 1992. In 1994, it points out, it invited sports groups to develop a first series of regulations governing soigneurs' activities. (Given the 39-year delay, this would hardly be a milestone in most people's book, but the UCI evidently thought otherwise.) Another series of norms for the sport's doctors was created, too, and on 1 January 1999 the regulations were enforced. The creation of a new position, that of the UCI anti-doping officer, was another step forward, even though when you read the small print it turns out their duties were initially hardly onerous or difficult to learn. Among the half-dozen bullet points for their obligations listed in the anti-doping pamphlet is 'organising a meeting with the relevant race organiser' – presumably not much more difficult than a phone call.

No matter how much a lost cause their anti-doping struggle might look from the outside, the UCI press office had no qualms about putting a positive spin on it, such as explaining exactly how it was possible its newly created Anti-Doping Commission (ADC) was not, in fact, always tough on doping. Early in the 1990s, the ADC insisted, as the booklet recalls, on the absolute need for the maintenence of three-month bans for first-time offenders in cycling. (These were often enforced over the winter months to soften the blow yet further.) This was despite being out of line with other federations, too – and notably less punitive compared with those that enforced a two-year ban for first-time offences. However, the UCI's document makes a vigorous defence that those penalties should not be changed, for reasons as vague as potential litigation, the difficulty doping offenders had finding teams after a long ban and an unexplained preference for a sliding scale of suspensions for different kinds of drug. If this were not odd enough, when it is revealed in an equally self-satisfied tone that in 1994 the penalties were in fact increased, from three to six months for a first-time offender against anti-doping regulations, there is no explanation why they were.

There were other advances, such as commissioning a study of the physiological effect of cycling on blood in the human body. This included an analysis of the long-term effects of EPO on healthy humans – among them heart attacks, as had happened to a suspicious number of young Dutch amateurs in the late 1980s and 1990s. There was also the hematocrit test, introduced in 1997, of which more later. Other measures included a high-profile congress on doping in 1994, and when a document outlining its conclusions was published it earned the UCI a letter of congratulations from CIO Juan Antonio Samaranch, praising it as 'a trustworthy testimony to your federation's care for its athletes'. And even as the 1998 Tour was unfolding, the UCI approved the introduction of a new system recording riders' physiological data in order to build up a record of an athlete's health – the *suivi medicale*. This was not, the UCI insisted, an anti-doping measure per se. But it nonetheless reflected growing concerns about riders' overall health, and could theoretically lead to short 'periods of rest' if there were any serious distortions in 25 different physiological parameters.

So it would be very wrong to say the UCI was entirely inactive on the issue of banned drugs. Yet it was clearly hopelessly outpaced by those exploring more and more effective ways of using them. But if its financial contribution to the struggle to keep pace was risible, the UCI did its public image no favours either by failing to be seen to tackle the issue head-on in a crisis. Verbruggen's absence from the 1998 Tour was a case in point. This tendency to avoid conflictive situations – like the 1998 Tour de France – did nothing to restore the public's plummeting faith in cycling as a sport as the race dragged on. Rather, it made it all too easy for a perception of tolerance towards doping inside cycling's governing body – if not actual tolerance itself – to flourish, particularly when the 'official version' of the UCI's anti-doping history in 2001 showed an organisation burying its head in the sand at best and operating with conveniently self-deceptive, skewed values. If *40 ans de lutte anti-dopage* reflects the official standpoint four years after the 1998 Tour – and its introduction is signed by Hein Verbruggen, UCI president, after all – then how detached from reality was the UCI before the storm broke?

The short answer to that is: considerably. In June 1994, *Cycle Sport*, one of the two leading English-language magazines at the time that specialised exclusively in road racing, ran its first ever mini-feature on EPO, asking if it represented 'a new power in the peloton'. For evidence, it pointed to comments by Belgian Cycling Federation doctor Chris Goessens, who told the newspaper *Het Belang Van Limburg* that the succession of Italian victories in recent months 'smelled dirty'. By this point in 1994 alone, Evgeni Berzin, racing with Italian squad Gewiss, had finished first in the Giro d'Italia (with Pantani in second place), Giorgio Furlan had won Milan–San Remo, Gianni Bugno the Tour of Flanders, Berzin had won Liège–Bastogne–Liège and Furlan, Argentin and Berzin had taken all three top places in the Flèche Wallonne for the same Gewiss squad. ('When I saw that at Flèche Wallonne,' Jean-Marie Leblanc said a few years later, 'it was clear what was happening.')

Goessens was more forthright: 'For some years now Italy have hardly had any important figures and suddenly they begin to dominate cycling. This isn't normal. Italian youth is neither in better or worse condition than the youth of other countries. So something else has to come into play.'

After pointing the finger indirectly at the untraceable drug EPO, Goessens argued that the arrival of much bigger budget teams in the sport, particularly in Spain and Italy, was actually pernicious 'because Italy and Spain are the only two countries where there's still big money for cycling and for teams with several million in their budget, it's not difficult to put aside 10 per cent for strict medical vigilance'. But it also skewed the playing field, given that, as an anonymous doctor told *Cycle Sport*, 'each dose costs around £2,000 which normal riders and teams cannot afford'.

An interview Verbruggen did in early 1997 with the same magazine reflects how close the UCI were to simple damage limitation when it came to certain areas of their anti-doping battle. Verbruggen came to the interview with the aim of convincing readers, many of whom were English-speaking pros, that a new blood testing programme within the UCI's health and anti-doping measures – testing riders for their hematocrit level – was necessary, rather, as interviewer William Fotheringham puts it, 'as a paint factory might take a blood sample from an employee to check for lead'.

Verbruggen put it this way to *Cycle Sport*: 'The whole doping fight is pretty ineffective and it's also unsatisfactory. Imagine that in future there's more of a move towards health controls, concentrating not only on doping but also on the health aspect. If there are certain products that enhance performance when taken in large quantities which are also dangerous to health, why not prescribe certain limits, check the blood and the urine and say that as long as you stay within determined limits where there is no risk to health, that's fine by us?'

When William Fotheringham asked the obvious question, that this was surely dangerously close to condoning doping, Verbruggen answered, 'concentrating on punishment does not solve the doping problem ... The fight against doping simply by controlling and punishing doesn't work. The cheats stay ahead.'

However, the UCI's creation of the 50 per cent hematocrit level as the one beyond which riders could not go without incurring a two-week suspension artificially introduced a point up to which those willing to cheat would consider themselves legally permitted to dope, principally with EPO. The 50 per cent threshold became a target to aim for, as Mario Traversoni, a sprinter with Mercatone Uno in the 1998 Tour, showed indirectly when, in a recent interview, he described his resentment that, as he sees it, changes in anti-doping rules made for a retroactive difference in attitudes to EPO that nobody could have anticipated.

Traversoni uses a series of rectangles to make his point. 'This,' he says, drawing the biggest rectangle, 'is the list of banned drugs in the 1990s. And this' – adding another, much smaller rectangle – 'is what they added later on, and this' – another, smaller rectangle – 'is what they added even later. So why,' he asks rhetorically, 'do they suddenly try to catch you now for something that was only illegal later?'

When it's pointed out to him that EPO was, in fact, banned in the 1990s, Traversoni instantly retorts, 'not if you were under the 50 per cent hematocrit level'. Twenty years on, the Italian still believes those later accused of doping were hard done by. They hadn't cheated, in Traversoni's opinion. Rather, the goalposts had been shifted afterwards.

Traversoni doesn't mention him directly at this point of the interview, but his team-mate Marco Pantani, whose possible use of EPO was revealed in the French Senate report in 2013 could be an example of one such 'victim' of the change of attitude . 'There is incontrovertible evidence that Marco's entire career was based on r-EPO abuse,' says Matt Rendell in *The Death of Marco Pantani*. With rules like the 50 per cent threshold in place, it's perhaps easier to understand why that happened.

Arguably, the one long-term benefit of the introduction of the hematocrit level as a health check was that it allowed blood testing to become something slowly but steadily accepted, without which the biological passport would not have been possible. According to Verbruggen, the people in the UCI who were working on the project were not at all convinced it could be so productive. 'Not according to our experts, no,' he said when asked if the hematocrit levels programme could have further long-term positive effects.

'A good job,' William Fotheringham later noted on the website *Cyclingnews*, 'that they got some new experts.'

That was particularly true given that one of the UCI's experts at the time was Dr Francesco Conconi of the University of Ferrara, Italy. Commissioned by the IOC to find an EPO test in the 1990s and a member of the UCI Medical Commission, in June 1996 Conconi reportedly proposed the hematocrit threshold testing to Verbruggen as an alternative, who accepted it as being a good idea.

At the same time it has to be asked how interested Conconi really was is finding a real EPO test. The answer is almost certainly: not very. He had undoubtedly received money from the IOC to do so, some of which was supposed to be spent on purchasing EPO for a group of 23 Italian amateur cyclists acting as guinea pigs for his testing, but it later emerged, when Conconi faced a police investigation for sporting fraud, that the only amateur in the 23-strong group was Conconi himself. The rest were top professional cyclists.

In 1994, Conconi agreed with the contention that EPO was being used by major teams: 'in theory, yes, it's a possibility.' He also, even at that point, had an idea which sounded remarkably similar to Verbruggen's 50 per cent threshold, arguing, 'you could say you are going to fix a certain level of haemoglobin and decide not to exceed it. It could be a safe procedure.' However, having run that particular idea up the flagpole, he then proceeded to deny he had done so, saying, 'I'm not suggesting it. I'm trying to suggest the opposite.' He also pointed out that people living at altitude did not die from having higher levels of natural EPO production.

Conconi's protégé Michele Ferrari, meanwhile, was equally ambiguous about the use of EPO, telling the Spanish daily newspaper *El Diario Vasco*, 'The sport at the highest level is not clean ... everybody wants to be at the limit of legality, the object is to win.' He denied administering drugs, but said, 'I would understand a rider who did ... if a professional rider knows that there is a product that will improve his performance, doesn't show positive and his rivals use it, would you use it?'

His words gained scant sympathy from the then head of Spain's National Anti-Doping Committee, Manuel Fonseca, according to *Cycle Sport*, who argued that EPO use 'was the same as if it were to prohibit you from having a piss in the middle of the Amazon jungle. Sure, we can prohibit you from doing it, but when it comes to enforcing it ...' Fonseca later worked as the head of Spain's National Sports Council before resigning in 2008.

It would be wrong to assume that the UCI had any knowledge of Conconi's allegedly nefarious dealings. But in the spring of 1994 Verbruggen was completely, and perhaps suspiciously, dismissive of Goessens' suggestions, writing an open letter to the cycling press in which he said that the claims had been partially retracted and that the reason the Italians were so successful was because of their greater organisation, better planned calendar and excellent training programmes. Frustration at a lack of success, he suggested, was partially responsible for the criticism of the Italians, while accusations without evidence were unacceptable. He finished off with some statistics showing that cycling carried out more tests than any other sport, but only ranked 14th in the number of positive tests. It may not have been an intentional smokescreen, but it might as well have been.

What is certain, too, is that well before Verbruggen spoke to *Cycle Sport* in 1997, a report into doping in Italy by another Italian doctor, Sandro Donati, whose publication had been mysteriously blocked for four years, had finally been published – and its effects were surprisingly hard to ignore. In that report, Conconi was named as being responsible for bringing EPO to Italy, and Donati was convinced that the traffic in EPO in cycling was worth millions of pounds, saying one pharmacy in Tuscany sold £60,000 worth of the drug in six months. As for the police investigation, it was concluded in 2003 without reaching a verdict after numerous delays and obstructions by Conconi's legal team. The judge overseeing the case, Franca Oliva, nonetheless described Conconi as 'morally guilty'.

Asked at the time, in 1997, whether the UCI should investigate the Donati report, Verbruggen claimed it was not necessary, saying it was 'an internal thing for the Italians'. He was equally dismissive of widespread EPO use revealed by professional cyclists in explosive whistle-blower reports in *L'Equipe* at the time, as well as claims by French professionals Gilles Delion and Nicolas Aubier that doping was widespread, responding, 'if you don't know, shut up'. (Aubier also told *L'Equipe* he could think of only one top pro at the time who was *not* using EPO or human growth hormone: Chris Boardman.) Later, Graeme Obree, who claimed his career as a European-based pro had ground to an abrupt halt, was given equally short shrift by Verbruggen.

'After I did that thing with *L'Equipe* it was difficult to go to a professional race because of the animosity from other riders,' Obree told *Scotland On Sunday*. 'I was almost scared to [use] the changing room in case I'd get beaten up. There was real tension. I remember reading Kimmage's book [*Rough Ride*] and there was lots of stuff about the problem of drugs in cycling in that book and I thought, "It can't be that bad, surely". But it was. It was a Pandora's box. If Verbruggen (then the UCI president) opened it, there would have been nothing left in the sport, so he kept it closed.' Verbruggen's wrath was not only directed towards Obree, but as the *Guardian* puts it he also 'effectively called Donati a crank'. As for *L'Equipe*'s story of a rider using EPO in the Tour de France, not to win, but merely to keep up, and because, the rider said, 'when you are fighting against men with machine guns, the least you need is a pistol', the *Guardian* said 'he [Verbruggen] did not seem perturbed, but saw the rider in question as a weak-bodied aberration.' As the paper summed up elsewhere, 'the response of the men who run the sport was to hide their heads in the sand.'

So good were the UCI at doing this that they also all but ignored what offers did exist of an EPO test, such as that developed by Canadian scientist Guy Brisson, an endocrinologist affiliated with the Montreal anti-doping laboratory and the Université du Québec. Brisson initially proposed the idea of a test to the UCI in February 1996 and a series of samples was taken from the peloton – after riders had refused to provide them at the Tour de Romandie in May – at the Tour de Suisse in June. (It almost goes without saying that anonymity and promises that the blood samples would only be used for research purposes were needed before any syringes could be produced by officials.)

However, the delays of almost two months were partly caused by the UCI themselves, given that one team, Polti, did actually agree to blood tests in Romandie. (By a strange twist, Polti was led at the time by Mauro Gianetti, later to be at the centre of numerous doping scandals, culminating in the multiple EPO tests for Saunier Duval, which he managed, in the 2008 Tour.) But reports say the UCI then 'backtracked' and the testing was rescheduled for the Tour de Suisse.

The tests from Suisse, rather than looking for EPO directly – not possible at the time – looked at indicators or markers, such as levels of both hematocrit and iron, the latter of which tends to be taken with EPO under the probably mistaken belief that it improves the drug's effectiveness. Both of these in the 77 riders tested were found to be unusual – the hematocrit averages and iron contents higher than should have been the case. But Brisson's work, despite such a promising start, quickly ran aground.

Why? As Brisson told the British magazine *Cycling Weekly* in July 1998, 'at repeated meetings with officials from the UCI and IOC, it became apparent that they would never accept any indirect test for EPO using antibodies such as he [Brisson] had developed, whatever its scientific merits'.

Officially, Brisson said, the reason was that the test was not able to stand up to legal challenges. But in fact, he told *Cycling Weekly*, it was a pretext for inaction: 'it was too easy for them to say that because then nobody is accused of using EPO. The arguments that they were using made it clear they didn't want to catch athletes.' The third, and probably the most conclusive, factor was that the man heading the UCI committee that decided on his test's fate was none other than Francesco Conconi.

'Putting Conconi in charge of that commission was like putting the fox in charge of the henhouse,' says Ian Austen, Canada correspondent and cycling journalist for the *New York Times* who wrote a series of investigative articles into the Brisson case in the 1990s for other publications. ('Verbruggen dismissed them as fantasy,' he wryly recalls.) 'But Conconi was intelligent enough to appreciate the political context of anti-doping at the time, because enough people working in anti-doping at the time felt threatened by these forms of anti-doping tests not to want them to go ahead.' Conconi, incidentally, had said as early as 1994 that a blood test for EPO would not be effective, in that it could not detect the 'surrounding glucose'.

To fully understand why some of those working in anti-doping felt threatened, Austen explains, it's necessary to rewind a little and remember that the introduction of hormones like EPO into the cycling world changed it radically. 'Up until then, cycling doping was designed to make you skinny, to increase muscle mass or to make you think you were going faster or could push harder. The actual gains were minimal and the organic chemists, who

113

were largely in charge of anti-doping, did tests for them that were in terms of absolute values – you were either positive for amphetamines or you weren't. The tests literally found the banned drug's molecules.

'When EPO comes on the scene, not only are the performance benefits for endurance sports far greater – one Scandinavian study put it at a 10 per cent improvement; the time difference between first and last at the Tour de France is often less than 10 per cent, even if it's many hours in a Grand Tour – but as a cloned hormone, it was not exposed in the anti-doping laboratory by the structure of its molecules. That testing needed to switch to being indirect, given that you are looking for a cloned genetic hormone. In layperson's terms, one format for this new testing process could be that you inject such-and-such a substance and if it produces x then you are positive for y.'

According to Austen, Brisson discovered that use of exogenous EPO produced levels of T-cell receptors – used by the bone marrow to capture iron from the bloodstream to combine with EPO and make red blood cells – 'that were ridiculously high, simply not possible by natural causes, and that there was a two- to three-week period where they remained in evidence'. However, urine testing was not possible, because the expulsion of T-cell receptors is largely through faeces: hence the need for blood testing.

'Conconi used two proposals, firstly that the idea of using blood cells was somehow invasive of riders' privacy, which was just ridiculous. Secondly he had the idea that without direct proof, a stack of litigation by the peloton would cause cycling to collapse. They were ethical and legal straw men' – but they looked convincing enough to the anti-doping authorities to allow Brisson to be defeated and his EPO project shelved.

Brisson, speaking later, put his finger on one of the key problems for the UCI, that they were expected to be both guardian of cycling's ethics and simultaneously promotor of the sport. He called for an independent agency with no ties to any sports body, 'like for horse racing in France'. As it was, the only positive effects of something like the hematocrit threshold test were almost accidental.

It is pure speculation to argue that a swiftly introduced Brisson test and a more aggressive UCI would have been sufficient to stop the 1998 Tour de France from disaster. What is certain is the UCI's tendency to believe the problems would go away if it looked hard enough in the opposite direction; its refusal to admit the scale of those problems despite the evidence to the contrary was never going to stop the sport from digging its own grave.

Meanwhile the Tour, now minus Festina, continued towards its first big showdown in the Pyrenees, with 20 riders from far down in the classification realising that with the mountains looming it was a question of now or never to make an impact on the race and getting in a break. The extreme heat and the high pace ahead whittled them down to seven, with two Frenchmen, Laurent Desbiens and Jacky Durand, sharing the day's spoils of the overall lead and the stage win.

While Durand had been on the attack every day since Dublin, neither he nor Desbiens were regarded by Ullrich and his team as a long-term threat. 'It was just a way for us to get rid of some work,' Aldag explains, 'if you want to win the Tour and need to do that, then get a Frenchman to wear the [yellow] jersey because they will ride until they die.'

This kind of pragmatic, 'business-as-usual' attitude jarred with the public's pro-Festina posters that appeared along the side of the road in increasing numbers. Apart from the now rather more symbolic '*Allez Virenque*' type, others referring to the abuse of Festina's 'right to work' and the more cryptic 'Bafoul' – conned – expressed a sense of outrage and loss. 'Why Festina and not the others?' asked another poster, most clearly. 'The Tour has ended up as an orphan after Festina left,' commented Banesto sports director Eusebio Unzué, while Pantani complained, 'there's only me and Jalabert left now to make attacks [on Telekom]'. 'Everyone knows that drug-taking goes on in the peloton,' said Festina manager Michel Gros. 'We are just the sacrificial lambs.' It was noted by several journalists that Desbiens had in fact tested positive for steroids in the past, as had Durand, although he had got off on a technicality.

The next stage, with victory for Holland's Léon van Bon from a group of three, was yet another classic transition day in the saddle, with Telekom and the other overall contenders saving their powder for the Pyrenees. Van Bon's victory reduced the pressure on his Rabobank team, winless in the Tour in 1997, but the number of pro-Festina banners, as Virenque's favoured terrain of the Pyrenees approached, did not decrease.

Meanwhile, the UCI's hematocrit testing programme continued unabated: Banesto, Saeco, Lotto, TVM, Riso Scotti on the Saturday, ONCE, GAN, Polti, Casino and Telekom the next day. The team doctors issued a joint communiqué insisting they were 'only there to look after the riders' health'. 'It would have been better if they remained silent,' *MARCA* commented darkly. There was yet more 'business as usual' as Mario Cipollini abandoned the race, allegedly with fever, as the mountains approached, for the fourth straight Tour in a row. 'The Festina case shows we are like abandoned dogs,' he insisted as a parting shot before boarding a plane, 'unable to defend ourselves.' Pantani, too, was in an equally sullen mood, complaining – as so often happened at the time – that 'the organisers always make routes for all-rounders; all I want is a bit of balance. I'm not here,' he concluded darkly, 'to save the Tour.'

8

The Pyrenees:
Two Cheers for Elefantino

Tuesday, 21 July. Stage 10: Pau–Luchon, 196.5 km

Wednesday, 22 July. Stage 11:
Luchon–Plateau de Beille, 170 km

Up as far as the Pyrenees, virtually nothing had been seen of Mercatone Uno or Marco Pantani in the Tour de France. Pantani's opening prologue performance had been unremarkable, to say the least, finishing 181st of 189 riders. Unaffected by the police raids – Mercatone Uno had no established direct links with Voet, according to team sources, or with the ongoing investigation into TVM – Pantani had adopted one of his favourite tactics for the first week: sitting as far back in the peloton as possible and staying out of sight.

The reasons for this were multiple. As the winner of the Giro d'Italia, in June Pantani had not been racing at all, preferring to rest prior to doing the Tour. His final decision to race there had only been made on 26 June, when long-term mentor Luciano Pezzi died suddenly. Pantani had promised Pezzi he would take part, and as a gesture of respect he did so – 'Pezzi was like a father to him,' recalled Roberto Conti, a Mercatone Uno team-mate. He was 'the only one [among the team's management] with a real understanding of *Il Pirata*, the only one who could bring him up a level, calm him down the most, provide serious advice he would listen to, really hard,' says Mario Traversoni. It did not seem to matter that his snap decision to race cycling's biggest bike race gave him a scant two weeks to get into solid form. 'His death inspired Marco to do the Tour,' Traversoni recalls. 'He spontaneously went for it, knowing he wasn't in any great shape, because he hadn't been training much at all, and with no idea of what could happen. He knew it would only take a little while to build up some base form, but from there to winning – he didn't believe it was possible at all. And I've always thought that it was only good luck that kept Marco in the right kind of position overall to be able to try to do so.'

When it came to staying in the front 30 or 40 of the peloton on the Tour's flat stages, as was – and still is – recommended to all modern-day overall Tour contenders, race condition wasn't the only handicap for the Italian. On top of that, Pantani didn't like being at the front of the pack, anyway: 'It was less stressful for him that way. He didn't have to brake-accelerate-brake all the time. He knew he had the whole team working for him, he could close a gap of 20 or 30 seconds. It was only the wind that was a real risk, because if you get 30 guys ahead doing turns in an echelon and just seven or eight guys chasing behind, then they can get a minute's gap in ten kilometres,' Traversoni recalls. 'As it was, in the sprints I was the only one who did remain anywhere near the front and the other seven Mercatone guys just surrounded Marco and tried to keep him out of trouble.' Indeed, several other participants in the 1998 Tour say their early recollections of Pantani in that year's race were that they couldn't see him – he was always at the centre of a little cloud of Mercatone Uno-clad riders.

In a sense the Italian had nothing to lose anyway, by racing the Tour, given that no matter what the result in France, Mercatone had already obtained a dream result for their sponsor in 1998 with victory in the Giro d'Italia, the Italian team's and Pantani's home Grand Tour. On top of that, Pantani was talented not only at racing, but at avoiding the pressure as best he could in all circumstances, not just when riding in the first week of the Tour. 'He had this great gift of being able to switch off the minute a race was over, and back on. He was more rested than guys who can't do that might be, coming into the Tour.' Where other champions might have been wracked with self-doubt, and find that acts as motivation, Pantani, Traversoni says, had a very different mind-set: of utter, unquestioning self-confidence. 'Physically he might not have been ready for it, but if he was convinced he could do something, he was unstoppable. The key thing was in his head, that he felt he was the strongest. Then his legs would follow.'

The pressure was also lower because Pantani, while watched closely by his rivals, was not considered a favourite. As a gifted climber, he was more at home on routes like those offered by the much more mountainous Giro, rather than the Tours of the 1990s – far less rugged, with much longer individual time trials. (Pantani once famously said he used to get bored when racing against the clock, and would like to be able to bring along a cartoon book to read while riding time trials.) Everybody knew, though, that historical precedent was hardly in Pantani's favour, either: in the Tour, the last out and out climber to win the race was Lucien Van Impe in 1976.

On this occasion, although the time trials played against him, he had one advantage which his rivals might not have expected. 'Back then in the Tour's opening stages, they were always all really flat, whereas in the Giro there's always a couple of hilly stages in that first week – and that would have wrecked him. So he was able to go for it and stay in contention, with about two weeks' hard training, the ten Tour stages before the Pyrenees, and with the Giro in his legs, too, as some kind of base form.'

It was true that like Richard Virenque and Mario Cipollini, the peloton's other two most charismatic personalities at the time, there was a lot of the showman about Pantani: his skull-and-crossbones bandana and *Il Pirata* nickname, the diamond nosepiece, the string of fast cars, the shaved head and predilection for karaoke and singing in musical gala shows across Italy. But the other favourites knew that, even if he was an outsider, Pantani could only be completely ignored at their peril. Festina's Alex Zülle had made that mistake in the 1998 Giro d'Italia, defeating Pantani in the opening prologue and the mid-race time trial only to be crushed by the Italian in the mountains. Yet unlike Virenque, who never won a stage race, Pantani knew how to race strategically as well as deliver dramatic solo attacks in the mountains. He was tenacious enough to produce comeback after comeback following terrible accidents, too. His nine-month recovery period following multiple leg fractures when he fell beneath the wheels of a jeep at Milan–Turin in October 1995 is probably the best example. But that career-threatening accident had been preceded and followed by very bad crashes in spring 1995 and in the 1997 Giro d'Italia, too – the latter caused, appropriately enough for the superstitious, by a black cat.

When he was not on the back foot, Pantani's climbing skills were second to none. Even by 1998, prior to the Tour de France, his mountain attacking was – and to a certain extent remains – the stuff of legend. As the website and magazine *Velonews* puts it, 'Though drugs may have coursed through his veins, nothing he could have taken would have created potential, flamboyance, and panache in the quantities that Pantani displayed.' It had always been like that. In the 1994 Giro d'Italia, as a third-year professional he won back-to-back stages at Merano and Aprica over the Mortirolo pass, even dropping Miguel Indurain, the dominating force in Grand Tours at the time. There were the two wins at

Alpe d'Huez in the Tour de France in 1995 and 1997 as well as a third place on the Tour's final podium that year. Then, in the 1998 Giro, his defeat of Pavel Tonkov on the Montecampione netted Pantani his first Grand Tour.

Pantani's wreaking such havoc in the mountains and his colourful life off the bike, contrasted sharply with cycling's previous big star, Miguel Indurain, the rider who had dominated the Tour in the early 1990s. If Indurain was all laconic detachment, strategic calculation and a dull but solid family life, Pantani had a tumultuous interior world and a constant sense of dissatisfaction at his own achievements, according to some close associates. Unlike Indurain, he was mentally incapable of forging alliances with other riders for longer-term gain. 'I remember Indurain because he was the man of the moment when I turned pro,' recounts Traversoni. 'Indurain was the last *señor* to ride a bike, because I've never known anybody as respectful as him to riders of all levels and types, towards journalists, first-year pros, his team-mates. He was more than capable of gifting stages to other riders. Marco wasn't like that, he was in a constant fight with himself and as part of that fight he had to be the first to reach the line.'

As a result of his success in the Giro, though, Pantani was almost obliged to go for the overall classification. Some top climbers will deliberately lose time in the early parts of a race if they feel they will then have extra room for manoeuvre. According to Traversoni, there was no point in Pantani's doing that, because of his fearsome reputation: whether he liked it or not, for Pantani the GC options, therefore, always remained on the cards. 'He might have told Ullrich all he wanted was stage wins, because he knew he wasn't prepared for the race. But he was never going to lose time intentionally. He wasn't ever going to be allowed to go up the road [by the GC contenders] just like that either way.

Marco was Marco. Even if he was 45 minutes down, they wouldn't let him get away.'

Pantani was therefore the man who mattered for Mercatone Uno in the Tour, and their man for the GC, even if he appeared to be sleepwalking through the race in the first ten days. That the squad was present to fight for Pantani was a given, 'because that was our only mission at the time,' Traversoni says. 'The whole team was built around him. It didn't matter what I won, all that mattered was Marco. The year before, we'd won around 40 races, but the Mercatone boss made a point of saying that while we'd done a heck of a lot, it was Marco's wins that brought the greatest benefits in terms of publicity.

'Being a sprinter, I was up there in the first week, fighting for a top place in the general classification for that first part of the race and a bunch sprint win if possible. But' – with the order of team cars following the peloton decided by the order of the overall classification – 'the only real reason was if I did well, our team car would be as high up as possible in the line for the climbing stages, being fourth or fifth, say, in the queue of the 25 team cars.' If, say, a rider punctures on a climb, having his team car close at hand can be vital.

Traversoni's role was far more limited, then, than his counterparts like sprinter Erik Zabel in Telekom, for example. Despite having two contenders in his Telekom team – Ullrich and Riis – Zabel had his own chance to shine through the race. But this lack of personal objectives was true of all of Mercatone Uno. Most of Pantani's team-mates in 1998 could be described as middle-ranking Italian professionals, the one exception being Dimitri Konyshev, a very talented Russian who had lived in Italy for many years and who had won stages in all three Grand Tours. Most were all-rounders, too, like Massimo Podenzana or Fabio Fontanelli, while Roberto Conti, a winner on Alpe d'Huez in

1994, was a strong climber. These riders formed a triumvirate to carry out Pantani's orders, according to Traversoni, and very occasionally – as when Pantani did not want the team to chase down a break on the road to Alpe d'Huez in 1995 – overruling him. (That they were right to do so was proved late on that day, when Pantani won on cycling's most mythical climb.) From then on, the triumvirate reportedly also took the bulk of the strategic, straightforward decisions on the road, rather than leaving that task to Mercatone director Giuseppe Martinelli, now working with 2015 Vuelta a España winner Fabio Aru. While a coherent unit with a clear objective – to help Pantani – Mercatone were by no means one of the top squads, then. Rather, the results depended entirely on, as he was dubbed in the English press, 'The little climber with big ears', or *Elefantino* – the Italian name for Dumbo the Elephant.

It was fair to say that, with the squad centring on Pantani, his presence 'lifted' the entire team, and his absence, given how little Mercatone Uno cared about anybody else's results, caused a big drop in collective motivation. 'We were all good professionals, but having Pantani there, that gave us that extra gear, it automatically boosted morale in the squad,' Traversoni says. The team's most unusual feature, perhaps, was that it lacked a 'negotiator' or 'team captain', usually a senior rider who would discuss working alliances with other squads. The idea that Mercatone could ally with other teams – as did happen occasionally – to 'burn off' mutual rivals was inconceivable. 'Pantani never liked talking to anybody, never made any deals,' he argues, 'so we didn't ever ask for help. The stages we feared the most were the ones like the 1998 Tour's stage 19 – a long, flat grind across eastern France – where the wind could split the peloton. There was a climb close to the end so the sprinters' teams weren't going to work and we wouldn't have any allies keeping things under control.'

Yet despite his lack of a strong team with other potential contenders, not to mention the unlikelihood of any collaboration, after the Giro d'Italia Pantani was not under any kind of external pressure – unlike Ullrich, say, or any of the other favourites. Internal pressure, however, was another story.

But if luck was on Pantani's side as he all but drifted in the peloton's slipstream down towards the Pyrenees, it was no plain sailing by any means – 'we had some really difficult moments as a result of his way of racing,' Traversoni says – 'and some near misses as a result of all this sitting at the back'. On the final part of the stage to Cork, Traversoni recalls, the peloton suddenly hit a patch of crosswinds and Pantani was one of those caught out, dropping back to the last of about eight or nine echelons. However, Mercatone Uno's leader struck lucky, because Boardman, the race leader, then crashed – and professional cycling's unwritten law that there is no racing while the *maillot jaune* is on the ground was respected. As a result, the peloton regrouped, and Pantani's time gap remained in place.

'Marco was very lucky on that stage that Boardman fell. I was the only guy up the front, but we didn't have any race radios to warn us what might be coming up. I saw that the Belgians and GAN were up the front despite the headwind and I thought that was odd because the route map said it was a straight line to the finish. Then suddenly there was a bend, the headwind changed into a crosswind and there were echelons everywhere. I was in the front and I could barely see our team's yellow jerseys, right at the back. After I dropped back, Mercatone and five or six guys who had been like dead men walking started to close the gap to the group ahead. But we only got back on thanks to Boardman's crash. If that crash hadn't happened, we could have lost 12 or 15 minutes.' The effect, curiously enough, was that such good fortune began to strengthen Traversoni's belief in the Italian's cause: 'It was moments like that, our getting back into the race when it had seemed so unlikely, that made me think it might be Pantani's Tour after all.'

For the first six days, Pantani's advantage remained at 43 seconds on Ullrich, his position in the overall classification a long way down. In the time trial at Corrèze, he finished 4′ 21″ seconds slower than Ullrich. Overall, as Matt Rendell points out in *The Death of Marco Pantani*, six more potential Tour winners – Abraham Olano, Laurent Jalabert, Evgeni Berzin, Luc Leblanc and outsider Bobby Julich all lay between Pantani and Ullrich. At that point, it looked like nothing but stage wins were possible for the Italian at most. Dire warnings were uttered by Luc Leblanc that Pantani was behind by a far smaller margin than in the 1997 Tour when the race had reached the mountains. But when Pantani finally made it on to the Tour's radar for the first time in the race, on the Col de Peyresourde climb in the Pyrenees, it looked to be no more than a symbolic reminder of the true identity of cycling's King of the Mountains. In terms of actual racing, Ullrich's strong ride on the first stage in the Pyrenees looked to be much more significant.

'Marco had not said anything about winning or attacking the night before,' Traversoni recalls. 'But he never would do.' Rather than table-thumping or gung-ho speeches, all Pantani would say prior to any mountain stage, in fact, was "tomorrow, I'm going to do my best". That morning [of the first stage in the Pyrenees], in fact, he was complaining about his breathing being rough. He wasn't that motivated and it was maybe too soon for him to tackle the first real mountain stage.'

While riders abandoned in droves – 17 went home that day, fuelling yet more speculation that illicit recovery products were notably absent by that point in the Tour – for the first two-thirds of the hardest stage of the race so far Telekom managed to keep their leader protected. Over the Aubisque and again over the Tourmalet, there was no question as to who was in charge: the pink-clad Telekom troops, with only Laurent Jalabert brave enough to test the waters close to the summit and then on the downhill section off the Col d'Aspin. The Frenchman's move caused some tension, but only up to a point: on the Peyresourde, as Ullrich himself came to the fore, Jalabert was reeled in. Then another top favourite, former World Champion Abraham Olano, who had crashed, also slid behind.

With several of the main challengers in difficulties, including 1994 Giro d'Italia winner and 1996 Tour leader Evgeni Berzin, Ullrich piled on the pressure. His margin of 59 seconds on Olano and 1′ 14″ on Jalabert by the time the race had dropped down into Luchon, the stage finish, was not a knockout blow. But there was no doubt the German had the upper hand. Most of the nine riders alongside Ullrich were mountain climbers, with Bobby Julich the only talented time triallist to survive the cull, which saw the German back in yellow following its two-day 'loan' to Desbiens.

As for Pantani, he had finished ahead of Ullrich, but his attack, a move around two kilometres from the summit of the Peyresourde, seemed inconsequential in the extreme. Too late to claim the stage win from fellow Italian Rodolfo Massi, Pantani's second place was enough to pull back 23 seconds on the German. But that was hardly a massive gain on a rider back in yellow and with a lead of nearly five minutes.

In fact the Tour's first mountain stage was seen as a major triumph for Ullrich. 'He's made a real advance,' argued Miguel Indurain. 'Pantani will have to attack on every mountain from here to Paris if he wants to win,' the *Guardian* observed. 'I'm going to attack every time I can, all the way to the finish,' Pantani said – but much later, according to Rendell, 'if I had won that stage, I'd have gone home'.

In the Telekom camp, meanwhile, Aldag says, 'there was a sensation after the time trial that we didn't know how we'd do it exactly, but we were going to win the Tour de France'. The first mountain stage had gone perfectly, too, with Riis and Udo Bölts working well as Ullrich's key climbing domestiques. It all looked to be going in the right direction.

However, Aldag was aware of two big weaknesses in the German team's plans. Ullrich was supported on the flat, by Aldag, Zabel and Heppner. But Telekom's Italian all-rounder Francesco Frattini was in bad shape – 'I remember him sitting on the bus one day, unable even to get out of his clothes, he couldn't move.' On top of that, 'it's fair to say Jan didn't have enough mountain support. Certainly there was nobody good enough to put pressure on Pantani's team.'

Aldag drew comfort, he recalls, from the fact that 'on average Mercatone Uno might be better in the climbs, but did they have guys who could stay with him [Pantani] until the last four, five or six kilometres of the last ascent? Nope.' The time gaps were hardly worrying, either. Pantani had moved up to 11th, 4′ 41″ back, but all of the big names were still in between the Italian and the German, now leading the race. Small wonder, then, that when Mercatone Uno sat down that evening to go over their plans for the second Pyrenean stage, to the summit of Plateau de Beille, Traversoni says, 'our only objective was to get rid of Riis and then see what happened'. The Dane, tenth overall at 3′ 51″, 50 seconds up on Pantani, was their only realistic target. However, once again, fate lent Pantani a hand.

Shortly before the foot of the day's final climb to the Plateau de Beille, in what proved to be a game-changing development in that year's Tour, Ullrich punctured. His tyre change took far longer than he would have liked and forced him to race hard to get back the group containing Pantani and the favourites. The

German overdid it, setting such a pace that by the time he got to the Pantani group, Riis was hanging on by the skin of his teeth and Bölts and all the rest of the Telekom squad were long gone.

Pantani, to his credit, respected cycling's unwritten law of not challenging a leader if he is unlucky enough to puncture, and so did not attack while Ullrich, the race leader, was returning to the front of the race. But with nine kilometres to go, as Pantani leapt away and Ullrich was left flailing, it was another story altogether. In the bigger picture, what had seemed to be Ullrich's serene progress towards winning a second straight Tour suddenly looked a lot harder.

To cap it all, Riis, Telekom's Plan B, was out of the equation. 'That year I wasn't good, I could have done with being a kilo and a half lighter, but I was using up a lot of energy in myself,' Riis says, with family issues also causing him a lot of difficulties at the time.

Riis remains adamant that there never was a power struggle between himself and Ullrich, but in any case, after Plateau de Beille and the Dane's collapse overall, the question became academic. Asked if he maintained any leadership status in stage races after the German had won the 1997 Tour, Riis now says, 'Yes, because I was strong, and when you've done your work, you were sitting almost there [at the front of the race] anyway. Jan and I never ever had a problem, anyway we had a huge amount of respect for each other. So that was pretty easy, I was eight years older. With my experience it was a case of "Stand by me, I'll take care of you".'

That day, though, Riis did not take care of Ullrich at all. Rather, Pantani made the running as he claimed his fourth Tour stage win, after catching and passing the one rider who could have beaten him, early breakaway Roland Meier. Meier had crashed on the descent from the Col de la Core, flying into a thicket after he spun over the barriers but was – amazingly – uninjured. It would have taken a sporting miracle, though, to stop him from being overtaken by Pantani, eight kilometres from the summit.

Ullrich briefly sitting up allowed the Dane to return to the group, but Riis was in no position to help. Instead, Pantani, by now past Meier, was steadily forging ahead.

Yet more work from Ullrich saw Riis go out the back again and whittled the chase group down to six riders – himself, Julich, Spain's Fernando Escartín, France's Christophe Rinero, Italian Leonardo Piepoli and Holland's Michael Boogerd. But it was not effective enough to start to reel Pantani back in, and the German, having spent so much energy chasing back through the groups earlier on, had no reserves left in the tank. Only Piepoli, giving some surprise assistance, and later Boogerd, enabled Ullrich to limit the gap.

Sitting in his team car, Telekom team manager Walter Godefroot was fuming at his protégé's strategic blunders but was obviously unable to rectify the situation. The Belgian was still livid with Ullrich later, arguing, 'Jan made some useless efforts on his own instead of waiting. Team-mates like [Georg] Totschnig could have been with him had he not ridden so hard. This could cost him dearly in the future.'

Pantani, meanwhile, was on a roll, for all he was grabbing Coca-Cola cans from fans and pouring water over his head in the intense heat. 'I'm not going that well,' he said after finally crossing the line, arms aloft, on the immense, empty, high plateau at the summit, 'but I kept my head and got over the difficult moments.'

Ullrich was still in yellow, then, but after Massi's victory for the second day in a row, the Tour had belonged to the Italians. It was not all celebration, though: at the start of the stage, the peloton had stopped en masse to pay their respects at the Fabio Casartelli memorial on the Col de Portet d'Aspet, where the

Italian had died in the 1995 Tour from terrible head injuries following a crash. But a victory like Pantani's must have seemed like a fitting tribute of another sort from Casartelli's compatriots.

Pantani had climbed from 11th to fourth overall. A margin of 3′ 01″ put the yellow jersey back within Pantani's reach, although the race's final time trial, Ullrich's strong point, would almost certainly swing the balance back in the German's favour even if he lost more time. However, at this point, with Olano quitting after a crash on the Aubisque had gouged out a lump of flesh the size of a golf ball from one thigh, several obstacles between Pantani and a possible assault on Ullrich's yellow had disappeared at a stroke.

He wasn't the only contender circling the besieged German leader, though: Julich, too, was clearly on the way up. Although the 26-year-old American had only regained seven seconds on Ullrich and was not such a great climber, the margin of 1′ 11″ made challenging for yellow feasible for Julich, too.

Pantani's interest in the yellow jersey, though, was seemingly minimal. 'Just thinking about it makes my head hurt,' he said, and he argued that he had used up too much energy at the Giro d'Italia. However, the daily presence of Felice Gimondi, the previous Italian to win the Tour de France back in 1965, in the Mercatone Uno team car as a guest of honour, was the kind of omen that the Italian media and the Pantani fans were keen to highlight.

Equally importantly, Pantani's Pyrenean stage win had given the usual massive lift to his Mercatone Uno team-mates. Suddenly, after ten days during which they had not been sure if they had been wasting their time looking after the Italian, their leap of faith had brought its first serious reward. 'Seeing Pantani up there on the podium and getting that win was a huge boost to the morale,' Traversoni recognises. 'It was as if the Marco Pantani of the Giro d'Italia had returned.'

At the same time, Pantani's success and two days relatively quiet from scandal put cycling as a 'pure' sport briefly back in the media limelight. There was no way of realising this at the time, but the fusion of sporting success plus a sudden dearth of drugs stories effectively pushed Pantani, albeit unwillingly, into a new role in the sport that was to prove a real two-edged weapon: that of the super-hero who 'redeems' cycling from its evil doping past and present thanks to amazing athletic performances. Rather than all the constant talk about drugs, here was a figure who superseded the scandals and fired up the fans by returning cycling to its former glory with gutsy attacks and no over-calculating of the risk involved. Ullrich might have youth on his side, but – put bluntly – the German lacked the charisma, the flair for improvising tactics, and the capacity for amateur dramatics best suited for this role. Rather, the idea of a 'cycling redemptor' was to be adopted and developed by numerous figures, many of whom, Pantani and Lance Armstrong among them, proved to have feet of clay, not least because, no matter how wonderful the performance, it was only a matter of time before the cloud of suspicion about how performance was achieved started to envelop it.

9

Ten Minutes to Midnight:
Strike One

Thursday, 23 July. Rest Day

Friday, 24 July. Stage 12:
Tarascon-sur-Ariège–Le Cap d'Agde, 222 km

Less than 36 hours after some spectacular Pyrenean racing had
returned a semblance of normality to the Tour de France, the event
derailed completely. On Friday, 24 July, the start of stage 12, the
peloton rode, albeit at a slow pace, as far the two-metre-high
inflatable tower that marked, as ever, the *départ réel*. This is the
point where each day's racing gets underway in earnest, in this case
from Tarascon-sur-Ariège in the Pyrenean foothills across the Midi
to the Mediterranean resort of Cap d'Agde. But when the bunch
reached the *départ réel*, the gendarme waving the flag to indicate
that racing had begun was ignored. Instead, swinging their legs
over their top tubes and leaving their bikes scattered across the
road, the riders, feeling increasingly besieged by events that had
unfurled earlier the previous day, sat down on the hot tarmac in
small groups, refusing to go any further. The 11.30 start time
passed and the Tour de France found itself in free fall, suddenly
metamorphosed into an empty, inert shell of a competition.

As the minutes ticked on and on, the crisis mushroomed:
never before in peacetime had the Tour felt so vulnerable, so close

to collapse. Officially there had been three such wildcat strikes in the past, the most recent in 1991, where Swiss rider Urs Zimmermann's refusal to travel on an official plane because of alleged fear of flying merged into a protest over the obligatory wearing of helmets. But 1991's 'industrial action' was fairly quickly resolved and in both the Tour's previous protests, in 1977 and 1966, the strike came at the end of a stage, with riders walking across the finish line rather than riding. In neither, nor indeed in 1991, had there been any suggestion they would not start the next day. 1998 was on a different level altogether, this was a deliberate sit-down with no obvious conclusion – and as the delay turned from minutes into hours it seemed the Tour would never move again. The show simply could not go on.

In spirit, the 1998 strike bore some similarities to the one in 1966 when the peloton downed tools over the imposition of surprise anti-doping tests. (Crossing the line with their arms in the air and shouting '*merde*', they claimed to be acting 'in the interests of professional dignity'.) Just as four decades before, drugs in the Tour were once again playing a critical role in why the strike took place, and – as in 1966 – the riders did not see it that way. Rather, they felt it was another question of defending their 'professional dignity', an expression of outrage caused by multiple sources, but with one outcome: stopping racing.

How had it come to this? First and foremost, the underlying stress and fear since Willy Voet's arrest had been present for nearly two weeks up to this point. The detention of Rijckaert and Roussel had rammed the message home that, for all the Tour might seem to be a self-governing nomadic 'bubble' with its own norms and codes of conduct (what other sporting event has its own bank and post office branches, for example?), the police could, and would, strike inside it, at any point and against whoever they wanted. But if that added another layer of tension, the organisers' expulsion of

Festina made it clear how merciless the Tour itself could be when presented with irrefutable evidence of doping, never mind a positive test. That it had had to do that was perhaps harder to understand for the riders, but what kind of precedent would it have set if the Tour had allowed them to continue?

Constant questioning from the press, relentless rumours of more arrests and raids, not to mention increasing numbers of roadside banners bearing pictures of syringes and/or support for Festina, made it impossible to ignore the cloud of suspicion rising above the Tour, and cycling in general. Factor in the innate stress, increasing exhaustion and occasional illness or injury caused by racing one of the hardest endurance events and the riders, as a profession, felt under collective attack as never before.

The straw that broke the camel's back in terms of galvanising the riders into making a protest was as the result of the events on the Tour's only rest day, coming straight after the second Pyrenean stage. When Virenque and his eight team-mates turned up at Lyon's main police station at around two o'clock that Thursday afternoon to make statements about the Festina case – Zülle's agent, Marc Biver, later claimed they had been informed they would be treated as witnesses – Virenque's first move was to introduce his team-mates, one by one as if they were a football team, to the police bosses. There were some handshakes and the riders stood, perhaps to attention, in a long line across the main hall. But rather than the strains of the French national anthem, the next part of the 'game' was not expected by these former national heroes: the handcuffs came out and the nine were arrested and escorted to separate cells. (Virenque's attempt to wave through a window at his supporters and the media outside a little earlier, without asking permission to stand up, earned him a sharp rebuke from the police officer keeping an eye on the nine.) Three members of the team staff, logistics manager Michel Gros, commercial manager Joel Chabiron and sports director Miguel Moreno had also been taken into custody – where Roussel, Rijckaert and Voet remained.

While Chabiron was quickly released for health reasons, the subsequent arrest of Virenque and his team-mates had one thing in common with the Tour peloton from which they had been wrested in Brive a few days earlier: an under-estimation of how seriously the police were taking these cases. Holding them for questioning allowed the police to keep them detained for up to 48 hours. National stars some of them might be, but that no longer mattered.

Placed in individual cells, forced to strip naked and allegedly subjected to cavity searches, this was a moment no rider had ever, surely, imagined their doping habits would see them experience. Virenque and other idols of French society, the rock stars of sport who had rubbed shoulders with the President, had been reduced to the status of everyday criminals, for some wrongdoing of which they seemed barely aware.

That was not the only pressure point on the Tour's peloton. While Festina's treatment at the hands of the police must have provoked a collective sense of 'there but for the grace of God', other teams were starting to feel the heat intensely. In the TVM case, where the investigation had suddenly radically gained in pace, manager Cees Priem, a team mechanic – who had already been detained once before, at Courcy that spring – and the TVM doctor, Russian Andrei Mikhailov, were all arrested at their Tour rest day hotel, the Rocade in Pamiers, and taken in for questioning. Riders' possessions in the TVM hotel were searched and bin bags of products, rumoured to contain masking agents, were taken away. When a second sports director and a soigneur were arrested in another police raid in the afternoon, it seemed as if TVM's time on the race was fast going the same way as Festina's. Needless to say, the TVM tradition of holding a mussels and frites party for the media on the Tour's rest day was cancelled.

In total that day a further 17 members of cycling's *gran famille* – as the sport's informal community of riders, journalists and management was often described – found themselves behind bars, in less than 24 hours. Such a huge acceleration in the rate of detentions made the race as a whole feel vulnerable. The question 'who would be next?' was unavoidable, particularly given the morass of collective guilt about doping lying just beneath the surface of so many individuals there.

Tour director Jean-Marie Leblanc repeatedly denied the possibility that this latest police action would see TVM expelled from the race, although his qualification of 'at the moment' brought back memories of his half-baked defence of Festina's continued presence in the race at the start of the Tour. His reassurance that 'the Tour is not finished' was hardly that, suggesting as it did that it actually might be. Equally troubling were the comments by retired Casino pro Frédéric Pontier, published in the papers that day, that he had used EPO in 1997. 'I'm not saying they're all doped,' he claimed, 'but a large number are.' Festina, he said 'were just unlucky'.

TVM, in any case, were nowhere near Festina in terms of importance. A minor Dutch squad sponsored by the Transport Verzekerings Maatschappij transport and insurance company in the 1990s, the team had first come into existence as a low-level outfit, sponsored by a snack foods company, Elro, in the 1980s. However, by the time TVM had morphed through a number of small backers into its 1998 format, its existence hinged almost solely on the interest of Ad Bos, TVM's owner and a cycling fan, in having his own professional team. Priem's talents as a director were notoriously haphazard, and Blijlevens' stage victory at Cholet was probably the maximum the squad could really hope to achieve in the Tour. The police, nonetheless, took the case as seriously as they clearly were doing with a top squad like Festina. They kept both Priem and Mikhailov in custody at Foix for as long as they were allowed to before transferring them to Reims for further questioning on Monday the 27th. No one, it seemed, be they big fish or minnows of the cycling world, was going to escape the net.

Back in Lyon, the effects on the Festina riders of being arrested and left in cells was not a long time coming, either. By early evening four had already confessed. Alex Zülle was the first. After seeing the three statements produced by Roussel, Rijckaert and Voet, he admitted to taking EPO, first with ONCE and then Festina. 'I am certain that most big teams will use EPO,' Zülle added.

After years of denial by riders, collective buck-passing by the UCI and ineffective action by race organisers, this admission by a former leader of all three Grand Tours and winner of two Vueltas could have caused huge shock waves – had the details been released immediately. Instead, with the story taking another two days to come out, what reverberated around the Tour that day was the humiliating treatment the riders were receiving. In Zülle's case, for example, alleged rectal searches, being forced to strip naked and making him hand over his glasses led to repeated accusations that the police were exceeding their brief. Even today, riders like Traversoni will highlight, in horrified tones, the treatment that their fellow pros were forced to endure at the hands of the French police that year, rather than focusing on why they were in jail in the first place.

With his cell next to that of Armin Meier, Zülle whispered to his Swiss compatriot that he had confessed and Meier duly followed suit. However, the Swiss rider named one Festina rider – Bassons, who wasn't riding the 1998 Tour – as racing clean. Meier, too, said that he had felt secure with Festina's use of EPO because 'riders were kept under close medical surveillance'. Finally, Laurent Brochard recognised his guilt, and the fear that lay beneath it. 'When I tried to stop using it, I worried about how my performance would be affected. I therefore didn't dare stop.' By the following Friday morning, just a few hours before the stage started, Meier confessed publicly to various TV crews he had doped. By 1 p.m., when the last of the Festina riders was released, only two were still maintaining they had raced clean: Neil Stephens and, crucially, Richard Virenque.

If the ill feeling and tension this wave of arrests produced was probably greater than ever before in the Tour, there were yet more grievances aired in a strike that seemed to do little more than express general discontent. Rather than protesting against excessive transfers and split stages, as in 1978, or a specific type of anti-doping strategy, as in 1966, some interviewed as they sat on the ground in sweltering heat did point at TVM's possible expulsion as a cause. However, others were angered by reports that two journalists had been caught a few days earlier rummaging through team hotel rubbish in search of banned products. Yet another group was particularly enraged by the UCI's announcement that it was bringing forward the start date for a new series of health checks. Not many, given how the press was regarded by this point in the race, would have gone on strike as a result of the editorial in *Le Monde* that morning, stating categorically that the Tour had to be stopped. But, ironically, that looked like the effect of the strike, given they were the only truly irreplaceable factor of the Tour.

That the target of the bunch's wrath was multiple made it very much harder to try and sort out a resolution that might save the race. So, too, did the fact that most who wanted to stop were following their hearts, not their heads. Those who fought the most persistently for the Tour to stop were predominantly the southern European squads: all of the Spanish and most of the Italian teams, including Mercatone Uno's and Marco Pantani. Pantani's influence at this point was key. 'He wanted to go home,' says Traversoni. 'He was very united to the riders' cause.

[His thinking was] if all the big shots had decided to head for home, then I am also going home as well. Even if I can win the Tour. This kind of cause is a cause that can unite everybody and if it does, then we go home ... [He believed] that we shouldn't be treated like delinquents, that you couldn't race if you woke up each morning and there were a load of policemen on top of you, looking through your stuff in the bathroom, wiretaps ... A situation had arisen in which the riders were like terrorists. And Marco said, "I have won the Giro and I'm here to win races, I'm not here to be treated like a criminal."

'We'd already heard at the team hotel that there had been problems, so our thought was that we should try to see what was going on when we got to the start.' As Traversoni recalls, 'Marco's reasoning was that he wasn't the race leader, but he believed that if the race leader had wanted to go home, then the rest of them would. It was always a question of everybody going, or nobody, otherwise those who did go home would have "dirty arses".'

Did the raids themselves affect the racing? Perhaps not, but they certainly affected the riders' performance, Traversoni argues. 'He'd suffered a bit in the first stage of the Pyrenees because it was half like he had bronchitis, but that was the hardest moment. The real problem for fatigue was the raids: when we were going to sleep, there'd be some kind of chaos, noise going on and suddenly we'd all be woken up, the tension would rise, they were watching us here, there and everywhere. It was like we were delinquents.'

There were also a few top French riders, headed by Laurent Jalabert of the ONCE squad – 'he was one of the most outspoken,' Traversoni recalls – as well as the Belgians and TVM themselves, most notably Blijlevens, who were in favour of the strike. Contemporary media reports say Max Sciandri, racing with a British passport but with strong Italian roots, was also an influential voice in favour, reportedly as was Vitalicio

Seguros' Prudencio Indurain, brother of the five-times Tour winner, who had retired 19 months earlier.

Yet if the division between those riders backing the strike and those against has been estimated as roughly three to one in favour, the ringleader among the directors wanting to end the Tour de France there and then was clear: ONCE's Manolo Saiz. Outspoken and uncompromising, Saiz all but came to blows with an equally angry and forthright Tour official, Jean-François Pescheux, while French police, already low in the popularity stakes in that year's race, did themselves no favours by trying to order team mechanics back into their cars. Some directors, perhaps mindful of their sponsors, believed that the Tour should continue. Martinelli's was apparently one such voice in favour of the race going on, even though his team leader Pantani was against it.

Jean-Marie Leblanc's response was first to offer Laurent Jalabert a chance to let off steam through the Tour's official channels: he allowed Jalabert, as an unofficial spokesman, to use his car's microphone and radio system to express the riders' disgust with 'being treated like cattle'. Jalabert also vented his wrath at the UCI, saying : 'They have turned up at the race ten days after they should have done and they have brought a whole load of new rules which mean nothing, which are meant only to make them look good in the eyes of the world.'

But when Leblanc then attempted to convince Jalabert and the rest of the field that, as he put it in his biography, 'good sense, respect for the spectators and the defence of their own sport's image' meant that they should continue, he was met with no sympathy at all. In order to attempt to create some kind of semblance of normality he drove down the route a few hundred yards in his red director's car, hoping that the riders, seeing the usual race vehicle ahead, would continue themselves. Instead, they did not move, and Leblanc was forced to order his driver to turn round and return to a position just ahead of the riders on the road. He tried this four times, to no effect.

After two hours – far longer than the 1991 strike – Leblanc was getting desperate. His final card was to tell the riders that unless they moved within the next ten minutes the stage would be cancelled. This finally had some sort of effect, with the first two of the 148 riders in the peloton to break the strike being two Telekom men: Aldag and Riis.

'When everybody was sitting on the road there, saying, "they treated TVM wrong, they did this wrong, they did that wrong", Bjarne and I started. There's this picture of us looking back at the peloton and no one would come,' Aldag recalls.

If the strike itself was, at the root of it, an indirect consequence of the drug use that fuelled such a high percentage of the peloton, it was ironic that the first breach in the dyke, by Telekom, was a consequence, pure and simple, of the peloton's unwritten code of silence about banned drugs. For Aldag, at least, staying on the ground would have been the equivalent of admitting they were as guilty as the other riders already facing condemnation for banned drug use. 'You all have different thoughts, like "maybe the best would be ..." but it is what it is, and what do we do? But it's so unreal and why would we do it? Everybody looks after himself at a point like that, and they say "they caught them, not us" and if we now all show [our feelings of] big sympathy for them, then we can directly admit we are all in that situation. Is that an option? On paper, yes, but realistically, no.'

'What do they want to do? What is their solution?' Riis now observes. 'They just sit there in the middle of the road and fight, and scream at each other, it's stupid. Starting screaming, having a huge discussion in the middle of the road, it will only make things worse, because you just get hysterical and you don't think. You need to stay calm and focused.

'[So] I talked to J-M. Leblanc, and he said "we need one of us to move". And I said, OK, I'll make the peloton move. And I said Rolf, OK, come to the start.'

Slowly, in dribs and drabs, the riders began to follow the two Telekoms: first the rest of the same squad and Casino's King of the Mountains Rodolfo Massi and then the bulk of the field. Little by little, the spirit of rebellion seemed to die. 'One team was riding because they had a Tour de France lead, the others because they were sprinters, then we were talking about maybe continuing for another day or even striking the next,' Traversoni recalls. Banesto and ONCE, the two biggest Spanish teams, were the slowest to start and at 13.37, more than two hours after its official start time, it got underway. The Tour, then, was saved, although, as Leblanc pointed out, 'we still might never have made it'.

'After the race started it was Jean-François Pescheux who was behind [in the second director's car] with the riders and we were lucky, in any case, because there were two groups, the hardliners, among them Jalabert, who all wanted to stop, and those who wanted to race. So I was with one group and Jean-François with another.

'Then Jean-François radioed through that they were all racing, albeit with ten minutes delay and we told the guys ahead, hey, lads, slow down, they're coming.

'We were lucky because we had a tailwind, a really strong one, it pushed us on behind. If we had had a headwind, I'm sure they would have stopped. As it was, on we all went.' But as an indication of how close the Tour was to disintegrating, it is there: 11 more minutes of arguing or a change of wind direction, and the entire 95-year-old structure could have been dealt a death blow.

Almost as if the racing itself that day could not be completed, or the Tour could not get away from the scene of its near demise fast enough, the stage itself, reduced by 16 to 190 km in length, turned out to be the third fastest in Tour history, with an average speed of 48.7 kmh. Just to add further flavour to the circumstantial irony, Laurent Jalabert, having acted as spokesman for the disgruntled riders, then carried out a devastating breakaway with his brother Nicolas and one of the riders from the troubled TVM squad, Bart Voskamp. Jalabert's attack was so effective, the three opened up a gap of five minutes. In the kind of surreal development which was becoming the norm for the 1998 Tour, two hours after he had led a rebellion that could have constituted a death blow to the Tour, the time gap allowed Jalabert to attain the honour of being the Tour's *maillot jaune*, albeit provisionally or, in cycling jargon, 'leader on the road'. 'I am proud of how Jalabert raced both off and on the bike,' said his director Manolo Saiz after the stage.

'I thought to myself, after the stuff we've had to put up with, we've got to show the Tour what we're made of, and when we discussed it with the riders, they all agreed,' Jalabert said. Voskamp being under threat of exclusion as TVM, too, made him a man with a point to make. After breaking the strike, Telekom, again, opted to quell this challenge to Ullrich's lead which – had it succeeded – would, with Jalabert as *maillot jaune*, have left the Tour organisers in an extremely embarrassing position. Instead the German team's counter-attack proved so effective it left Pantani, again, on the point of losing the Tour, as crosswinds and high speed combined to see the Italian squeezed out of the back of a third echelon. Finally, though, Ullrich's most serious challenger returned to the main bunch without anybody noticing – again. It was that kind of race.

'Laurent had got pissed off, with himself and with everybody and when the peloton got going, it was like "right, well you want to race and have a fight, well let's have a fight",' Saiz adds later.

'Then the bunch started chasing hard, the time he would normally eat at during a stage had changed, too, and he half got the bonk. It was all a bit too much' – so Jalabert, after 90 km as race leader, threw in the towel – waving his little brother and Voskamp ahead as he eased across the road. But they did not last much longer.

The searing heat did not discourage yet more suicidal breakaways, but TVM, perhaps aware they might not be in the race for much longer, opted to send their entire squad to the front of the pack. Combined with Telekom and Mapei's hard work, that all but ensured a bunch sprint, with Steels outpowering François Simon (GAN) and Stéphane Barthe (Casino) for his second stage win. 'He won, but to be honest nobody really was that bothered, that wasn't what mattered that day,' Traversoni commented. 'It had been a completely fake stage, I think the only bit that was raced full on was the last 30 or 40 kilometres.'

The final chapter of the most troubled day in the history of the Tour was as inconclusive as any of the previous ones. Jean-Marie Leblanc, who had probably given more press conferences in two weeks than in his previous decade as Tour boss, once again swept into a press room after the stage. Rather than announce that TVM, like Festina, would be packing their bags, he opted to blame the press for provoking the riders' wrath and that if they had opted to cancel the stage, then the race might not have continued, which both the peloton and the fans wanted it to do. If his observations about the riders seemed dubious at best, his argument about the fans was impossible to disprove. As for his criticism of the press, it simply acted as a smokescreen for any deeper analysis of how a race could have come to a point where it all but self-destructed.

10

The Communication Breakdown – Media and the 1998 Tour

Saturday, 25 July. Stage 13:
Frontignan-la-Peyrade–Carpentras, 196 km

In the 1998 Tour de France Jean Montois of the AFP newsagency was one of the most popular men in the press room. Reporting, on the 1998 Tour de France, pre-internet and with mobile phones still relatively low-fi affairs, constituted a fair amount of following your nose, judging which rumour could be correct on instinct as much as on actual information. It was a risky business. Teams might be overnighting in different hotels 100 km apart, leading to fruitless, lengthy car drives looking for the latest raid if the hotel receptionist was unwilling to admit that there were an awful lot of gendarmerie vehicles sitting in their car park. Contacts within the squad could rarely be trusted, either, given it could be assumed that teams, knowing it was not in their interests to reveal police interest, would keep silent until the search warrants appeared.

One of the few options available to reporters to try to save time and petrol was to find out what leads the agencies were following. That included Montois, whose contacts both inside and outside the Tour organisation were said to be second to none. Journalists would therefore wander over to the agency desks, and appearing just to chat, sneakily glance at whatever story Montois, or the writers from Reuters or AP, had on their computer screens.

But essentially, as one raid after another took place, the cloud of rumour and paranoia was so thick over the press room that it was all but impossible to distinguish the truth. It reached the point where, if a group of journalists was gathered, they were automatically assumed to have a story. That was seldom the case. Editors keen for more and more copy on the biggest team sport doping scandal of the century found that their journalists had less and less concrete, trustworthy news.

There were considerable differences in attitudes to the doping issues, too. A wave of new journalists, parachuted in to make the most of the biggest banned drugs stories in organised team sport, attempted to build up the hype. Meanwhile, the older generation shared a mixture of cynicism, depression that 'their' sport was now considered little more than a corpse to be picked over for the juiciest bits of scandal, and in some quarters a feeling of guilt, too, that they had not done more to stop it. Finally, there was an ongoing, if limited, interest – greater among those nationalities whose riders were making the running, of course – in the outcome of the race itself, which would, in radically different circumstances, have had everyone on the edge of their seats.

At the same time, usual contacts dried up, both within teams and the race organisation. Whereas before it would be normal to sit in the *village départ* with one or another group of riders and chat over coffee, suddenly journalists were unwelcome. Old acquaintances would refuse to communicate. Riders were less and less willing to take calls from journalists in their hotels and others were convinced their mobiles were being tapped by police, and refused to talk in anything but their broadest local dialect. When they did talk about doping, it was invariably to say that they were clean.

'During the Tour, it was stressful, journalists kept on asking ...' Aldag recalls. 'It became a routine to repeat a lie constantly, which is not too much fun. Before you leave the hotel, in the morning, in the evening, the press would constantly be asking, "what are you doing, what are you taking?" So what do we do?' – he asks ironically – 'All stand up and say "yep, we all did it?"' That was not, he says, an option. 'There was no other way' except to continue lying.

Even so, the breakdown in communication between riders, journalists and organisers was clear. The channel broadcasting the Tour in France, France 2, found that its mawkish post-race chat show *Vélo Club* was sporadically boycotted by the riders. Team buses offered refuges from intense questioning, quite apart from providing, as was the case with the Polti vacuum cleaner, useful hiding places for certain substances. That fluid, close relationship between journalists and organisers was no longer in place either: the 1998 Tour was the last time, for example, that a journalist from *L'Equipe* was given a place in the Tour director's lead vehicle.

The line, at the time, between friendliness with riders and teams and direct complicity with doping is a hard one to define, but that does not mean it did not exist. There is no doubt that many journalists were not harsh enough in their condemnation of doping before 1998. But to assume the journalists tacitly accepted cheating en masse, as has been claimed, is an accusation too far. Most of them muddled along somewhere in the middle, some justifying their lack of aggression concerning the issue in the belief that they were at least doing more than the authorities. But with the 1998 Tour, they were all too aware that their world was changing very fast. Or, as Montois puts it, 'This was the year when the masks came off.

'Just as there was a before and an after in terms of doping in cycling in 1998, there was a rupture between riders, teams and journalists in 1998, too,' says Montois, who started working in the early 1980s and is still reporting today. 'From then on, we were seen as adversaries.

'But that increase in mistrust replaced something that wasn't "trust", in any case, given the peloton was living a lie [regarding doping] at that time. This isn't nostalgia: I'd say the breach of real trust came about at the end of the 1980s, with the arrival of blood doping in the peloton. Up until that point, it was normal to be able to interview a rider during his massage or in his room. After that, it wasn't. All of the interviews shifted down to the hotel lobby. And, curiously enough, that tradition is only just beginning to appear once more: from about 2012 onwards, we've started to be able to interview some riders in their rooms again. That's a gap of more than 20 years, and I hope that healthy relationship, which we had in the 1980s, is now returning.'

The breakdown in trust was not a simple process, on either side. Montois recounts that it was no easy matter for the journalists to believe professionals when the riders had been, at times, so adamant they were not doping. 'One top Swiss rider I knew was prepared to swear he was clean on the heads of his children, for year after year. That was the problem, they were prisoners in a chain of lies. They had no choice but to say that.' The effect, he says, too, was 'that a lot of journalists left the sport, moved on to other jobs. They had had the feeling that they had helped something completely artificial, riders that were completely artificial.'

The journalists' relationship with the riders and teams became much more difficult, but handling the reporting itself on the ground also changed radically in the 1998 Tour. What had been a structurally predictable event – as is any sport, although few, like the Tour, last nearly a month – mutated into something 'where you just couldn't tell what was going to happen. Nobody, the riders, the organisers, the journalists, knew that at all. After the Festina team were expelled, Jean-Marie Leblanc and the organisation thought it would all calm down,' Montois recalls. 'But instead it all blew up again with TVM.'

Working under such conditions, 'the pressure on us from [our agency headquarters] in Paris was enormous. We were constantly being asked to write more. I can remember having an argument with the AFP night editor, quite a violent one, after I'd written up the expulsion of Festina, which happened very late anyway and that meant I got to my hotel at 3 a.m. He called me again to ask me to write an early morning piece on the ethical implications of their expulsion. And I told him I wouldn't do it, because we'd got the next day to get through as well.'

The problem, as one seasoned 1998 Tour de France rider observes, was that 'everybody was telling different things but it was all different situations. It's only been with time that we've been able to find out what was really happening. Nobody knew what the truth was.' At the same time, Montois perceived that the Tour represented another unwelcome landmark in the nature of sports reporting. Although the media have always been opinion makers, it was during the 1998 Tour, he says, that he first observed a phenomenon that has become depressingly familiar, thanks to the Internet – that a leading newspaper considered the publication of its own opinion, let alone its content, a newsworthy event. 'It was when *Le Monde* ran their editorial about stopping the Tour de France. Their main headline was the usual "carnage at the Tour", and then the second headline underneath ran "*Le Monde* demands the Tour be cancelled", as if what mattered was that it was their opinion, not what it said. I still find that disturbing.'

Among the cycling establishment there was a general awareness, Montois argues, that doping had existed in their sport, and had done so for decades. 'But the crucial difference was that it had modified the results in cycling beforehand, but it hadn't distorted them totally in the way that blood doping did from the 1990s onwards. We had riders becoming the number one rider in the world in the space of two months flat, others coming out of nowhere to win Milan–San Remo or suddenly becoming a favourite for races like that in no time at all, and yet others, whom we'd never heard of, suddenly winning the Giro d'Italia in the 1990s. It was an aberration of the sport. Some riders, I'm sure, like Lance Armstrong or Laurent Jalabert, would have had a palmares with or without doping. Others, and there were lots of them, not at all.'

As Montois says, it wasn't as if when the Tour 1998 started that nobody knew doping was going on. '*L'Equipe* had run a week-long enquiry into doping earlier in the decade and in France I can think of several regional newspapers which took the issue very seriously. When Moser got his Hour Record in the 1980s, there was lots of talk about blood transfusion.

'But nobody really wanted to know too much about the subject. The attitude was very similar to how people think about tennis or football now. We all know that doping exists in these sports, but we're not that keen to find out too much about it. The same issue – whose lawyers had the deepest pockets unless you had what Lance Armstrong used to call "extra-ordinary evidence" of doping – was one journalists had to face as well. 'We did our job, did the articles and the doping enquiries and then moved on to write about something else,' Montois recalls. He knows, for example, that 'it was a tip-off from inside the sport that led to Willy Voet's arrest', but refuses, even now, to go on the record as to who provided it.

Having lived through the Festina and written dozen of articles about it, Montois is convinced that Roussel not only attempted to limit his knowledge of exactly what doping took place – which was up to the doctor – but also tried 'to organise things in such a way that it didn't get out of control, by using things like the doping "kitty", to which all the riders contributed. But it didn't work as he hoped, and he was overwhelmed by the riders' demands for more and more doping. The top names formed a gang, and Roussel's role was simply that of coordinator, rather than director. The only rider of the top echelon in Festina who remained fully under Roussel's control was perhaps Alex Zülle. He just didn't have the same kind of power-hungry personality as the rest.'

With France's top team out of the race, and the Tour itself all but reduced to a sorry caricature of itself, did it reach the point, for Montois, when he thought the Tour should have stopped, to make a clean break with the past? 'What would have been the point? It's a nice idea intellectually, but would that really have changed anything? Would the penny have suddenly dropped en masse among the peloton that EPO was bad for the sport? How many riders are going to sacrifice their chances of winning because they realise that cycling's very survival is at stake? It wouldn't have worked.

'Some would have stopped, and some riders did stop, on their own initiative, but it wouldn't have stopped the system in general. And how could anybody have really checked it had stopped? The authorities – neither the UCI nor, had it been their responsibility, the Tour de France organisation – had no way of checking up on them. It's as if, from tomorrow onwards, they suddenly dropped the motorway speed limit to 100 kmh. But without any police radars.'

Over the border in Spain, meanwhile, while stage 13 was unfolding in the Tour de France, Festina were taking part in their first race – the GP Ordizia in the Basque Country – since the expulsion of the squad. The increasingly jingoistic, anti-French tones within certain influential sectors of the Spanish media – many of whom agreed with the riders that the police actions were an abuse of human rights (thus offering a convenient moral smokescreen about the doping issues) – struck a chord with the public on the other side of the Pyrenees. Although the race was won by young Belgian Frank Vandenbroucke – talented and wayward, VDB's tragic entanglement with doping is worthy of a book in itself – the Festina riders drew the loudest cheers. 'Everybody is free to think what they want, but the only thing we're trying to do is work,' said Spanish Festina rider Félix García Casas. 'We don't want to be judged for things which we didn't do.' If he meant doping, there was plenty of evidence to the contrary, even though to this day the argument that riders would 'confess to anything' given the pressure put on them by police still occasionally circulates among some Spanish journalists.

Even as the news trickled out that all bar three from Festina – Stephens, Virenque and Hervé – were now known to have confessed, a meeting was held before the stage with some top riders, organisers and the UCI's vice president Daniel Baal. Among them were Riis and Jalabert, as well as Marco Pantani. An agreement was hammered out that the UCI's new health checks would be postponed, but little else was decided.

As the Tour moved eastwards for its second of three transition stages, the racing itself saw Ullrich comfortably retain his overall lead. The stage's one classified ascent, the second-category climb of the Murs, saw a brief move by Luc Leblanc, sixth overall, gain some 30 seconds' advantage but Riis kept to his promise that he would work for his team-mate Ullrich and quickly chased him down. The stage win itself, with two talented Mapei riders – Italian national champion Andrea Tafi and his younger compatriot, gifted all-rounder Daniele Nardello – in a break of six, looked certain to end going the Italian squad's way. And so it proved, as Nardello outpowered Banesto's Txente García Acosta for Mapei's fourth victory of the 1998 Tour, following three barren years in the race.

By then, Montois says, he was noticing a new feeling among the public, 'and the increasingly large rupture between the fans and the riders. Up until then, you'd almost only ever see signs and posters on the roadsides of the Tour saying *Allez Virenque* and *Allez Jalabert*. They would support specific riders. And from 1998 onwards, there would be far less. Instead they would say *Allez le Tour, Vive le Tour*. Up until then, it was the Tour that they liked, even if they didn't like the riders.' Whether the race would survive at that point was still not yet certain. Thanks to the Tour's rumour mill remaining in overdrive, Montois' popularity, at least in the short term, was still guaranteed.

11

Out Here in the Middle: Frankie Andreu, the White Lady and Handling the 1998 Tour

Sunday, 26 July. Stage 14: Valréas–Grenoble, 186.5 km

In a race in which the predictable and the outlandish regularly rubbed shoulders – images of finishes with ecstatic riders raising their arms in victory one minute, organisers expelling riders, police arresting team managers and riders downing tools (or bikes) the next – events following stage 14 could be considered as business as usual.

After stage 14's breakaway to Grenoble had seen a victory for Australian Stuart O'Grady, when the head race commissaire, Martin Bruin, swept into the press room, it was widely assumed that the Dutchman's presence indicated another serious problem for the Tour. After all, Bruin had been at Jean-Marie Leblanc's side during the Festina expulsion press conference, had been back in action again during the riders' strike and had been photographed, looking as serious as ever, after Saturday, 25 July's emergency meeting to thrash out the details of postponing the UCI's new regulations.

Bruin took a seat at the end of a table and was instantly swamped by a sea of microphones, all anticipating the latest dramatic development. The tension mounted with the temperature, already

40 degrees in the shade. Was this to be the point at which TVM – a squad with serious credibility issues following arrests among the higher echelons of team management and ongoing investigation into the banned drugs seized in April – suffered the same fate as Festina?

But this time round any journalists expecting to witness the latest episode in the Tour's disintegration were to be disappointed. Instead, Bruin read out a statement informing them that Giuseppe Calcaterra, the rider who had finished second in the recently completed stage, had been demoted to sixth place for an apparently dangerous late manoeuvre. For a moment, all seemed normal on the Tour: this was a sudden reminder of what the UCI commissaires' top priority had, up until two weeks earlier at least, always been – ensuring that race regulations, be it in on an epic trek through the mountains or on a fairly unexciting transition stage, were always respected. In this case Calcaterra's demotion was, the *Guardian* said at the time, 'as if to show that the Tour's disciplinarians are only able to deal with minor offences'. The bigger ones – like doping – got handled rather differently and even the fans seemed to view them differently: EPO, one roadside banner on stage 14 informed, 'is like Pastis'. 'If so,' the *Guardian* wryly observed, 'it is going to leave this year's Tour with one hell of a hangover.'

Like Nardello on stage 13 and O'Grady, now enjoying his day of glory on stage 14, in the 1998 Tour de France Illinois-born rider Frankie Andreu was just another fairly anonymous, middle-ranking member of the poor bloody infantry in the Tour's long battle to reach Paris safely. Racing with the US Postal team, at that point pre-Armstrong's Tour comeback, a solid but definitely second-tier squad, Andreu's role was that of a top domestique. His best results were a respectable number of top five placings in Tour stages, a win in the Tour of Poland and Tour of Luxembourg, a seventh in Het Volk and a ninth in the ultra-tough edition Paris–Roubaix in 1994. As such he was working for the American team's leaders of the time, Frenchman Jean-Cyril Robin and, following his first week time trial success, Tyler Hamilton.

'We were a small team, trying to get through and hunting for stage wins,' Andreu recalls. 'But once that Festina thing happened the stress level was immense – and the shock, too. EPO was around and everybody kind of knew that other people were taking this product, and I was taking this product and stuff like that. But the thing that shocked people was the amount of crap that this guy Willy Voet got caught with. It was unbelievable. Holy cow, this was a whole 'nother ball game here.'

That Andreu was so impressed by the scale of Voet's medical armoury confirms there was a doping 'hierarchy' inside the Tour peloton. Some super-rich teams, like Festina, were using products and operating with a degree of sophistication that other, smaller fish in the pond like US Postal were not able to do. Quite apart from individual riders' reactions to certain substances – Hamilton, for example, could not use some substances for that reason – the 1998 playing field, then, was not at all level given each team had a different level of access to the illegal medicines cupboard. 'Then the next thing you realise', continues Andreu, 'is if there are teams doing that much, then there have to be other teams doing it, they're not smart enough to be doing it on their own. So it was a big eye-opener, as to how much crap and risk people were willing to take to be able to do well.'

Yet some, like Andreu, were simply using the drugs to save their own skins, to get through races which had increased in velocity through the 1990s to what Andreu calls 'warp speed'. In her autobiography *The Race to Truth*, Postal soigneur Emma O'Reilly confirms, indirectly, Andreu's belief at the time that doping was necessary merely to keep up. 'It's ridiculous,' she remembers him commenting one day on the way to a start. 'I did my first Tour on spaghetti and water but it's impossible to do it like that now. You just can't. Maybe this will clean it up?' Yet O'Reilly, too, was as surprised as Andreu by the sheer amount of illegal drugs found on Voet. The Irishwoman, herself to play a well-documented part in the revelations of organised doping in later years at Postal that led to the downfall of Lance Armstrong, argued that Voet 'was carrying enough drugs to look like a dealer. Heads were going to roll.'

Although there have been rumours that Postal had to 'flush stuff down the toilet', Andreu says he 'never saw that or was aware of it'. But people on other squads, he recognises, 'were freaking out. I was never in a situation, though, to be that nervous.' The reason being, he says, 'I didn't have that stuff. A lot of times you'd do it [take banned substances, such as a course of EPO to raise hematocrit levels] leading up to the Tour, and then at the Tour they have the tests and all that kind of stuff, so I didn't have anything to worry about. I had nothing illegal.'

Yet that was almost certainly not the case across the board, and, as Andreu was to discover the following year, when Armstrong and certain other Postal riders received 'preferential treatment' for their doping, the 1998 Tour highlighted those internal divisions between the haves and the have-nots – by reducing all the riders to the same level. As the police raids on the Tour continued, O'Reilly recalls in her autobiography that 'suddenly there was lots more space in the cupboards and fridges and all the plain cardboard boxes had vanished into thin air. I'd never need to tell a rider off for leaving dirty needles in hotel bins again. Whatever had been going on underground before had now dug down a whole lot deeper.' Some of it indeed went underground – literally: according to O'Reilly she heard that £15,000 worth of drugs were flushed down the team bus toilet into a field during one of the time trial stages. Other areas, such as team vehicles, became more inaccessible. The door to the Postal team camper, O'Reilly recalls, now remained closed all the time. Indeed, when Postal rider Jonathan Vaughters once tried to invite me inside the camper during the Dauphiné Libéré of 1999 for an interview, US Postal sports director Johan Bruyneel at once urgently bellowed 'No!' We were reduced to sitting on the pavement to talk instead.

Postal themselves were never searched, and, as Andreu reiterates, 'I didn't have anything to worry about them busting down my door. But the mood of the peloton was anxious, tense, all that kind of stuff.

'Anybody who had anything in reserve from the Tour made it disappear for sure, after Festina and then even more in the case of TVM, when they were treated like delinquents.' Nonetheless, rumours about raids and arrests 'were constant. It was hard to keep track. You'd hear stories about camping cars and team cars getting searched or guys jumping out of hotel windows in case they were going to get busted.' (During the 2001 police raids on the team hotels at San Remo during the Giro d'Italia, when he believed the carabinieri would be knocking on his door, one Italian rider did exactly that.)

The mood among the teams regarding the possibility of leaving early varied radically. Although at other moments it was clear Postal was going to stay, the night before the Tour's strike at Tarascon-sur-Ariège, Andreu says, 'It reached the point that we were all going to quit. All the teams were going to go home.' His personal dilemma, he said, was trivial in one sense, but it reflects perfectly how the effects of doping raids were reaching into every last corner. 'At the time, I can remember debating on whether I would have a *dame blanche*, a big old ice-cream sundae, because if we wouldn't be going on racing after that day I could eat that no problem. Johnny Weltz was saying we should still be prepared to ride and yada yada. And everybody was like, "hey, we don't know if we're going on or not" and I was like, "dammit, I don't know if I should have the sundae or not, I don't know what I should do".'

Inside the squad, though, US Postal were not in general – apart from one or two days – a team that clearly and definitively wanted to go home early. 'That never even came up. We supported the protests for the riders who were being held prisoner or whatever till two in the morning, keeping them and searching them. The riders had no rights at all. So whenever people said we should have to protest and sit on the ground, I was like, "OK, we'll sit on the ground". And then we'd be sitting around saying, "what the hell are we doing, how long is this going to last, when are we going …?" There were riders going up and talking to the organisation, but I was just a small [low-level] rider, I didn't even know what they were figuring out.'

Andreu said that at the time it did not sink in that this might be the end of the Tour – possibly indefinitely. The riders' resentment at their mistreatment was centred more on the here and now, rather than the 'effect was, or could have been, us stopping the entire Tour or the sport. We were more like, "this is not right, this is not good, we're in a protest, we're not going to race". At the same time, I didn't want the Tour to stop.' With the exception of the Tarascon-sur-Ariège strike, Postal were, he said, 'always going to keep going'. His feelings on what action should be taken were contradictory rather than clear – which in his case and for so many others only intensified the tension in the peloton. Given the unprecedented nature of the 1998 Tour, nobody knew which way they should turn for sure, which course of action was the correct one. For Andreu as for the rest of the peloton, this was a voyage in the dark. As he points out, for many riders in the peloton racing the Tour was a chance 'of a lifetime' to take part in the sport's showcase event. Nor did he much trust what he was hearing, and, given the degree of self-interest that had been shown when Festina were thrown out, perhaps he was wise not to do so. 'When you [the riders] decided not to do the race, there were a lot of personal interests going round, and there were those who talked in the interest of the peloton. The ones who were really trying to talk in everybody's interests were very, very few.

'So there would be times when some of us would say we weren't going to race, and the others would say, "fuck you, we're going". So, like, Jalabert and his little brother [on stage 12 after the strike] had taken off, and we ride easy and then somebody starts riding tempo and ends up chasing, and then you end up having the race at the end. There was never a cohesion.' Yet the anger and resentment at the gendarmes' handling of the cases was not so easily forgotten. 'We were treated like meat. Anybody could do anything to you, we felt humiliated, violated.' Yet curiously, even though the goalposts had shifted so radically in terms of what some riders thought was acceptable and some didn't – as with Mario Traversoni – Andreu did not feel that the police activity in itself was wrong. It was more the way in which the operations were carried out. 'A lot of people were taking EPO and a lot of riders limited themselves to that, a lot of riders branched into a lot of other stuff. We knew what we were doing was kind of skirting round the rules, so for all of a sudden the hammer to come down – no.

'Because for me, besides it being cheating and being wrong, you didn't want to get caught. I was scared to death – always, from beginning to end, forever – of getting caught, because then your name is there, my reputation is ruined, my name is ruined. It was a huge worry for me.' He is, along with Aldag and Riis, one of those who believes that even if the methodology used by the police during the Festina Tour was wrong and the end did not justify the means, the end in itself was the correct one. 'Doping was so prevalent. You know, they did all these raids against people and they found stuff, it's not like they were raiding against innocent people, they were guilty. It's like being a robber and you're bitching about being arrested.'

Andreu believes that if there was one division in the peloton between those who could afford or were willing to use more expensive brands of drugs, another was the depth of remorse that different nationalities would feel about doping. 'I thought it was more of an American thing than a European thing. For the Europeans it felt like they'd say, OK, you're caught, you do your two years, and that's it, you come back, nobody cares.

'We were surprised at Voet, because nobody, at that time in Italy amongst us [at US Postal], did group doping. For sure there were individuals who did bad things, but it was individual. This amount of products and that all of the Festina riders were involved ... was a team thing, precalculated, premeditated.'

As several riders have observed, once the stages themselves got underway the racing was full on – which, given the strain the riders were under off the bike, must have contributed to their usual state of exhaustion. 'The tension didn't affect the racing that much,' Andreu says. 'Either we were doing the race or we weren't. If it was happening, there was no time for discussion except for maybe in the first few kilometres. So the race was a real one, except when TVM won and when Steels won at Cap d'Agde and we only did 40 kilometres.'

For Andreu, O'Grady, Calcaterra and all the domestiques in the race, it should be stressed that the raids were only one of several concerns. Even if careers and reputations were not necessarily on the line; even if, like Andreu, riders had no illegal substances on them, for all the exceptional events surrounding it in 1998 the Tour was no easier to handle than in any other year. After three days of extreme heat as the race moved across southern France, with temperatures reaching the low 40s in the afternoon, the Tour's next big set-piece challenge was about to begin. Three days of hard riding in the Alps were about to test Ullrich – the race leader since the first stage in the Pyrenees – Julich, Pantani and the rest of the overall challengers. For riders like Andreu, however, such stages were all about surviving as best they could – with or without banned drugs.

12

Pantani Turns the Clock Back

Monday, 27 July. Stage 15:
Grenoble–Les Deux Alpes, 189 km

In *The Death of Marco Pantani*, Matt Rendell describes the moment when the Italian launched his main attack on the rain-soaked, mist-shrouded stage 15 of the 1998 Tour de France as 'a brushstroke of saturated colour in the grey'. Indeed, for many observers at the time, after weeks of doping scandals in the Tour and years of clinical domination by time trial experts of the calibre of Ullrich and Miguel Indurain, Pantani's exploits over stage 15's four brutally difficult Alpine climbs truly felt like a ray of sunlight. Just as the race seemed to be on the point of collapse, the Mercatone Uno rider raised the Tour's sporting stature to a higher level than it had been for decades. 'He has breathed new life into the sport ... his charisma and genius send us back to the legend of the lone climber in the storm, the legend of Fausto Coppi and [1958 Tour winner] Charly Gaul, the Luxembourg rider who tore up the rulebook and who inspired him,' as *L'Equipe* put it after the stage. If that was the French take on Pantani's exploits, the more partisan Italians outdid them, turning their man into an idol. Internationally, as Rendell puts it, he 'became a global sporting icon'.

Today, with the benefit of hindsight, it's hard not to view that era of cycling from a new perspective. But what is the correct perspective? On the one hand, unqualified condemnation of doping in the 1990s and noughties not only erases dark chapters of sporting history but simultaneously makes a mockery of whatever human endeavour and athletic achievement that they also encapsulated. On the other hand, unqualified praise, like that of Pantani from a 2015 Sfide documentary on Italy's RAI 3 TV station, for example, seems tacky at best, hypocritical and exploitative at worst.

It is true that the air Pantani breathed back into the near-comatose Tour turned out to be tainted by doping. At the same time, however, you could say that Pantani's exploits on stage 15 of the 1998 Tour de France represented one of the race's greatest and most exciting post-war dramas ever. That Pantani's performance was very probably fuelled (how much we shall never know) by the very drugs that brought the Tour to the edge of extinction is, as it were, a bitter pill to swallow. But it cannot be avoided.

***

Inside the Ullrich camp, even before the hardest single mountain day of the 1998 Tour and with a Marco Pantani increasingly on the rampage, everything looked to be on track. 'It all seemed to be under control' is how Rolf Aldag recalls it, and Telekom certainly seemed to have the race in their pocket. With Pantani more than three minutes behind and a third week time trial yet to come where the Italian would, on previous form, lose around four minutes to Ullrich, the Mercatone Uno rider might be Ullrich's greatest threat – but he would need to take well over seven minutes on the German in order to win the Tour. The chances of such a huge upset were slim, to say the least.

However, at Mercatone Uno management and riders had been doing their own calculations. 'The thing that we'd really come to understand that day at Plateau de Beille was not so much about Ullrich, it was more about Riis,' Traversoni recalls. 'We'd seen that

Riis wasn't in good shape and wasn't having a good Tour at all. That was crucial [because] we knew that Ullrich needed Riis to take any kind of important decision and that, if we could isolate Ullrich from Riis, Ullrich would be much easier to beat.'

At the same time, with Pantani lying fourth overall, tied on time with Laurent Jalabert, and Julich less than two minutes ahead, a podium placing in Paris was, Traversoni says, 'something we thought was sure to happen. Ever since the Plateau de Beille, the team had nurtured the hope that Marco would do something similar on the Galibier.' At the start of stage 15, when speaking to the outside world, Pantani himself sounded deliberately vague and neutral about his chances. 'It depends,' he told TV journalists. 'It all depends on my legs.'

But that was not actually the case. Mercatone Uno knew, Traversoni recalls, that Pantani was pretty gung-ho. This time there were no chest infections to worry him, as in the Pyrenees. And the night before the stage – contrary to one of the many legends that would later spring up about that mythical day in cycling – 'Marco told us exactly where he was going to attack on the Galibier. Nobody else thought of it, nobody. Attacking there, exactly there, was all Marco's idea.'

Conditions for the stage itself were hardly inspiring. Stage 15 of the 1998 Tour was a classic high mountain trek, with two *hors catégorie* climbs, the Croix de Fer and Galibier, as the day's first and third challenges, and the second category Télégraphe and first category ascent to a summit finish at Les Deux Alpes the other two difficulties. But after a start in a deceptively warm Grenoble, the increasingly foul weather – freezing cold, heavy fog on all the mountain summits and torrential rain showers, cloud cover so low the usual helicopters retransmitting TV imagery were replaced by a plane – was hardly typical Alpine summer weather. If nothing else, however, some of the grainy and in some cases all but obscure images sent back by the aircraft that day helped viewers of the Tour imagine they were watching cycling from an earlier, simpler, less troubled age.

Still, for the first third of its 189 km, the stage played out much as expected with an early break containing Aldag and Zabel, on paper two of the weaker elements for Telekom in the mountains, keeping Telekom at the forefront of affairs as far as the foot of the first climb. Then, as the front wave of the bunch rolled up and over the summit of the Croix de Fer, a new group of 40 riders containing all the favourites slowly sheared clear, with Pyrenean stage winner Rodolfo Massi bridging across to the lead break and picking up maximum points to add to his lead in the King of the Mountains classification. The Tour had, in fact, stuck to its usual script of the top contenders keeping a steady, rather than explosive tempo on the first of the big climbs of the day – weeding out only the very ill, the sprinters and the weakest of the climbers.

Massi was once again first over the stage's second climb, the Télégraphe as the front break shrank to three – Massi himself, the talented young Christophe Rinero, in place as Plan B after Julich for Cofidis' options for the overall, and Spain's Marcos Serrano. Then, on the five-kilometre climb, the yellow jersey group thinned out behind. This was largely due to Banesto's José María Jiménez, himself a hugely gifted if eccentric climber. Jiménez provided another footnote to the long-standing rivalry between Spain's two top teams, ONCE and Banesto, when his attacks on the second category climb stretched the bunch repeatedly to the point that ONCE's leader Laurent Jalabert cracked.

As a result, Jiménez effectively worked as a support act for Pantani, considerably softening up the opposition in a way which the Croix de Fer had failed to do. Even in the unlikely event that the general classification was to remain unchanged, with Jalabert gone Pantani's podium place was looking increasingly secure. As yet, the Italian had not had to move a finger. Instead, he could watch and observe how Telekom's support cast for Ullrich was now down to just two riders: Udo Bölts and Bjarne Riis.

Events on the first half of the Galibier raised the stakes even more. Well aware this was the day when Ullrich would be at his most vulnerable, two other climbers, Luc Leblanc and Fernando Escartín, the latter by this point Spain's top rider overall, tried their luck. Each time, though, Riis brought them back. The overall effect did not directly damage Ullrich. But with no other Telekoms in the front group as a result of these accelerations, Riis had become the one protective layer left for Ullrich.

The point came, as it was bound to, where Riis could do no more and dropped behind, and Ullrich immediately feigned an attempt at domination by setting the pace at the head of the group. Nobody was fooled. It was only a few minutes before Escartín – like Jiménez before him unintentionally smoothing Pantani's path just a little more – broke away again. Although it remains unclear whether Pantani attacked at the precise point where he had told Traversoni and company he would do so the night before, the Spaniard's repeated digs certainly had one crucial effect on the Mercatone plans. They helpfully ensured that Riis, who might have been able to give Ullrich the support he needed had the pace been a little lower, was permanently out of the game.

'I was aiming for the podium, because Bobby Julich was there, too, and I wanted to see if I could get rid of him,' Escartín now says. 'Ullrich and Pantani were out of my league, I thought, but I wanted to move up as best I could.

'This kind of long, grinding climb was exactly where I could do that the best because I had to get as big an advantage as I could on Julich before the final time trial, which was always my weak point. I could see that Ullrich was on a really bad day, but it was kind of by chance. He wasn't my big objective.' However, for another out and out climber in the race, watching and waiting for his moment to go clear, the German most certainly was.

Just before that moment came, a flurry of attacks by Michael Boogerd, and Luc Leblanc – again – caused Ullrich to respond personally, with Pantani close behind. By this point the race began to move above the Galibier's tree line, with even riders like Dariusz Baranowski of the US Postal Service briefly taking a turn at the front of the pack. Yet despite the uneven pace, the Tour's leader looked just as exposed as the mountain's increasingly rocky, scree-lined surface, dropping back and forth in the group of some dozen riders. So Pantani duly delivered the blow he had designed to test Ullrich to the limit – and bounded off up the climb.

'It was really slow-motion when we got to the steep part,' Julich now recalls. 'I asked [Cofidis team-mate] Kevin Livingston to do a good tempo and he went full gas into this turn. And after he did so I said, "Kevin, slow down" and he got mad at me for asking one thing and then another, and I retorted, "I said, hard but not that hard – we've still got eight kilometres to go."

'It was at that moment that Pantani heard me, and sprinted on his big ring, down on his drops, for like 50 metres. Then he turned, stopped pedalling, looked back and smiled. And I said' – presumably because the pace would then drop – '"thank God". And then he went, again.

'There's a whole bunch of us behind, and we're like sitting there, waiting to see what Jan is going to do. That was when it hit me, it was like, "shit we're climbing at ten kilometres an hour, and who knows where Pantani is?"'

It was, in many ways, a typical Pantani attack, sloping away out of the right-hand side of the pack with his usual bizarre mixture of a fluid pedalling style and an almost painfully hunched upper body, seemingly hooked over the frame with his hands stretched out on the drops. But there was one difference: the total of 47 km that remained to the finish made his move, by the standards of the day, an exceptionally long-distance attack.

Pantani had, in keeping with his customary bad luck, already crashed that day, on the Croix de Fer. Yet there was nothing to show that it had really had any effect as the Italian darted up the road after Escartín, looked briefly back at the flailing Ullrich, who could not even respond to a counter-move by Leblanc. Then, as the fog and rain closed in again, Pantani was gone.

But if the Italian appeared to be having an inspired day, Ullrich – his face puffy and ashen beneath the usual pro cyclist's tan – his legs turning ever more stiffly, and skimming from the front end of the group to the rear, was dipping in and out of a complete crisis. At a point where older pros might have settled into their own rhythm, his lack of experience suddenly began to tell. At this point it should be remembered that, although he'd won the Tour at 23 in 1997, Ullrich was still a comparatively new professional – just 24 and in his third full season. He had no idea what was coming, either, given that he had never been up the Galibier in a race. (The closest had been in 1996, when its ascent was cancelled because of a snowstorm, and Ullrich and the rest of the bunch were driven over it in a team car.) His lack of awareness of what he was facing, with no Riis or team car to ask for information, and a language barrier that meant he rarely talked to rivals, all left him even more exposed. The German's racing cocoon had collapsed just when he was most vulnerable.

Pantani, meanwhile, was going hell for leather up the climb, Fernando Escartín recalls, 18 years on. 'I tried to talk to Marco as he went past me, to see if he would be willing to reach some kind of a working alliance so we could get to the last climb together. But he was way too strong for me, I couldn't follow him at all. He just shot away – pff, like that. I was lucky because [team-mate]

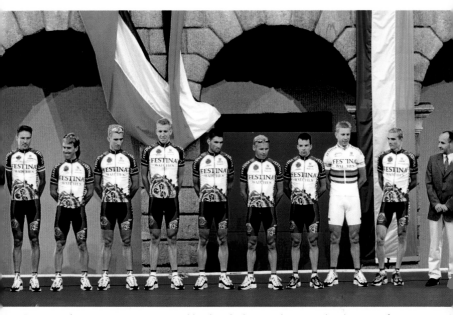

Festina at the team presentation in Dublin, by which point they were already aware of Willy Voet's arrest. Sports director Bruno Roussel stands on the far right. © Offside/Pressesports

Two Banesto riders warm up for the opening Dublin prologue. © Alex Livesey/Getty Images

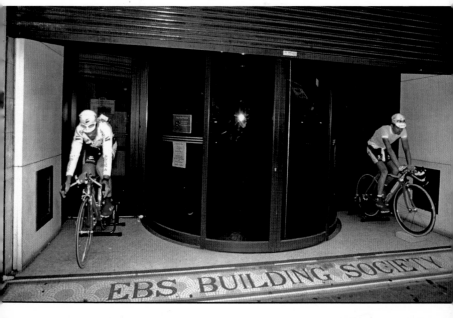

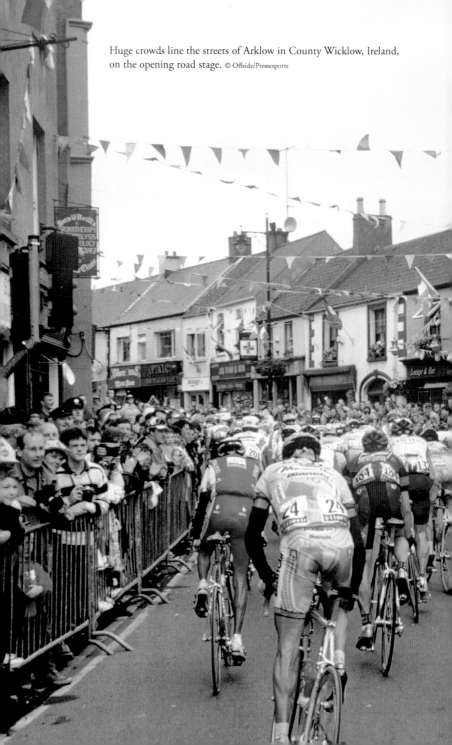

Huge crowds line the streets of Arklow in County Wicklow, Ireland, on the opening road stage. © Offside/Pressesports

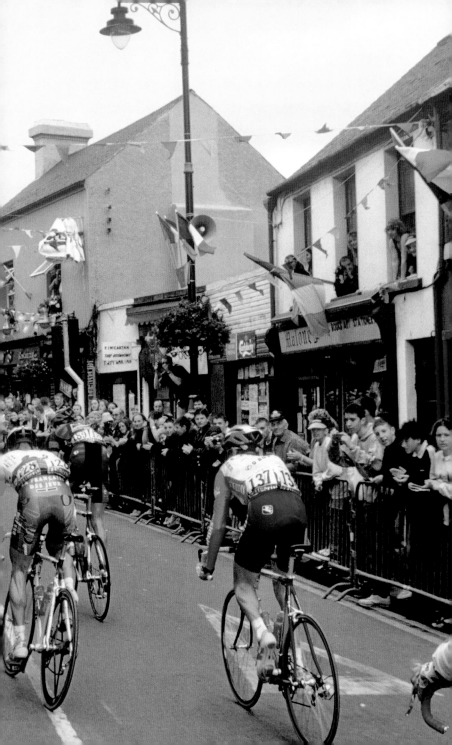

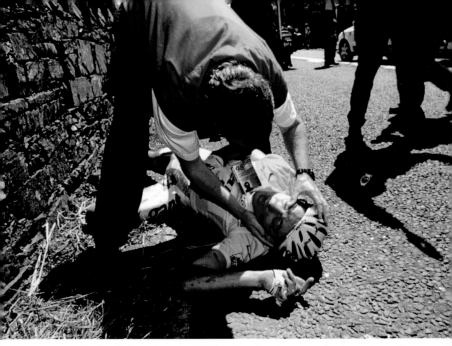

Tour medical staff check the extent of Chris Boardman's injuries after he crashes and abandons on stage 2, the first yellow-jersey wearer to have to quit during the race since Luis Ocaña in 1971. © Lars Ronbog/Getty Images

15 July: French police surround the Festina car as director Bruno Roussel faces questioning. © Joel Saget/Getty Images

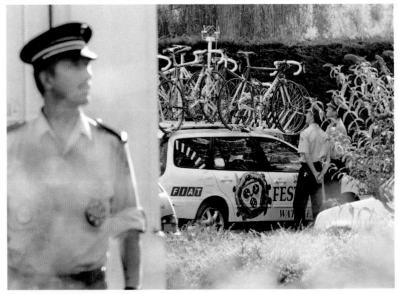

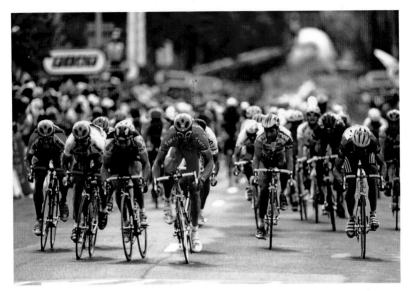

17 July: Mario Cipollini, in red Saeco kit, wins the stage 6 bunch sprint into Brive-la-Gaillarde against fellow Italian sprinter Nicola Minali (left), whilst former race leader Erik Zabel (far right, in green) has to settle for fifth. It was arguably the last normal event on a day which rocked the Tour's foundations to the core. © Alex Livesey/Getty Images

17 July, the end of the road for Festina: Jean-Marie Leblanc announces the expulsion of the team. © Offside/Pressesports

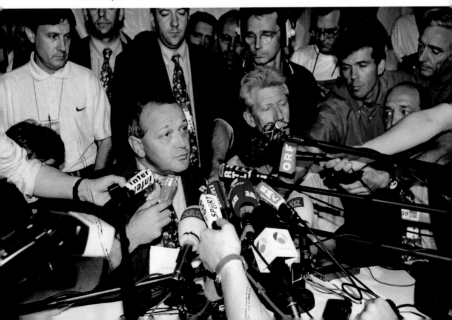

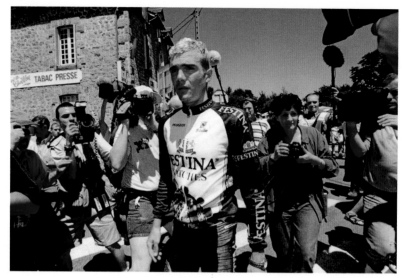

18 July: Richard Virenque leaves the Chez Gillou café after confirming the Festina team will accept their exclusion from the Tour. © Andreas Rentz/Getty Images

Telekom rider Rolf Aldag during the stage 7 time trial – even as Festina were preparing to quit the race, for the rest of the peloton it was business as usual. © Graham Chadwick/Getty Images

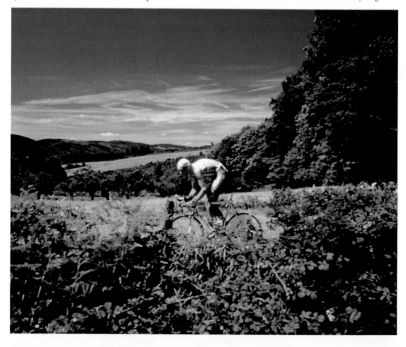

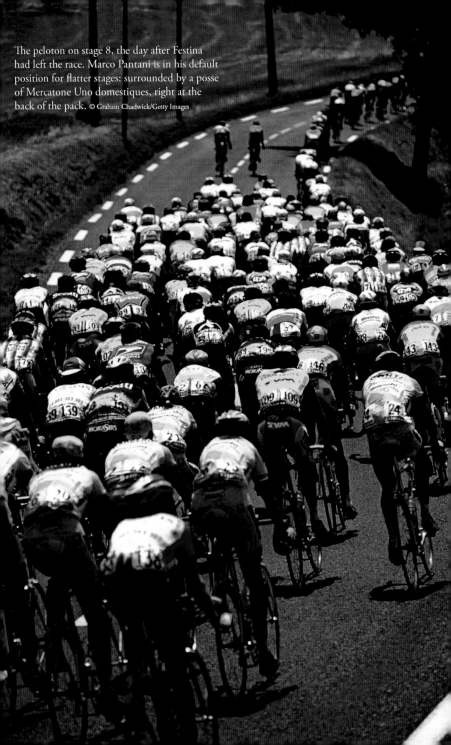

The peloton on stage 8, the day after Festina had left the race. Marco Pantani is in his default position for flatter stages: surrounded by a posse of Mercatone Uno domestiques, right at the back of the pack. © Graham Chadwick/Getty Images

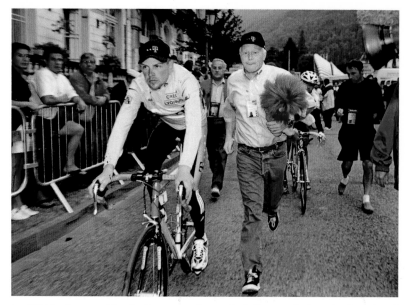

Jan Ullrich after stage 10 to Luchon, team director Rudy Pevenage by his side. On a day of 17 abandons as the Tour headed into the mountains, Ullrich's hold on yellow would never look stronger. © Andreas Rentz/Getty Images

The stage 12 strike: Laurent Jalabert and other riders discuss possible courses of action.
© Offside/Pressesports

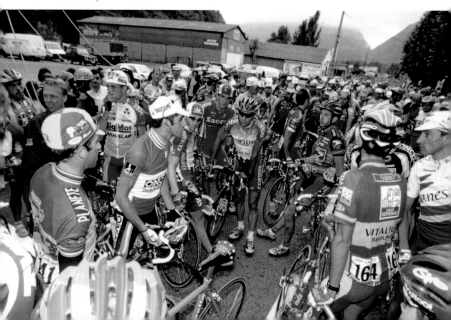

Marco Pantani during the Tour's first strike, at Tarascon-sur-Ariège.
© Joel Saget/Getty Images

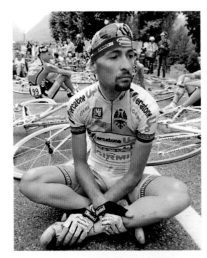

Laurent Jalabert uses the Tour's official race radio, via Jean-Marie Leblanc's lead car, to express riders' reasons for striking.
© Bongarts/Getty Images

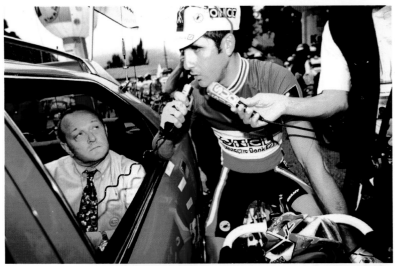

Anti-doping graffiti during the 1998 Tour.
© Andreas Rentz/Getty Images

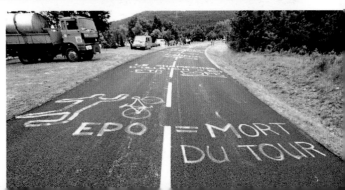

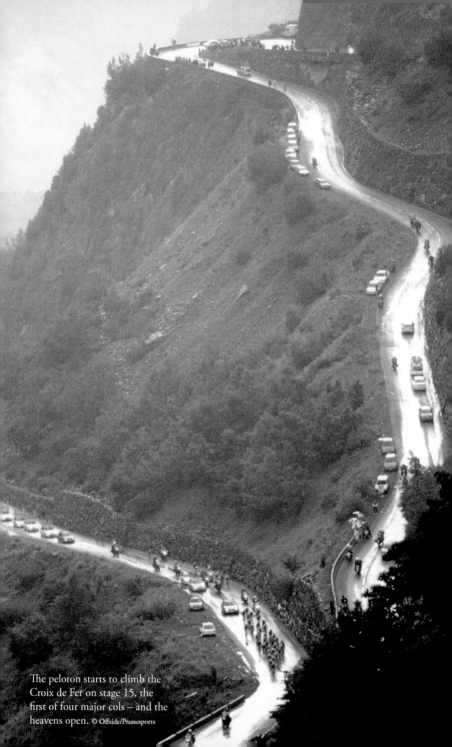

The peloton starts to climb the Croix de Fer on stage 15, the first of four major cols – and the heavens open. © Offside/Pressesports

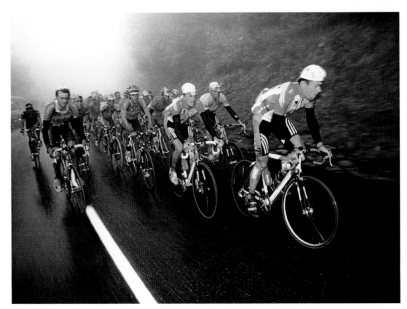

On the lower slopes of the Galibier on stage 15, and race leader Ullrich is already down to just Udo Bolts and Bjarne Riis for protection. © Alex Livesey/Getty Images

Marco Pantani heads for stage 15 victory in Les Deux Alpes – a win that would lead, ultimately, to overall victory in the Tour. © Offside/Pressesports

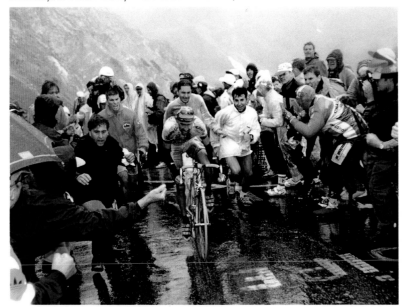

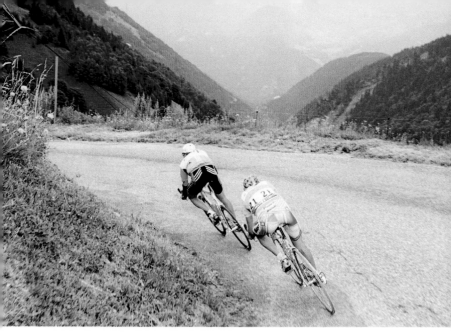

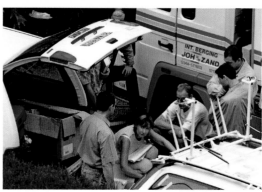

28 July: the day after losing the Tour de France at Les Deux Alpes, Ullrich leads Pantani en route to a stage victory. If the stage win was a gift from Pantani, it also sealed Ullrich's second place overall. © Offside/Pressesports

28 July: plain-clothes police officers and other French justice officials register TVM vehicles near Albertville. © Pascal Pavani/Getty Images

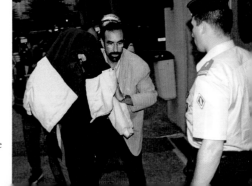

28 July: TVM riders are escorted away from their hotel by the police late in the evening. © Offside/Pressesports

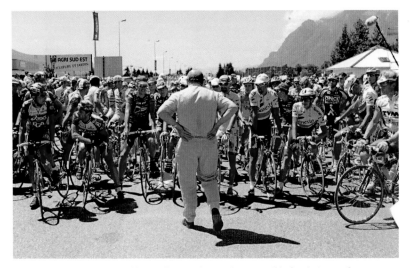

Race director Jean-Marie Leblanc talks to riders as they assemble for the start of stage 17, where they briefly protested against the TVM raids of the previous night. Far more serious protests were to follow. © AFP/Stringer/Getty Images

Strike two: riders resting under a tree and answering a call of nature during their sit-down protest on stage 17. © Offside/Pressesports

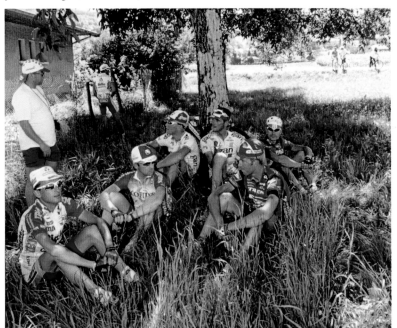

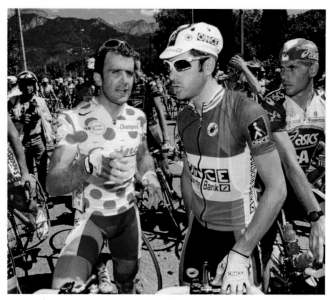

Rodolfo Massi and Laurent Jalabert exchange opinions during the Tour's second strike, on stage 17. Jalabert pulled out shortly afterwards along with the rest of his team, ONCE. Massi continued but was later arrested.

Bjarne Riis (with Telekom team-mate Rolf Aldag to his right) negotiates terms between riders and Tour management during the strike.

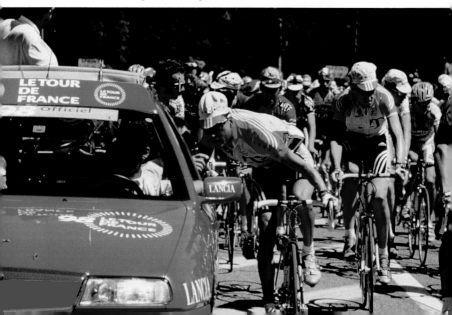

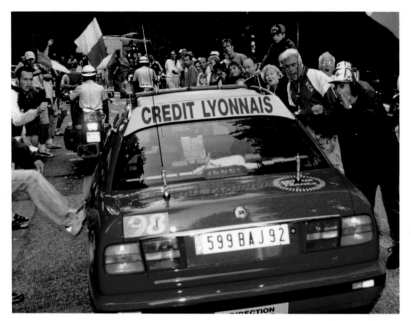

Irate fans take out their frustration on the Tour's lead car as the delays and strikes mount up on stage 17. © AFP/Stringer/Getty Images

29 July: Gendarmes surround ONCE's team hotel. The team had already abandoned the race earlier in the day. © Offside/Pressesports

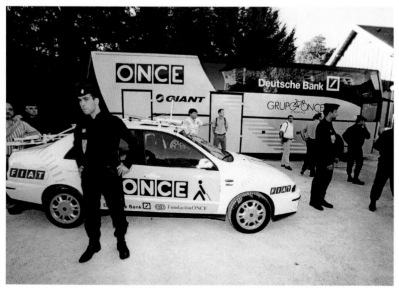

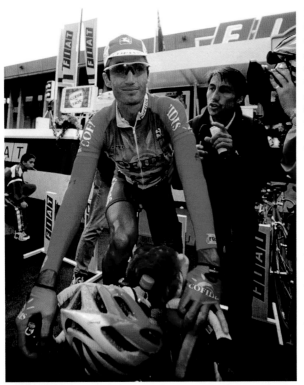

Bobby Julich at the Grenoble stage start of the 1998 Tour de France. Julich finished third overall, the best finish for an American since Greg LeMond won the race outright in 1990. © Andreas Rentz/ Getty Images

The peloton on the rain-drenched Champs-Elysées, with Marco Pantani in the middle of the pack. The end of the most turbulent Tour de France in history is finally nigh. © William Stevens/Getty Images

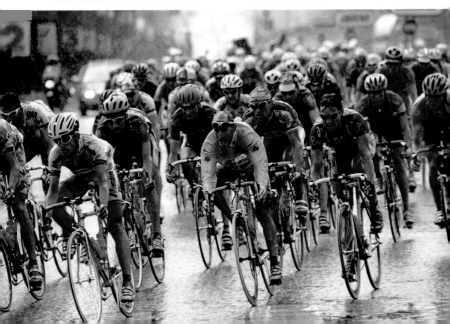

Marcos Serrano was up the road, and between the two of us we could get back to Marco on the descent.'

Never at his best in the rain and cold, the plummeting temperatures did Ullrich no favours. But his team's strong-arm strategy had caused Telekom to burn up their support riders too quickly, too, leaving him isolated and liable to panic. Pantani's attack inspired a general rebellion against the team which had dominated the Tour for two and a half years, with Julich, for one, making his own assault by piling on the pressure rather than an all-out attack and briefly leaving Ullrich behind as the German struggled to put on a flimsy, sleeveless rain jacket just before the summit.

Pantani, meanwhile, had reached and passed a breakaway group consisting of Massi, Jiménez, Serrano and Rinero, the Frenchman in turn making a solo bid and only being reeled in almost within sight of the summit. By this point Pantani had wrenched open a lead of well over two minutes on the Tour's highest mountain pass of the year, 2,645 metres above sea level. But the Italian then made his own decision to grab a rain jacket (as flimsy as Ullrich's but much larger and allowing him to keep warmer) before indulging in some perilous-looking showboating as he freewheeled down the highest slopes of the Galibier.

Pantani's decision to stop on the side of the road to put the rain jacket on properly has added inordinately to the legend surrounding that 15th stage. 'When I saw him appear,' said Orlando Maini – one of Mercatone's second directors, who sprinted alongside to hand over the cape and who recounted the experience in *The Death of Marco Pantani* – 'I was afraid I wouldn't be able to give him it, because I was more tired than him. He was doing something great, something important and I felt unable to do it. The moment I passed him the cape I felt liberated.'

But for all the fanciful nature of such tales, the ever-pragmatic Traversoni, for one, gives those stories short shrift. 'There's all this stuff about the mythical rain jacket which somebody managed to give to Marco just at the right moment on the top of the Galibier,' he recalls. 'What isn't remembered is that nobody else [in the team] got the rain jacket there and half of the rest of the team was on the point of going home because we didn't have anything to wear. So if Marco gets the yellow jersey and half the team get sent home, what good is that?' 'Neither me nor Marcos Serrano stopped to get a rain cape,' Escartín recalls, 'and it was the coldest stage I ever spent on a bike. Three degrees, raining at the summit and all we had on was a usual jersey.' 'I was frozen, locked up,' Luc Leblanc said at the time. 'It was as if I was cross-eyed, when other riders passed me at 80 kilometres an hour, I didn't know where I was any more.' Several riders, like Banesto's José Luis Arrieta and Italian sprinter Fabrizio Guidi, abandoned with hypothermia.

Such tales are indicative, too, of how, in a race which was sinking into disrepute, Pantani was somehow managing to become one of the sport's greatest legends. As in Maini's case, it had reached a point where individuals no longer questioned his status, but used the Italian as a way of measuring their own achievements or failures, as if Pantani had become the focal point of a new religion.

If we look beyond the undoubted hero-worship a little, Pantani's decision to stop and don a rain cape indicated a rider who was acting anything but impetuously. His attack on the Galibier had been premeditated, so too his decision to stop. This was the complete opposite to Ullrich. He had tried desperately to keep Pantani within range, but with the cold eating into him was already suffering due to a lack of appropriate clothing and, possibly, from the longer-term consequences of having lost weight too fast in the build-up to the Tour, too.

On the long descent to the foot of Les Deux Alpes, the Italian was joined by two of the three following Spaniards – Escartín and Serrano – as well as Rinero and Pantani's friend Massi. Rinero, scooting away off the front and with team-mate Julich close behind, was probably the least interested in working with the Italian. But initially there was little collaboration. The gap, which had risen to 2′ 47″, was now squeezed back to 2′ 02″ as the sodden riders came off the steeper parts of the Galibier's descent and Serrano – on paper the rider who should have been working, given that Escartín was his team-mate and leader – at least at first did not help the Italian. Pantani had gained the upper hand on the climb. But on the descent the race stabilised into stalemate.

Behind, Ullrich might have been physically weakened, isolated and forced to do all the work in a group of five riders – which contained no Telekoms and rivals of the calibre of Julich and Michael Boogerd – but, contrary to those accounts which suggest the stage was all over by the summit of the Galibier, Ullrich was not yet entirely out of contention. At one point his speed was such that he shot past a fast-descending TV motorcycle, clearly determined to prevent Pantani's advantage from increasing. Not only did he initially succeed in holding the gap, with the long time trial yet to come, Ullrich could still have regained control of the Tour and won it.

However, such high-speed downhill pedalling by the German on the shallower descending slopes as the road turned on to the main A-road from Briancon to Grenoble came at a cost. Unaided, suffering in the cold and forced to devise his own strategy, Ullrich's energy levels were running dangerously low, as became clear by a very risky tactical decision – to drop back through the group of chasers to the team car and stock up on food and drink rather than squeezing the gap down still further. This illustrated the German's dilemma: he could not afford to risk tackling Les Deux Alpes, the last climb of the day, without some attempt to restore his strength. Yet as a result of going back to the car, his pursuit of Pantani lacked the relentlessness that might have turned the tables, even so late in the game.

With 23.7 km to go – 14 km of descending and nine of climbing to the summit Les Deux Alpes – the difference had increased once more to 2′ 11″. However, what really made the difference was the decision by Marcos Serrano and Massi to provide assistance at the front of Pantani's group on the long, sweeping descents and tunnels in the wide, jagged, tree-lined gorge leading to the climb. Three kilometres later, as Ullrich dropped back once again for more supplies, the TV cameras showing him easing through the chase group with a red bidon clenched between his teeth, the gap had risen to nearly three minutes. With 19 km to go, it was exactly 3′ 01″ – the precise difference between the two overall. Then, one kilometre later, with an advantage of 3′ 13″ for the break, the words *Pantani maillot jaune virtuel* flashed up on TV screens in the press room for the first time. Ullrich's lead was on a knife-edge.

But if Pantani's newfound allies had ended the stalemate between the two giants of the Tour, then an unpredictable setback left Ullrich reeling even further off the lead. A front-wheel puncture in the teeming rain just a few kilometres short of Les Deux Alpes meant more lost time, particularly as the Telekom mechanics changed the wheel very slowly. More time lost and another blow to his already poor morale.

'The puncture made me lose heart,' Ullrich would say later, '[although] in any case I was freezing cold and my legs wouldn't work.' Just as much as the ascent off the Galibier had weakened him, the chill factor on a 45-minute descent engaged at top speed, with part of his body soaking wet and overexposed to boot, had made his already unwilling and tired legs even less responsive. His morale would have sunk even further had he known, as Escartín recalled, that Pantani, with his lead on Ullrich now up to 3′ 58″, had gone clear of the other riders in the makeshift alliance at the foot of the final ascent.. 'We'd caught up with Pantani on

172

the descent, there were five of us there, and as soon as we got to the Deux Alpes climb he shot away. By this point he was going for the Tour, of course, and the way he went up that climb, we couldn't follow him.'

By that point, too, Ullrich was close to breaking. As 1988 Tour winner Pedro Delgado, commenting for Spanish TV on the stage, put it, 'the cold, the wet and above all the change of pace on the last climb threaten to destroy your legs'. Just after the foot of the climb, as he tried to accelerate and simply ended up going even slower, one gesture spoke volumes about Ullrich's state of mind. Discarding his sleeveless yellow rain jacket of Tour leader, Ullrich threw it down on the road, not even bothering to hand it in to his team car. 'It was,' the *Guardian* reported, 'the act of an utterly defeated man.'

By that point, Udo Bölts, the closest chasing Telekom rider, had just reached and passed him and was soft-pedalling a little further above on the climb. But it was all Ullrich could do to maintain his momentum to reach Bölts. Therefore, the damage wreaked by Pantani, by now irrevocable, continued, utterly demolishing Ullrich's domination. Les Deux Alpes is not an excessively steep climb, reaching a maximum of 9 per cent – less than 1 in 10 – in places but normally with a fairly unchallenging 7 or 8 per cent and a flattish final kilometre. But in freezing weather, with steady rain and after two massive Alpine climbs, and in a state of total exhaustion, to Ullrich the nine-kilometre ascent must have felt as if he was trying to ride up the side of a house.

What was, therefore, already a major defeat for Ullrich then became a rout. Four kilometres from the summit, Pantani's advantage of 5′ 17″ was steadily increasing, for all that another 'tow truck' in the shape of Riis had now regained contact with Bölts and Ullrich. It's worth remembering that Bölts was widely credited with saving Ullrich's Tour in 1997. This time round there was nothing either Riis or he could do but offer his team-mate a wheel Ullrich could barely follow.

Pantani, meanwhile, was on what *Cycling Weekly* later called 'a stairway to cycling heaven', all but sprinting on the climb's numerous more gently rising sections, and still hammering out a ferociously fast pace whenever it steepened slightly. With three kilometres to go, with his advantage now at 5′ 43″, both the stage and the yellow jersey were his for the taking. The only question was how much time Ullrich, now dropped by Julich as the American finally went clear for good, would lose.

Comparative bystanders in the German's battle with Pantani, like Cofidis' Roland Meier, or even another theoretically exhausted rider, one of the stage's early breakaways, Lotto's Peter Farazijn, now could pass Ullrich. Like someone sitting upright and trying to fight sleep, the German's head slumped down to the bars again and again. Riis and Bölts were, for the umpteenth time, forced to slow their pace, resisting what must have been an overwhelming temptation simply to push their leader. Support from German 'Devil' Didi Senftt, the eccentric inventor dressed up in his red and black horned rubber suit and cheering on one corner of the climb, was of no assistance. By this point even if Ullrich had made a Faustian pact with a real representative of the Underworld, it would not have been of any help. As the rain continued and some fans, regrettably, booed the race's fallen leader, Ullrich finally crossed the line nearly nine minutes behind Pantani. He was 25th on the stage and all but unable to pedal, completely crushed by the Italian's performance.

Right up to the finish line Pantani showed that for all the praise he garnered for his passion, this time round – and in keeping with his calculating style earlier on the stage – he was keeping a very cool head. Knowing he needed to gain as much time as possible before the final time trial, there were no celebrations on his part that would have risked him being slowed down, no kisses blown at the camera, no tears or histrionics of the type favoured by the likes of Richard Virenque. Instead, clearly keen to wring out as much time as possible on Ullrich and Julich, Pantani continued rising and falling out of the saddle, half-sprinting whenever he could towards the finish line.

There was no way for Pantani to know, as he finally raised his arms to the heavens and crossed the line, his face contorted with relief, pain and joy, how deeply this solo victory, nearly two minutes clear of closest chaser Massi, would become etched on the Tour's history. For the first time since 1976 and Lucien Van Impe, a rider who could be described as a 'thoroughbred climber' was now in a position to win it. In a Tour that had been bedevilled by its own troubled history, 'drinking poisons of its own making,' as *L'Equipe's* Philippe Brunel once memorably wrote of doping, this victory had journalists of all nationalities, not just Italian, hugging each other in delight at the finish. 'What an amazing Tour this is turning out to be,' stated British television commentator Phil Liggett, which, given all the scandals, was also a fairly amazing thing to say.

In broader terms for the Tour, the sense of the stage's importance in its history quickly emerged thanks to Pantani dedicating his victory to Luciano Pezzi. After all, Pantani's mentor had been behind the steering wheel of Felice Gimondi's team car, directing the Salvarani squad, when Gimondi had won the Tour in 1965, the last Italian to do so.

Not only that, but a victory in the Tour, now just six days away from its conclusion in Paris, could also net Pantani an extremely rare Giro–Tour double, the first for Italy since Fausto Coppi's in 1952 and making him one of just eight riders ever to win two Grand Tours in the same year. But if, thanks to Les Deux Alpes, comparisons between Pantani and Italy's greatest ever pro were making headlines in the following day's newspapers across the country, when it came to Pantani's seizing of the yellow jersey, in fact, only one moment in more recent Italian cycling history could be comparable.

The lone attack to Sestriere in 1992 by Pantani's predecessor in Italian climbing folklore, Claudio Chiappucci, has been described by Richard Moore in his *Etape: 20 Great Stages from the Modern Tour de France* as 'one of the most extraordinary, almost unbelievable, performances in Tour history'. It is true Chiappucci's move was far longer – over 200 km – although the first part was in a joint break with other riders. But it was nowhere near as ambitious as Pantani's move, given that Chiappucci knew he could not win the Tour that year, only that he had nothing to lose against race leader Miguel Indurain. Nor did it come after winning the Giro d'Italia just six weeks earlier.

With Julich and Escartín now Pantani's closest rivals, but with two more big mountain stages to come, the battle was not completely over. Julich's disadvantage of 3′ 53″ to Pantani still left the Italian a little vulnerable, not least because the American had already shone in one Tour time trial and could well shine in another. But the collapse of Ullrich, now nearly six minutes behind and in fourth place overall, left Pantani firmly in the Tour's driving seat for the first time in his career. The Tour was not over, but his team were convinced that the most decisive corner had now been turned.

It was not only Pantani's team who were convinced *Il Pirata* had it in him to capture the Tour. 'Ever since Plateau de Beille, we'd all been expecting him to do something important,' confirms Escartín. 'That was the point when I personally thought he had it in him to win overall. The thing was, Ullrich let a rival who was really dangerous pull back a lot of time. And that's something, if you're going to win the Tour, you can't let happen. At the same time, his weak point was that Riis was weak that year. Ullrich depended on him. And on top of that, Telekom was too fractured as a squad. They didn't have enough mountain riders, just four or five guys for Ullrich and instead they had maybe two or three guys to work for Erik Zabel, and I think that was a mistake. They weren't built around the one leader.'

Pantani had also turned in a performance which surpassed his own limits. Up until then in his career, normally his attacks had been made on the last climb of a mountain stage. This time, rarely for him, he gambled on a much more long-range move. Pantani's strategy on the Galibier therefore did not just indicate he was a nonconformist when it came to the domination of the time triallists. He was also acting outside his own comfort zone. 'Today I showed that I can attack from far out, I probably risked blowing up, but it's too easy to stick to what you know you can do,' he argued in his winner's press conference. 'Often it's simply impossible to think of everything that might lie ahead of you. I rode myself into the ground today.'

He was uncertain, he said, of whether he could hold on to the lead. 'I'm not going to worry about the time trial, I just want to enjoy the most beautiful day of my career. It's the most beautiful win I've ever had, because I've suffered in this Tour, I took a long time to get going after the Giro, it took a lot of courage to come here six weeks on and put everything up for grabs again. I will try to hold on to the jersey, but this already feels like too much to think about.' He waxed lyrical, too, about the consequences for Ullrich, and hinted again at how his struggle with the German symbolised a conflict between Latin passion and German calculation, emotion versus logic, heart versus head: 'His strength was to drain the race of all its emotion. But my ambition cracked him.'

Pantani's win also represented a victory of perseverance, triumph against a series of misfortunes and crashes which had plagued his career. 'This man was forged out of suffering,' claimed *L'Equipe*. 'He has broken his fingers, his collarbone, the bones in his feet, his tibia and his perone, twice fractured his skull, dislocated his shoulder, crushed his vertebrae in his lower back, injured his knee. He lost the Giro 1997 when a black cat ran under his bike. In October 1995, while racing, his body was all but destroyed, his leg ripped into shreds. He wasn't far from death, and yesterday [on stage 15] he brought cycling back to life.' (Ever faithful to the hardcore cycling fans, *L'Equipe* also pointed out that his bike, with a frame weighing just a kilo, was the lightest in the entire peloton, and had first been ridden by him in the Dolomities earlier that year to one major success, the Giro d'Italia.)

The triumph of Mercatone Uno that day was also the triumph of the David of climbing against the Goliath of time trialling, the Indurains and Ullrichs who had dominated the racing scene for years and years before. In comparison with the huge budget, patrician Telekom, Mercatone Uno were the scrawny kids from the wrong side of the tracks, sponsored, not by one of the world's biggest telephone companies, but by a local supermarket chain from northern Italy.

As the Italian fans who had poured over the border cheered and waved outside the Tour's makeshift – and freezing – press pavilions, Pantani's team-mates, too, were more than appreciative of his greatest achievement. 'It was perishingly cold on the descent off the Galibier and then when we got to the last climb, [fellow rider, the late] Franco Ballerini came up to tell me Marco had done so well.' Crucially for the remainder of the Tour, Ballerini also told Traversoni that if they had had thoughts of a mass abandon, now 'there was no way we'd be going home'. At this point, even the typically sage Traversoni permits himself a moment of sentimentality: 'When he got going, Marco would write some beautiful pages of cycling.' The one fly in the ointment, he recollects, was in that the absence of Festina, Pantani felt that he had not inflicted a full defeat on the complete list of rivals.

Even so, on the other side of the fence, the feeling within Telekom was that the war was now over bar the shouting. Their defeat had come as a result of the simplest of errors on Ullrich's part – tipping over into physical exhaustion as a result of some very straightforward miscalculations.

'He didn't wait for me. He should have waited for his team-mates' is how Riis now analyses the Galibier in conversation with the author. 'And we knew it was going to be shit weather. So I said in the morning to [Telekom team sports director] Rudy Pevenage, "do we have someone on the summit of the Galibier with warm clothing?" And he said, "Nooo, we don't have, it's too much."' Riis repeated the question to Pevenage, 'Do we have somebody?', the implication being that they ought to have had – and got the same answer. Even now, nearly two decades on, Riis insists that Telekom's error be made absolutely clear: 'Just mention that.

'We lost the Tour there,' Riis states categorically. 'Nobody was there. And he [Ullrich] was going down [the Galibier] alone, the idiot, without waiting for his team-mates. He froze. No jacket, and then we caught him, and' – as Ullrich hit total exhaustion, his lead of the Tour was over. Or, as Riis puts it: 'he was gone. I mean, Pantani would probably have won the stage, anyway, by a lot of minutes, but Jan would not have lost the Tour.' 'Even during the first part of the stage, it seemed that everything was under control,' Aldag recalls. 'I was on a pretty good day, I remember [Álvaro] González de Galdeano (Vitalicio Seguros) attacked on the Galibier and I could bring him back. At that point there were maybe 30 guys left, and then I got dropped. '

But when Aldag reached the finish line, 15′ 33″ down on Pantani after descending the Galibier alongside former Tour leader Stéphane Heulot, the Telekom domestique did not need anybody to tell him that Ullrich had lost the Tour. 'As soon as I got to the finish,' he recollects, the writing was on the wall because,

'Jan was still there, he'd suffered so much with the weather situation. He wasn't expected to have that problem. If he'd worn a [thermal or full] rain jacket or eaten something, then it would not have happened. I think it was just that, not wearing enough clothes.' If Ullrich had been sick, as Aldag points out, then the Tour would have taken a very different course afterwards.

'In principle,' Telekom's team manager Walter Godefroot said, 'the Tour is lost. We have to be realistic. He's not going to get six minutes back on Pantani.'

One Tour had been lost. The critical question for the German's long-term future – given he was just 24 – was more if Ullrich had cracked mentally, rather than physically, that day. However, Aldag says both short-term evidence and Ullrich's historical development as a rider indicate that wasn't the case. 'That evening after the stage at supper, Jan said he was sorry, that he had made mistakes, but that tomorrow he would be back, he would get into the game. That doesn't indicate mental weakness, just the opposite.'

This might have been a way of building up his own self-confidence, of course – talking the talk in order to oblige himself to walk the walk, as it were – but Aldag says Ullrich was not so complex. 'I believe he did not think too much and that made his life easier. He did not ever think too much about different options, he kept things relatively simple and that's why he succeeded. He didn't get super-stressed.'

For example, Aldag points out, 'In 1996, his second place [overall in the Tour] was a huge surprise, but in 1997, the only reason Jan attacked [and effectively won the Tour] at Andorra was because Bjarne told him to go. Jan was looking round at Bjarne, and Riis told him to go and attack, otherwise he was a loyal kid. If [Ullrich had] looked backwards he could have won the Tour in 1996, too, if he'd raced in his own interests. But he was a simple guy.' And in 1998, although Aldag says Ullrich was 'changing from being the red-haired kid he'd been when he joined the making more demands, but that's normal', he is nonetheless adamant that for all Ullrich panicked after Pantani attacked, underlying nervousness was not the real issue that day.

Beyond the immediate question of failing to eat enough – ironic, given his weight issues throughout the build-up to the Tour – Ullrich's problems, in fact, can be traced to over dependency on his team-mates and his squad when it came to making crucial decisions. Once isolated, given the limited number of responses he seemed to have to changing race scenarios, Ullrich was almost bound to run into difficulties.

There's even a theory that Ullrich's lack of personal initiative has historical roots in his upbringing and education as a sportsman in the former GDR, where athletes were indoctrinated always to think in terms of the collective good. That may or may not have been true in Ullrich's case. But anyway, on top of the Galibier, isolated from his ringmaster Riis in the sodden, foggy terrain, weak and hungry, Ullrich was unable to regain any kind of grip on solid terrain for a counter-attack. Crisis negotiations with rivals, of the type at which Riis excelled, were never really an option for the uncommunicative Ullrich. 'I got on fine with Marco but I don't think I ever once spoke to Ullrich,' Escartín – the kind of rival who might have helped – says. 'He was not good at talking.'

If Telekom can be criticised for two things as a team, the first was a sense of collective complacency, a group refusal to recognise that Pantani could seriously threaten Ullrich's lead. In a sense, this went with the territory, given one element which often irritated non-German journalists: an air of superiority among some of the German staff on Telekom, typified by a firm belief that they would sweep their disorganised southern European rivals into the sea. 'Going into the 1998 Tour and while we were racing it, we were always going to compare it to 1997 and 1996,' Aldag argues.

'We expected to win everything.' However, as Pantani himself had said in the Pyrenees, 'I can win if Ullrich has one bad day.' With Pantani underestimated by Telekom across the board, once the Italian opened up a gap there was little they could do.

The second criticism of Telekom was that this was not the first time Ullrich had fallen seriously foul of bad weather in a major stage race – and Telekom should have been more prepared. In the 1997 Tour de Suisse, a break early in the race containing unknown French rider Christophe Agnolutto had gained a 12-minute advantage over Ullrich and the rest of the field. Although Agnolutto clung on to the lead, Ullrich, clearly the strongest rider, regained huge swathes of time on his rival with a lone win on stage four hoisting him from 57th to third overall, and a second place on the stage five time trial pushing him even closer.

But then on stage six, an immensely difficult mountain stage which was slashed to half its length because of snowstorms, Ullrich suddenly floundered in plummeting temperatures, finishing 13th on the stage. His best chance of regaining more time on Agnolutto had been lost in a single day, a lesson not learned by Telekom.

While gloom reigned in the German camp, for Italian cycling and sport in general Pantani's victory had a huge impact. As Matt Rendell writes, in Italy on RAI 3, the Tour's broadcaster, the news opened with his win, while a diplomatic mission for Italian prime minister Romano Prodi was relegated to second place. 'Quite right,' Prodi is reported to have said, 'his exploit is unique.'

On a more positive note, for journalists and the fans the sudden explosion of interest in the racing overshadowed the ongoing anti-doping raids. Even the Tour's near-collapse a few days earlier briefly seemed unimportant. Pantani, it was felt, had single-handedly dragged the sport out of the doping crisis. That he failed to receive recognition for that long term – and despite the fact that he also left cycling with even greater associations to banned drugs – is something his diehard fans and closest friends continue to resent. As one of them put it off the record, 'Pantani did what he did, and then the Tour told him to get stuffed, just when he needed them in return. He was betrayed.'

The counter-argument against that is not hard to find. With the benefit of hindsight, of course, all Pantani achieved for cycling that day was subsequently buried under the colossal weight of the doping scandals which followed in the years to come. But as William Fotheringham, the *Guardian*'s correspondent on the Tour, put it recently, 'his reputation is mud now but I liked the guy a lot, I loved the way he raced'. He was not alone in his sentiments, not by a long chalk.

But the Tour's doping crises, regrettably, were not going to go away just because sport had – for once – reasserted itself as the main news of the race. The same day Pantani won at Les Deux Alpes, Cees Priem and Andrei Mikhailov of the TVM squad had completed their long journey from the police station in Foix to the Palais de Justice in Reims and, by midnight, Priem, following three hours' interrogation, had been charged with transporting toxic substances and transporting dangerous goods. The next step would come in the small hours of the following day, when Mikhailov was charged with anti-doping offences.

It was also reported that the prosecuting judge in Reims argued that the riders were not responsible for the drug seizure, an odd statement in view of the events to come, and perhaps more indicative of the relentless series of rumours spewed out by the Tour as it lurched from one uncertain battle over doping to another. It's often said that the truth is the first casualty of any conflict, and at the time, cycling's war on drugs was no different at all.

13

The Exception to the Rule

Tuesday, 28 July. Stage 16:
Vizille–Albertville, 204 km

A former news agency reporter used to make an odd boast about Jan Ullrich. The journalist would claim that every early spring at Ullrich's start-of-season press conference when the 1997 Tour winner outlined his objectives for that year, the German's comments would be so predictably similar to those of the previous January that he would write up the entire event, complete with quotes, beforehand. Two minutes after the press conference was over, much to the bewilderment of his competitors, he would have stepped outside the auditorium and filed his copy.

That was when Ullrich was racking up one runner's-up or podium spot after another behind Lance Armstrong, alternating them each January with increasingly unlikely claims that the following July he would be defeating Armstrong. Back at the start of his career, however, Ullrich was still occasionally able to take the world by surprise. That was, arguably, never so true as on stage 16 of the 1998 Tour. Twenty-four hours after suffering what amounts to possibly the worst ever defeat of his career, on the Tour's second to last mountain stages Ullrich launched what would prove to be, in hindsight, one of his most courageous attacks. Although the move seemed more designed to prove his own strength to himself and his team after a stinging setback on stage 15, outside Telekom the question of whom it would affect the most of the overall contenders was the main point of interest.

Crucially, Ullrich's comeback, launched on the hardest climb of the stage, the Madeleine, was not damaging to Pantani although it proved a severe test. The Tour's new *maillot jaune* was able to follow Ullrich's move although the Italian admitted later that it had been touch and go. 'He told me that if Ullrich had gone half a kilometre an hour faster up that climb, he'd have cracked,' Traversoni recalls. Instead, the day after Pantani had left Ullrich without his yellow jersey, on stage 16 the Tour's top two adversaries formed an alliance. Their collaboration strengthened Pantani's overall domination and simultaneously regained Ullrich time on the two riders who had eased Ullrich off the two lower steps of the podium on stage 15 as well: Julich and Escartín.

Once Pantani's ability to retain his overall lead had been tested and not found wanting, albeit by a very narrow margin, Ullrich's move developed into a classic example of how the old adage 'if you can't beat 'em, join 'em' can play out in high-level stage racing. It was, essentially, an open admission that a second straight victory in the Tour was no longer possible. Six days out of Paris, rather than oust Pantani from the game altogether the fight for the right to stand next to the Italian on the final podium had begun. What was so unusual was that here was Ullrich, a rider who had hammered out a reputation for his time trialling skills and for entrenching himself behind his support riders on all but the most set-piece of mountain attacks, opting to tear up the script. For a second day, too, it appeared that the Tour had been able to put the next instalment of its doping soap opera on hold – after which the bubble promptly burst.

Ullrich's stage 16 move was probably the least expected major attack of any of the top contenders in the Tour, but it was preceded by a more predictable opening gambit for his team – Telekom placing Aldag in the morning break, just as they had done the previous day. Keeping a man ahead was only to be expected of all the major teams, but it was particularly important for Telekom given Ullrich's collapse the previous day in the mountains and the fact that stage 16 was a 204-km Alpine trek.

Examined in more detail, the stage featured five classified climbs, one more than stage 15, opening with a difficult first category ascent, the Col de Porte, in the first hour of racing. But the next three climbs were second category, and with rolling terrain for most of the middle section. As a result, the 18-km Madeleine, classified *hors catégorie*, averaging a daunting 7.6 per cent and the final climb of the day before a long drop down into the town of Albertville, was all but certain to be decisive.

For the first three hours of racing, and perhaps unsurprisingly following the extreme difficulty of the previous day, the stage quickly settled into a fairly dull routine. The six breakaways, including Aldag, ground over climb after climb of the Massif de la Chartreuse – the Porte, the Cucheron, the Granier. The drama, if it can be called that, was provided courtesy of riders like early breakaway Andrei Teteriouk skidding off the road on the descent from the Porte, to be followed by Lotto team-mate Rik Verbrugghe, all but coming off his bike as he veered into the same grass banking a few seconds later. Thankfully, neither was seriously injured.

On the Madeleine, though, that scenario changed completely. Ignoring team tactics yet again, Ullrich opted to storm out of the pack at the foot of the climb, 18 km from the summit. Telekom had been setting the pace with a small cloud of pink-clad jerseys dotted across the road at the front of the pack, when suddenly their leader, helmetless and all but sprinting uphill, thundered out of the left-hand side of the bunch. 'I couldn't have done it better myself,' Pantani later said approvingly. Indeed, the distance from the finish in the 1992 Winter Olympics town of Albertville around 39 km to go, was only slightly less close to the line than the point at which Pantani had made his bid for Tour victory on the Galibier.

Early speculation by the media that new sticking plaster on and behind one of Ullrich's knees indicated that the German was set for a second troubled day and perhaps suffering from a form of tendinitis had clearly proved to be incorrect. German television reporters had even said in informal conversations to their British colleagues that morning that they thought Ullrich would not start the stage. But as Ullrich galloped uphill on the Madeleine with Pantani bouncing in and out on the saddle behind, for all the world like a yellow-clad rider trying to rein in a large, temperamental, pink horse, that theory was evidently incorrect, too. The better weather, too, must have been to the German's liking: no wind, warm temperatures of around 20 degrees, in stark comparison to stage 15's three degrees on the Galibier summit, and, despite initial cloud cover, staying dry. But in a lot of ways the real explanation for the attack was a question of sporting pride, pure and simple, on Ullrich's part.

'I had been thinking and thinking and thinking last night, and I came to the conclusion that I had to attack to thank my team because I knew they would be disappointed in me if I didn't,' Ullrich said later.

It was an attack of such brute force – and ambition, given the distance remaining – that only one rider was able or willing to latch on to his back wheel for more than a few hundred metres: Pantani, taking a swig from his bottle fractions of a second before Ullrich had attacked, but finally able to respond. Escartín did attempt to move across, as did Saeco's Leonardo Piepoli, but after a kilometre or so they found it impossible to keep up. Bobby Julich and Christophe Rinero, second and fifth overall, moved into damage-limitation mode. But all that could be seen of

Michael Boogerd – lying sixth overall – was his name, written repeatedly all over much of the climb in huge letters.

'You could tell by the way Jan was racing that the previous stage had just been a bad day,' Escartín recalls. 'He blew us all apart, it was like it was another story altogether. He just drove off and dropped us all apart from Pantani.'

'He was supposed to wait for me to drive for a kilometre, and then I was going to turn and nod at him so he would know he should go,' Riis commented afterwards. 'Instead, he just went for it.' Although letting him up the road would have been far too risky, Pantani had something to gain by collaborating with the German, too – the greater the gap on Julich for both of them, the better. After a few kilometres, the two settled into a steadier pace, with Ullrich constantly looking back to see where the others were. Apart from Pantani, they were all out of sight. Either way, the German seemed utterly indifferent to the Italian's presence just behind his back wheel. Their two styles could not have been more different – Ullrich grinding away seated, churning a huge gear, Pantani dropping in and out of the saddle as he punched at the pedals.

Assistance came briefly at one point for Ullrich, but, given the German's speed and evidently much better physical condition compared to Monday's stage, it was more symbolic than realistic. Dropping back from the other earlier attackers, Aldag led the duo of overall favourites for over half a kilometre before a steeper hairpin meant he lost power altogether.

'After the Galibier [stage] we [Telekom] had got a bit lost and that evening everybody had been in a superbad mood. But Jan had promised to attack and we adopted our strategy for that,' Aldag recalls.

'I was in the front break with three or four other guys and we heard, "Jan is coming, only with Pantani". So I had to wait and wait, then pull like hell for 700 metres on the big ring. When I saw them coming up behind me, I was like "Shit, they're coming fast. But then comes the next [big] right-hand corner, me using the big chainring and I just go pffff ..."' In a flash, the two were gone, Ullrich bounding past him and Pantani glued to Ullrich's back wheel. For Telekom, following such an appalling defeat, Aldag might have felt exhausted – and the way he grits his teeth as Ullrich and Pantani line up behind him is painful even to look at – but his underlying reaction to how Ullrich was racing on stage 16, regardless of the result, was typical of that of his team-mates: 'Pantani was too strong for him [Ullrich], but everybody afterwards had a lot of respect for Jan.'

Such was the speed of the race as the two romped through the tiny village of Saint François Longchamp and past rough Alpine meadows that the closest chase group, led by a reappearing Boogerd, along with Escartín, Piepoli and Rinero and Roland Meier from Cofidis, all but disintegrated. By halfway up the Madeleine, only half a dozen riders remained, with Julich, not enjoying a good day after his strong performance in considerably worse weather conditions on stage 15, suffering to stay on. Still, after losing their nominal leader, Francesco Casagrande, on the first day in the Pyrenees, Cofidis collectively had stepped up to the plate in impressive style, to the point where they were not only with three riders in the top ten, but also leading the teams classification.

'When Ullrich attacked, I was more worried about holding on than following him,' the Cofidis rider said later. 'Today I thought I might get dropped, so it was others who did all the work. I suffered, but I kept on thinking about the people on the roadside waiting for me, cheering me on. I thought, I can't let them see me this way, let them down and get dropped.'

After catching and shooting past France's Stéphane Heulot, the last remnant of the early break, the two passed over the Madeleine's peak two minutes and six seconds ahead of the pack.

Had that lead been maintained, it would have been enough for Ullrich to rise from fourth to second overall.

Come the summit, despite much warmer weather Ullrich was clearly determined not to make the same mistake as on the Monday, when he did not have adequate protection against the freezing wind and rain. A much heavier jacket than on stage 15 was duly donned by the German, together with arm warmers and a cap, while Pantani, seemingly less affected either way, just rammed some newspapers down his jersey.

The descent to Albertville was somewhat longer than the 35-km drop off the Galibier, but it was far less vertiginous, with the duo able to reach speeds of 90 kmh at times without any of the risks of stage 15. Although Ullrich was a talented descender, he lacked Pantani's slightly reckless edge and a few conversations ensued as the Italian – finally – began taking turns on the front and keeping the speed at around 90 kmh.

The final sprint in Albertville bordered on the farcical. Pantani, realising that there was no point in trying to humiliate Ullrich at this stage in the game, and recognising the German morally deserved the win, eased back as best he could without making it overly obvious. However, it was touch and go that Ullrich was able to sprint hard enough to take the stage on offer and the win seemed more than a shade forced.

Having reached a point where presumably he felt close enough to the finish for there to be no risk of Ullrich subsequently dropping him, Pantani's scant collaboration effectively sealed the battle, barring disaster, for the overall classification. Thanks to the German, his advantage over Julich, still clinging on to second, had stretched to 5′ 42″, while with Ullrich it continued to hover at just below six minutes.

'Our big fear, from this point on, was the [final] time trial,' says Traversoni. Their nerves were not eased by their leader's apparent lack of calmness prior to such crucial stages. 'Pantani would get to the day before a time trial and still be fiddling around with his bike, saying the saddle had to be a little bit higher, a little bit lower and so on and so forth. For goodness' sake, you can't be doing that when the time trial is just a couple of days away.'

But if his team knew that Pantani had his weak points, on Tuesday, barring Ullrich, his rivals had been too concerned with ensuring they did not slide even further down the ladder after Monday's trouncing. If they had been in awe of Pantani before, by this point in the game they felt even more impressed. 'The Tour is lost,' Ullrich recognised after calling Monday's previous stage his worst day ever on the bike, 'but this has enabled me to bounce back mentally, and that's what counted.

'I had never expected Pantani to race so well after the tough last week in the Giro, there's no doubt, he's the best mountain climber in the world. His win [at Les Deux Alpes] was incredible.'

Although the Tour overall was no longer realistic, Ullrich promised he would 'try to give Pantani a fight all the way to Paris'.

Julich had suffered but managed nonetheless to hold on to second, albeit by the bare minimum, after taking third on the line at the end of a day where he had been racing on fumes. 'I was cramping up a lot and for about five kilometres on the downhill I could hardly pedal, but I pushed the pace at the end to save my second place.

'I suffered a lot, but I tell you, I was hanging on to the wheel. All I could think about were all the people with American flags, the emails that I've been receiving, the positive vibes that everyone's been sending, and there was no way I was going to get dropped,' he recollects.

'This race isn't over,' he argued at the time – although later, the after-effects of battling against the cramps made him noticeably less optimistic, at least privately. 'A guy like Ullrich loses [nine minutes] yesterday, takes two back today. You never know when it's somebody's time to take time. It's not over until the final time trial, so stayed tuned.'

Despite losing 1′ 18″ to Ullrich in the first week's long time trial, Pantani was adamant that the race was not finished yet.

'I don't think it's over – not by a long shot,' he said. 'Ullrich was very strong, and he deserved to take the stage. I tried to stay with him, and he reacted like a champion.' It was a feeling that was, given the scale of Ullrich's comeback, not just limited to Pantani. The German had proved that, rather than take the soft option of throwing in the towel, he still wanted to show that he had the staying power to attempt the impossible and try to dislodge Pantani. He was never to know how closely he had come to achieving that target, but his status as a leader in Telekom was hugely reinforced. And a podium position in Paris, his third in three years, was close to being attained as well. For a 24-year-old, his status as a Tour favourite, so badly diminished after the debacle of Les Deux Alpes, had quickly been repaired – if not for 1998 then certainly for the years to come.

The much older Escartín, on the other hand, was not at all optimistic about his chances of pushing his way back in from fourth – already a career best in the Tour – to third, saying, 'had I stayed with Ullrich any longer or even tried to, I would have cracked. If I can do something tomorrow, I will, but I don't know if I can.'

Escartín's circumstances, though, and the Tour's, were to change to the point where that was no longer conceivable. Everybody on the Tour's final Alpine stage, from the Tour director downwards, found they had far bigger and less digestible fish to fry than 'just' the outcome of a bike race.

14

Nobody Listens to the Weak: The Second Rebellion

Wednesday, 29 July. Stage 17:
Albertville–Aix-les-Bains, 149 km

Sixteen years on, Manolo Saiz, former director of the ONCE team, sitting in a restaurant in his home town of Torrelavega, is at pains to explain why he should not be viewed as the man who wanted to wreck the 1998 Tour de France.

As the most outspoken manager of all the 1998 Tour's 'rebel' teams, those that left the Tour on or after stage 17 of the race, he became their unofficial spokesman almost by default. As such, Saiz was not one to pull his punches. His resounding comment that summer that 'we have stuffed our finger up the Tour's arse', in particular, continues to haunt him. That he was one of the most high-profile arrests in 2006 during the Operación Puerto anti-doping probe – in a case in which he has only recently been cleared of all charges – has only contributed to the myth of a wayward, iconoclastic figure from the wrong side of the tracks. For some Saiz was a necessary revolutionary, for others the 1998 Tour was where it all started to go wrong. As Jean-Marie Leblanc describes him in his autobiography, 'The cynical, Machiavellian and authoritarian figure we got to know well in the years to come began to make his presence known [in the 1998 Tour].'

Impassioned and deeply engaged with his sport are perhaps two ways of describing Saiz with which everybody would agree. The photograph of the ONCE team manager, livid with rage as he and top race official Jean-François Pescheux engaged in a shouting match at the riders' first strike in Tarascon-sur-Ariège, remains one of the most expressive of the divisions that ripped through cycling's number one race that summer. In the left-hand corner of their verbal boxing ring, Pescheux: one of the most long-standing and widely respected officials working on the Tour. In the right-hand corner: Saiz, who may have been one of Leblanc's least favourite figures, but who was also one of the most successful team managers of the 1990s, charismatic, articulate and dynamic. His team was held to be at the vanguard of technological development, new training methods and better organisation: yet, unlike more modern behemoths of the sport, Saiz insisted that ONCE had retained a human face. As he put it to *Cycle Sport*, 'ONCE is different to all the other squads, because this team has a soul.'

Both Pescheux and Saiz were (and are) passionate fans of cycling, both well-known figures. But whereas Pescheux was determined that the Tour continue willy-nilly, Saiz and his riders, like French national champion Laurent Jalabert, had felt the treatment the peloton had received from the gendarmes was unacceptable and it was time to pull down the curtain. At Tarascon-sur-Ariège in the Pyrenees, Saiz, Jalabert and those in favour of quitting had lost the battle. The Tour had continued. But when a second, massive crisis rocked the Tour in the Alps on the night of Tuesday, 28 July and deep into the stage on Wednesday, would it be a different story?

In the Pyrenees, the immediate causes of the strike were partly police action against the Dutch TVM squad and partly the Festina confessions and the way that team's riders had been treated during their interrogations in a Lyon gendarmerie. This time a much bigger raid against the Dutch team, with no added news on the Festina affair itself was all that was needed to light the fuse. The new element, and the one which probably provoked a much more dramatic reaction, was that, rather than team staff or riders who had already been expelled being taken into custody, this time it was the riders competing in the Tour itself who were targeted by the police. They could be in custody and on their bikes on the same day: barring taking them off to a police station by stopping a stage itself, the dividing line between police and Tour de France had never been so narrow.

None of the six members of the TVM squad to whom this happened after stage 16, with the exception of stage four bunch sprint winner Jeroen Blijlevens, had been significant players in the 1998 Tour de France by that point. Yet when the French police following the trail of the EPO stash, which had been seized from TVM vehicles in March near Reims, moved into the TVM team hotel in Albertville on the evening of stage 16, the domino effect of the fallout was to come close to destroying the Tour de France itself.

Outside the leafy, stone-walled hotel Le Million, the police first made a thorough search of the TVM team bus. On finding nothing, they then entered the building itself and began knocking on team riders' doors. Taken away by 12 plain-clothes officers, TVM's six riders left in the race by that point – Steven de Jongh, Servais Knaven, Sergei Outschakov, Blijlevens, Bart Voskamp and Sergei Ivanov – were detained for six hours, before being driven to hospital for blood, hair and urine samples. 'We had to sign an agreement to appear before the judge at a later date or we faced prison for 48 hours immediately,' Blijlevens later recounted. 'We could only eat when we got back at midnight.' All of this after one of the hardest stages of the entire Tour and with a third Alpine stage coming the next day. 'The police were acting like Nazis,' one anonymous TVM rider said the following morning.

At the same time, the investigation's net spread far wider. The French Big Mat team truck was pulled over at a service station by two police motorbikes and two police cars, and searched for 40 minutes. Two team soigneurs were questioned, as was one from Française des Jeux, and Casino respectively. Events the following day concerning the latter two teams would show to what effect.

With the Tour already suffering from a barrage of constant questioning in the media, the impact both inside and outside the race of the dramatic TVM raid, combined with the lower level check-ups against the French teams for good measure, was huge. For the newspapers and TV channels, after two days where sport had once more dominated the news thanks to Pantani and Ullrich, this story revived interest in the doping angles. For the Tour itself, after six days of relative calm, in fact, it was wrenched back to where it had been on the first rest day: embroiled in a huge crisis of credibility and with no idea how to avoid it. Only this time it was worse. More teams than ever were now seemingly involved in the police investigations – and there was no knowing where the trails of information might lead after that. Furthermore, compared to the Pyrenees the mental and physical exhaustion that always sets in as a Tour progresses had had another six days more to drain the riders' dwindling reserves, making them much more prone to knee-jerk responses as a way of dealing with unwanted problems or stress. With the police's investigative strategy now reaching down to the riders on the Tour itself – picking them out, questioning them and then expecting them to continue racing the following day – something had to snap.

The key shift compared to the first Tour de France strike was the attitude of the teams, which was in more significant numbers, much more uncompromisingly on the side of the disgruntled elements in the peloton. For why this matters so much it is worth recalling a given tenet of bike racing: if any race from the Tour downwards cannot function without riders, riders, in turn, are wholly dependent on their teams, for everything from sustenance to clothing to transport and a hotel in which to sleep.

Therefore, no matter how unhappy a group of riders may be, the practical elements of downing tools and stopping racing, in locations sometimes thousands of kilometres from home, wearing nothing but race clothing and with any money they might have in the team hotel are considerable. They depend almost wholly on their teams' backing. There's also the long-term consideration that roughly 80 per cent of their income (if not more) comes directly from the squad. A stage race might stop for a day, therefore, if all the riders pulled over to the side of the road. But for moments of tension to turn into all-out, definitive rebellion lasting more than a couple of hours the teams hold the whip hand. This perhaps helps to explain why teams pulling out of a Tour in protest is extremely rare and why it caused such a huge impact: before 1998, in fact, the previous 'mass exit' was in 1950, when Gino Bartali, believing himself under threat from spectators, insisted that two Italian teams – the national squad and the national 'espoirs' team – quit the race en masse on stage 12.

At a point when the Tour was reaching general meltdown, the teams' relationship with the race, therefore, was crucial. According to Saiz as he discusses the 1998 Tour, even before the Festina scandal erupted a significant percentage of the teams were already in the process of falling out with the Tour organisers. This was less likely than it sounds: in a sport depending wholly on commercial backers, a successful relationship with the Tour, as the showcase event, all but guarantees a team's economic survival. Put simply, it ensures sponsors gain maximum bang for their buck.

Although it does not make sense to bite the hand that feeds you, the teams' dislike of their dependence on the Tour has led, over the years, to many attempts to 'restructure' the sport, from the ProTour and WorldTour through to – arguably – the latest bids to create an independent, Formula One-like, calendar of events and league. 'It's clear that the Tour has always been supported by those who will suck up to it, who are so sold on the idea of the Tour de France that they say yes to everything the Tour demands,' Saiz – later to be one of the key voices behind the ProTour – claims as night falls in Torrelavega. '[But] the years of [long-standing Tour bosses Felix] Levitan, Jacques Goddet and so on had passed, the times when they used to say one word and everybody would jump, but after that, when the lower ranking management began to take over from them, an across-the-board debate began to open up. In that general debate, everybody wanted to be a part … the teams had been very generous to the Tour at prior historical points in the race and they wanted that favour returned.'

You can accuse Saiz of having his own axe to grind. That said, his opinion is corroborated by other insiders in the sport and claims that the Festina affair accelerated an already deteriorating relationship between the Tour and the teams of the time. Furthermore, Saiz was influential enough to be elected president of the teams' association, the AIGCP, after the 1998 Tour de France; at the time he was a heavyweight in the sport. Even if his personal relationship with Jean-Marie Leblanc, prior to the Tour de France 1998, had been, he insists, 'good,' in a later point in the interview Saiz says he felt that the Tour, 'rightly or wrongly, always spoke to the same managers – [Roger] Legeay (GAN), Marc Madiot [FDJ], Patrick Lefevere (Mapei), [Gianluigi] Stanga (Polti) a bit, Francis Lafargue (Banesto public relations officer and point man between the Spanish team and French cycling in general). ONCE wasn't in there. That's not a criticism, it's just the way it was.' But it mattered in the 1998 Tour. When the raids began and the tension started to build, there was no direct line of communication with the Tour's two most high-profile ringleaders of the rebellion – Laurent Jalabert and Manolo Saiz.

'When me and Leblanc talked about cycling, we got on fine,' Saiz says. 'Leblanc, in some ways, was the part of the Tour's organisation who knew about cycling the most, he was an ex-pro, the rest of the management weren't so well-rooted in the sport. [But] when he wanted to act as organiser, he displayed the slightly more "totalitarian attitude" that the Tour de France organisation sometimes tended to have.' This is not an opinion shared widely, but, rather than a comment to be taken at face value, it's perhaps more an indication of how Saiz viewed the Tour.

What is clear is that no matter how well Saiz got on with Leblanc on a personal level, the underlying disputes remained. But on top of that, in 1998, even before the Tour, Saiz had already witnessed what he took as another assault on the teams from the French police. As he now reveals, full-scale, specifically targeted police raids in France against bike teams did not start, as has been widely thought, in the Tour 1998: they had started in March that year, with ONCE.

'Governments always hide the reality behind the stories. But the Thursday before that year's Milan–Sanremo, ONCE experienced the first major police raid of 1998. We had finished Paris–Nice, and were training as usual on the Costa Azul and on the Thursday before Milan–Sanremo we headed over to do the last few kilometres of the race as a reconnaissance with Jalabert. The team bus had already gone from the hotel and we left a little bit later and then I got a call through to me: "Manolo, we've been stopped by the police in the last rest area before crossing the frontier."

'Logically, as the team manager I went there. The police find the suitcase where we had all the medication – we had nothing to hide there – and we, the bus driver and I, are escorted to the Pasteur [government medical research centre] in Nice.

'The team went on to the hotel. It would not be accurate to say we were arrested but all our medication was tested. We said they could test whatever they liked, we had nothing to hide. And they analysed absolutely everything, product by product, and, as could have been expected, they didn't find any kind of doping product at all.'

Saiz argues that the ONCE police raid was deliberately ignored by the French media – certainly it was not reported and even in 2014, some of the best informed 1998 journalists, like Jean Montois, had no idea it had happened. 'At the time I didn't really think it was that important ... There were occasional check-ups on vehicles by customs at frontiers, like they had always done, which I think is absolutely normal ... But then the police checked over the TVM vehicles, too' – although slightly earlier than ONCE, that was a result of a routine customs check rather than a full-on investigation – 'and the French press began ... to run stories that EPO was being used in amateur teams'.

So what was the problem with the police raids in the 1998 Tour and why did Saiz take them so badly? Saiz claims that, rather than the raids per se being an issue, it was the way they were leaked to the press – and which had *not* happened with the March investigation at Nice – that infuriated him and the ONCE riders in general. 'All the Tour wanted to do was to save its own skin. Cycling required something as simple as respect. We knew that things could have been done differently, that the police could behave normally in such raids. After all we have police forces because they're necessary, they're there to defend normal citizens. What we couldn't understand at the Tour was the press getting the tip-off that the raids were going to be made and turning up as well. It wasn't that the police were looking for drugs [that angered me], it was the way they did it.' In other words, Saiz's beef was with the presence of the media, filming and reporting – as he saw it – every moment of an investigation. But he roundly rejects the idea that he disliked investigations per se. 'Why should I be pissed off if they do the first big raid of 1998 on us and we're clean? How am I not going to defend police raids? That March raid was covered up.' Saiz had no problem with that, because that meant it had been done discreetly. 'But the police shouldn't have gone in there doing the [July] raids with the TV cameras following every move. The media found out first about what raids were going to take place and where and that was what we didn't approve of, what we didn't understand. And I still don't understand it.'

Therefore, when the rules of the game changed and the media's level of prior knowledge about the raids was too high in Saiz's eyes, 'I felt I was in the right when it came to talking as I did during the 1998 Tour.' Had the teams been closely united to the Tour organisation across the board, of course, they might have called their riders to order. But with one key segment of the 20 Tour squads – rightly or wrongly – already feeling alienated and at odds with the Tour, they were always going to lend a more sympathetic ear to their riders' complaints. The standoff had already reached its head in Tarascon-sur-Ariège and then did so again, but in a much more serious format, in the Alps. Faced with a situation of such extreme unpredictability, Saiz said he had told his riders 'not to wander too far away, because we needed to stay in radio contact. There was a sense that day, basically, that everything was going to end badly.'

Not that Saiz, or anybody else for that matter, needed to stoke the flames much on the morning of stage 17. For many of the riders – but, crucially, not all – the police action against TVM had crossed another boundary they were not prepared to accept. In the case of sports directors like Saiz and like those of the Spanish teams, unlike in the Pyrenees where the management was seemingly more fractured, this time the riders found they got a more sympathetic response from their bosses.

At 149 km, the stage was not one of the hardest in the Alps, with the first category climbs of the Le Semnoz after around an hour of racing, then a third category, the Col de Prés, at 97 km and the Col du Revard, 30 km before the finish in Aix-les-Bains. (Conspiracy theorists argue that in an attempt to keep the events of the 1998 Tour buried for as long as possible, Le Semnoz and the Col du Revard took a very long time to reappear in the Tour's route, only featuring once more on the last stage through the Alps … in 2013.) But after two tough days in the mountains and nearly two and a half weeks of racing, it could well have taken its toll.

As it was the riders made an unspoken agreement that stage, after a brief, two-minute halt at the start as their first show of solidarity with TVM, to go slow at least as far as the foot of the first climb. 'We are only here for the public,' Luc Leblanc said at the line, but to judge by the whistling and booing as the riders set off the fans on the roadside were not impressed by what they saw.

Once again, the peloton was far from united in their slow-pedalling protest. Telekom had already expressed their desire to continue racing, as had Rabobank. But, either way, the TVM riders' comments at the start village or in the team hotel that morning, on how they had been eating at midnight and had got to bed at 2.30 a.m., had struck home. 'The police started searching all cupboards, suitcases and bags,' a haggard-looking Blijlevens recounted. 'All our personal letters were translated by a police interpreter. They searched the hotel from top to bottom … and we woke up at 9 a.m. because we were so hungry, so that was a very short night's rest. And today we have to perform at the peak of our form so we will see what the result is. This is a witch-hunt of our team and I think when the other riders see what has happened to us, something will be organised. What has been done to us beggars belief, it's like we were outlaws. It's just a shame.' With that call for action in mind, Pantani had himself been approached by Sergei

Outschakov at the start line and was asked, as Tour leader, to provide some show of solidarity. Saiz, meanwhile, was sitting on the bonnet of his team car, waiting for the race start and proclaiming loudly and clearly: 'This family is heading for a divorce.'

Even now, Manolo Saiz speaks rather cryptically when discussing the 1998 Tour. He wishes he could call Jean-Marie Leblanc, for instance, and have a private meeting, because 'There are things that he doesn't know that I do know and which he can be sure that I'm not going to tell; I love my sport too much to hurt it.' What those things are he will not say. Some parts of his description of events in the 1998 race he is happy to make public, though, such as his insistence that nothing illegal was found in ONCE's medical chest during the Tour. (This was confirmed later – up to a point – in the Spanish press, with the most dangerous product apparently one for fighting colds. However, given that the French Senate report directly named some ONCE riders as possible positive EPO tests, plus the events surrounding the Spanish anti-doping probe Operación Puerto in 2006 and the fact that by this point in the Tour de France much of the illegal material in other teams had been thrown away, it's possible to argue that this squeaky clean medicine cabinet was only to be expected.)

Saiz sees it very differently, however. His interpretation of the teams' reaction in Dublin was that they were concerned, but only because 'the amount of drugs that they had found in the Festina car was a load far greater than normal', not because doping was widespread in the peloton at that point. 'Then when we came back to France, there were more raids. Logically, at least in our case, nothing was found, but that means you end up vulnerable, it feels like you have' – and here he starts speaking cryptically again – 'you have feet of clay.

'However, in the ONCE team at least, our clay had been baked properly and we could take things more calmly.' He brushes aside claims in the French Senate report that at least one of his riders, Laurent Jalabert, was on EPO. 'It doesn't make sense ... they [the French Senate] have their issues.' With Voet in the police cells, Saiz argues, 'Everybody tried to find out what was happening. [But] then Willy Voet writes books ... and in that moment it was said that he had material for more teams.' However, he then returns to his favoured, more mysterious sounding analysis of events: 'But when you don't know what's really going on, what you do is avoid a discussion that might compromise a lot of other people.' They had had meetings with the Tour management, 'but nothing had come out of them'.

The other angle on Saiz's mind in Dublin was, of course, the race. It is clear that even with a top pro like Jalabert, fourth overall in the 1995 Tour after a spectacular collective attack by ONCE en route to Mende, 'we knew that we didn't have a Tour winner in our ranks. But I think that even knowing that we did not have that winner, our history in the Tour de France was always one of trying to create scenarios which would favour our team as a whole. From [1991 Vuelta winner] Melcior Mauri to [1995 Tour de France leader and later director for Lance Armstrong] Johan Bruyneel, they weren't winners [as riders], but they were very important figures and they helped the collective to win. So we went to that Tour,' he insists, 'with the usual philosophy of honesty and sincerity, to try and be as provocative as possible inside the race.'

What was unexpected, perhaps, was that Laurent Jalabert should be so close to Jan Ullrich in the long time trial at Corrèze. Fourth on the stage, just 1′ 24″ back, the reigning French national champion moved from outside the top 30 on GC into fourth overall. However, always an uneven performer in the mountains – he had won the 1995 Vuelta a España and at the Covadonga Lakes in 1996 – Jalabert started to haemorrhage time in the Pyrenees and even lost 23 seconds on Ullrich when the German was on an off-day, at Plateau de Beille. Three minutes down on Ullrich as they started the Alps, Jalabert was dropped on the Télégraphe on the crucial mountain stage, even before major hostilities had commenced. He finished well out of contention, 15 minutes down at Les Deux Alpes. 'We were pretty much where we expected to be in the Tour,' Saiz says. 'I do know that we felt extremely proud to have a French national champion in our line-up and I'd even say that we felt more attached to that achievement than – at times – we'd felt when we'd won the Spanish nationals. Jalabert was a very special rider for us, and as a born attacker, he stood out in the team.'

There was no sensation of any kind of 'mutiny', Saiz explains, prior to the expulsion of Festina. However, after France's top team had left, 'a sense of fear began [to spread]. Each team began to withdraw inside its own shell, became much more individualistic in their approach.' There was, he agrees, a general sense – as Gaumont has corroborated – of self-interest being more important than collective interests, or, as the Spanish saying (quoted by Saiz) goes: *cada uno barre para dentro* – everybody acts in their own interests first.

But at the same time, as the Pyrenees grew closer, Saiz says, 'individual riders from other teams started to come and talk to me. They knew that I was always closer to the riders than I was to the squads. And that's where things begin to brew towards something' – that something being the collective withdrawal from the Tour. Those doing most of the talking to Saiz were the other Spanish teams – Vitalicio Seguros, Kelme, ONCE and Banesto. Even before Aix-les-Bains, the four did agree, Saiz said, 'that if any one team suffered a police search, then we were all going home'. The question of whether they would actually do so, however, was debatable prior to the Alps, given that a Kelme team car was searched 'and as [Kelme owner] Pepe Quiles didn't seem too bothered, we didn't get too bothered either'.

By the Alps, though, the situation had changed radically. At km 32 of stage 17, just at the point where riders should have been accelerating for the points and bonus seconds on offer in an intermediate sprint, instead they slowed to a halt. On a straight, flat section of road in the small, lakeside town of Saint-Jorioz, flanked by a wood on the right and low hedges on the left, the second big strike of the Tour de France 1998 began. Overhead camera shots show the lack of coordination in the stoppage. As one rider from Telekom – probably Riis – continued to talk to race officials in the red lead car, one arm holding on to the driver door, some 50 to 100 yards behind him forward-placed riders in groups of two or three suddenly coasted to a halt, most with one foot out of the pedal and scraping along the ground to act as an extra brake. The bulk of the bunch, grouped around the second race director's car, also halted.

Suddenly, the sense that the Tour had reached the end of the road, a definitive point of no return, was palpable. Some of the riders might want to race, but unlike at Tarascon-sur-Ariège they could not – or would not – influence their team-mates. After the Pyrenean protest, and all the fear and tension caused by police raids, this new strike could perhaps have been predicted; but this time, rather than at a start or even on a neutralised section where riders standing around looked relatively commonplace and might seem understandable, this was a decision to break the race apart *during* the event itself. In a moment the glory, the history and the spectacle of the Tour had been reduced to this: 100-odd men in their twenties and thirties in shorts and coloured jerseys, standing around disconsolately on a back road leading out of a small Alpine town. After 95 years, after surviving two world wars, the Tour de France, the biggest annual sporting event in the world, suddenly had nowhere to go.

In blistering heat, some riders sought the shade of trees; others simply plonked themselves down by their bikes in the middle of the tarmac, in Ullrich's case looking back down the road. Pantani, meanwhile, remained standing, straddling his bike's top tube as photographers scuttled around, shooing spectators – who mixed freely with the peloton – out of the way for better pictures. A few minutes later, while Jean-François Pescheux spoke volubly to Pantani's team-mates, the race leader stood a little to the side, his familiar other-worldly air even more marked than usual. In what was an uncoordinated, undirected protest, someone was going to grasp this particular bull by the horns; it clearly wasn't going to be the Tour leader, or Ullrich, the previous race winner. Yet with the entire race on the point of collapse, nothing seemed able to move forwards.

The discontent, though, was palpable. 'It was ridiculous what the police did to TVM last night,' Julich said to TV cameramen as everybody waited for somebody – anybody – to make a decision and gaggles of bare-chested fans in cycling caps and mothers with children in their arms wandered past him on the road. 'It wasn't right. If that happened in America, there would be lawsuits and it'd be hundreds of millions of dollars' worth at stake. You can't just barge into people's rooms and demand they go down to the police station to give urine and hair samples, blood samples, whatever they had to do, in the middle of the night. That's ridiculous.' Jacky Durand, who would go on to win the Tour's most combative rider award, said bluntly they were being treated like child rapists, 'and that's what hurts. If there's an underlying problem, we should resolve it – but at the end of the race.'

A second landmark for the day's strike quickly followed the first. Up until then, it is likely that some of the professionals who had quit the Tour for official reasons, such as feeling under the weather or being ill, were simply looking for a way out. But that first halt on stage 17 saw the first abandon of a rider from the 1998 Tour as a clear expression of outrage. Laurent Jalabert pulled back to his team car, dropped his bike behind for the mechanics to put on the racks and got in the front co-pilot's seat, next to ONCE's Saiz. Photographers craned in at the French national champion as he worked his way through a chocolate ice cream. Right behind the team car, two or three heavily built ONCE domestiques were close by, just as Saiz had instructed. 'It's not a personal protest,' Jalabert spoke into a microphone from radio station RTL thrust through the open car window, 'it's because we just don't know what's going on and it's about showing that we seem incapable of making a decision. Well, I've made my decision, my conscience is clear and I'm sure I have nothing left to do in this Tour. Given the situation, it's better I stop and there it is, I've stopped. The police have no scruples, they will go after every rider and I don't think all the riders are aware of that.'

He made stronger comments to Spanish sports daily *MARCA*, saying he felt as 'affected as any rider in TVM or Festina by what's happened. I understand that others may not want to quit, because if they [team management] tell you "either continue or you're going to be sacked", then what are you going to do? I'm well paid, I can take that risk, but others cannot.' His description of the Tour was, according to *MARCA*, very direct: 'This Tour is shit.'

Not even the arrival of another, more powerful figure could convince Jalabert to change his mind. 'Jean-Marie Leblanc came over to talk to Laurent Jalabert but I stayed out of it,' Saiz recalls. 'I think whoever the rider is, when he stops in a situation like that, he feels relief. It's very difficult to be in the TV news, and feel defenceless.'

Ironically, once one of the most outspoken protestors had actually taken the final step of quitting, the peloton, hovering between the exit door and the road ahead, found themselves more easily swayed by the Tour director's entreaties that they continue. By this point, as Leblanc recollects, he was clutching at straws to try and suppress the mutiny. 'I wasn't surprised when they stopped after an hour of riding at a snail's pace alongside the Lake Annecy … things were hanging by the thinnest of threads, was the Tour de France going to go down with all hands in a tragic finale?' Leblanc wrote later in his autobiography.

By now all that mattered for Leblanc was for the Tour to regain some sort of semblance of racing – in other words to go on moving, no matter how slowly, from point A to point B. Astonishingly, one of the Tour's publicity stunts of inviting VIPs and figures from the French establishment to sit in the back seat of Leblanc's car ended up saving the Tour that day, and perhaps, given subsequent events in the stage and that evening, from extinction altogether. One of Leblanc's guests in the car that day, watching as the Tour went into meltdown, was a civil servant from the Ministry of the Interior – a high-flying police force representative. As Leblanc recalls it now, 'he was sitting there and he saw that everything was falling apart, and he said to me, "Mr Leblanc, if I can help you, from what I've heard, there will be more investigations this evening, but not against the riders." And so immediately I passed that information on to the riders. More investigations, but not against the riders. And in fact, he hadn't lied, and soigneurs and doctors were questioned, but the riders' – at least not en masse, although that was not the case for one high-profile individual – 'weren't affected. The civil servant in the police force said that, but it was on a knife-edge, and I had to bluff a bit, too, it was not in any sense official.' Whether it was true or not – 'and there were no mobile phones back then, you see?' he adds – Leblanc was forced to make do with a scrap of information that he could then, in best spin doctor fashion, turn into a firm-sounding promise that police action would cease. As he puts it, it was couched in generalisations … 'I said to them "I think I can tell you that …"' is how he recalls his semi-official language. 'I was bluffing.'

Although the Spanish in general and Saiz in particular were convinced that he had direct contact with the Ministry of Sport or the Ministry of the Interior, Leblanc argues that is not the case.

'It was a much more dangerous strike than in Tarascon,' Leblanc says now. 'In the first one, we convinced them to move very quickly.' In Tarascon, no carrot of the type waved at the riders thanks to his friendly police guest 'insider information' had been necessary, 'in fact [at Tarascon] I can't even remember what I said'. But would it work this time, when the Tour was on a knife-edge? Leblanc's 'puffed up' argument, delivered to knots of riders around his car, was that he was 'seeking guarantees that any further investigations are carried out in a manner appropriate for the dignity of athletes of the highest level'. And slowly, as one rider after another slung his leg over his top tube and began moving down the road, the Tour moved into some semblance of action. The race now was not to see who was first, though, but who would be left racing by the end of the day.

Once Jalabert had gone, with their leader sitting in a team car yards behind the riders still in the peloton, the only question was how soon ONCE as a team would follow. It took a very few minutes, given that in the Jalabert interview with RTL, Saiz, sitting next to the Frenchman, can be heard telling the mechanics over the phone in the background, 'load up all the bikes, and let's get out of here'. *MARCA*, once again, was on hand, lending the Spanish team their van to put their bikes in and following the squad to their hotel. But as Saiz explains, the final decision for the Spanish squad to cut their ties with the 1998 Tour was not one that had been planned, not even when they started the stage that day. 'We had no intention of going, it was a spur-of-the-moment decision.' So why quit? 'Because it was so unclear as to what was happening,' Saiz said. 'Nobody knew anything, whether we were going to keep going after the climb or before the climb. One moment we were stopping, the next we were going. Were we going to do the last 20 kilometres of a race? What the hell were we doing there? What was happening to those professionals who deserved all the respect in the world, sitting on the side of the road? The bunch stopped, I was in the team car, and Laurent directly came back and sat in the car. One or two other riders were there, we all realised it was pointless [to continue]. Nothing was going to be won and a lot was going to be lost. Riders were sitting down all over the road. We didn't feel like people, we felt like cattle that were being herded from one city to another. And this was supposed to be sport.'

Saiz will not be drawn, even now, as to who actually opted to stop ONCE as a team en masse. He will not even reveal if it was a rider or the team. 'The decision was taken by the situation' is all he will say cryptically, his standard defence mechanism. However, he is equally insistent that he did not tell the team to halt. 'They want to look for a guilty party when there really isn't one. The guilty party was the situation. It's not a single person, nor a group, nor anybody in particular. The proof that it was a collective decision [to quit] is that I am stuck with the label of [deciding to quit], when arguably I was the least involved of all of them. I only knew that when that decision had been taken, it was me that has to deal with it. That's what the captain of a ship does.

'We were the first team to leave because we were the most protected by our [sponsor's] president, José María Arroyo,' Saiz also avows, before insisting that, as a team, ONCE could not have been better supported by their sponsor whatever decision they took. 'And because we felt we were so well supported, that was an enormous advantage. Before making the final decision to quit, I called him by phone to tell him, but the responsibility was not his, in any way.' Saiz is at pains to explain that he had not masterminded an attempt to sink the Tour. As he sees it, his team's abandoning of the race was done, he insists, with the long-term interests of the sport at heart. 'They see me as the leader of the rebellion and, it's a mistake, I wasn't. I wish there had been a leader, I really wish that. Because if somebody can be followed, somebody could have transmitted the truth to all those people. But there were no ringleaders. There was no real analysis of what was going on. The people who should have been the ringleaders, failed to be; those who had the direct contact [with the authorities, although Leblanc denies this] should have been [i.e. the Tour]. They tried to protect their own interests and they forgot that we are their own interests, too. It was a disastrous Tour.'

If Leblanc's spin-doctoring of an off-the-record comment and pleading with Pantani and the rest had one effect and got the peloton moving, ONCE's departure suggested that the race was, despite all this, on the point of folding. When the pace refused to pick up, to a backdrop of wolf whistles and boos from spectators frustrated by waiting in blazing heat for the Tour's painfully late appearance, Pantani himself showed that he was not prepared to race, at least for a day. As the peloton ambled along, a team-mate riding alongside the race leader very slowly peeled the Italian's number from the back of his jersey. Once that was done – symbolising that the race had been neutralised – other riders, most notably the Italians and Spanish, began to do the same. Having keeled over so far it looked like the 1998 Tour would sink with all hands, and from the outside it now appeared as if Pantani was living up to his nickname. *Il Pirata* was giving the race no quarter.

Inside the Mercatone Uno squad, however, a collective decision had been reached – albeit by a hair's breadth – to continue. 'We were very close to going home,' Traversoni now recalls. 'It was something we decided during the stage. Marco would have gone home, even if he was wearing the leader's jersey.' However, he argues that Leblanc had 'talked to Pantani and begged him to save the Tour and bring the Tour with him to Paris. Leblanc said, "Please don't you go home, let us finish this Tour."' (This then fostered resentment, still lingering today, that when Pantani asked for his team in 2001 to have a wild card, Leblanc did not return the favour. Or, as Traversoni puts it bluntly, 'Leblanc slammed the door in his face.' Leblanc himself says the decision was based purely on sporting criteria.)

Traversoni himself was part of the Mercatone camp, if in a slight minority, that would have preferred to down tools, 'and if it had been 50 per cent on one side, and 50 per cent on the other, then we'd have gone home. But if my team leader doesn't decide to do that, then I can't decide to do that for my leader.' Mercatone Uno themselves were not raided at any point in the Tour, something which Traversoni says shows that the police action was based purely on 'intercepted messages', rather than Pantani or others performing so well in the sporting arena. 'One rider gets caught, or it could be a masseur or a doctor and the rest would get hauled in. One mistake or a wrong call, and then suddenly the whole lot get nailed. Then it [the doping trail] would cross over to another team.' Traversoni says he has no proof whether his theories are right. But his way of thinking is indicative of how Pantani's riders perceived the police actions. 'But if they wanted it to be fair, they should have raided every team, not just a few.'

If Mercatone were divided, ONCE had now quit, and simply getting through the stage seemed to be the order of the day, the mood in the peloton was turning sourer by the moment. 'A Vitalicio Seguros rider started ripping the race numbers off riders' jerseys,' Jaksche recalls. 'They started lifting the numbers [saying], "I don't care, we can't go on any more."' Jaksche describes his conversation with Prudencio Indurain, a rider who wanted to quit, as 'a discussion'. If so, it certainly belonged in what politicians would call a full and frank exchange of views.

'He said I should be like my "boss" – Luc Leblanc – 'because he was going to quit' – something Luc Leblanc did later in the stage. 'I was shouting at him in English or in German to get the fuck out of my way. But it was a typical problem. A huge part of the peloton is not well educated. They did not reflect. They thought, "if we pull out, we can change the situation". They did not understand that we created the situation. It was not the police that created our failure, but they blamed the police. Jens Voigt said, "they should just let us race", but, no, doping was an illegal act in France, and I was fed up with the self-protection of the riders. I was really angry, it was, "get out of my way or I am going to hit you." I was really aggressive. And then they blame the police. If you play with fire, then you can get burned.'

Although some will point to the anti-doping investigations of Operación Puerto constituting irrefutable evidence to the contrary, Saiz to this day argues that his anger was not directed at the police raids per se and the fact that they were searching for banned drugs with a ferocity the Tour had never experienced before. Asked directly if ONCE had something to hide in the 1990s, Saiz responds, 'Never. I'm telling you it and I'll sign a paper to say it. ONCE never had anything to hide in its entire life as a team. And I'm telling you loud and clear.'

'The riders in' – and he names a top modern-day team – 'last two or three years. The riders in ONCE lasted 16 years. It's just a question of one word: sacrifice. I'm telling you that clearly. [Alberto] Contador was with me when he was 17 and is still winning now. Zülle lasted for an age. Jalabert as well. That's not by chance. That's a question of sacrifice, hard work and humility. It's one of the things I most miss about this sport now.'

With ONCE gone, and with Mercatone sitting on the fence if not edging towards quitting – other team managers confirm Pantani wished to abandon, but only loyalty to his team-mates and concern for their financial wellbeing kept him from doing so – Bjarne Riis stepped into the breach as unofficial spokesman for the peloton and negotiator with Jean-Marie Leblanc. But there was a crucial difference between the Dane and Jalabert. Unlike Jalabert, Riis was determined that the Tour should continue. Rumours, particularly among the Spanish and Italian cycling communities of the time, abound to this day that Riis wanted to leave and then changed his mind during the stage. But the evidence from the Pyrenees, where he and Aldag acted as 'strike-breakers', contradicts this completely. As Riis puts it, 'I'm not a quitter.'

'He was the lord and master of Telekom, so it made sense he talked,' Traversoni argues. 'Plus he was talking because he was still convinced that Ullrich could win the Tour. Ullrich had really turned things round in that previous stage to Albertville' – after which Pantani had told his team-mates that if Ullrich had gone 'just half a kilometre per hour faster' he'd have been dropped.

Riis says now there was no pressure from his team sponsors or directors to act in one way or another, never a point when he wanted to go home early from the Tour. 'No. That is not in my character. It is not in me to give up. It's not going to solve the problem just by going home. I'm not a quitter.' He confirms he wanted to go on to keep on trying to win the Tour with Ullrich. 'Yes. Of course it was special and there was a lot of shit going on. [But] you resolve it and definitely the things you couldn't take care of right then. You say, "OK, this has to be resolved in another way, another time".'

Photographs of Riis riding for minutes at a time with one arm clutching the open window of Leblanc's car, thrashing out some kind of deal as the peloton inched its way up the Col de Semnoz, became some of the most well-known images of the entire race. Their conversation gained weight because, as Leblanc has said, the Frenchman felt he could relate to Riis – multilingual, belonging to French and Italian teams at other points during his long career as well as Telekom's undisputed decision-maker and a former Tour winner, too. 'I was there trying to be the middleman for the peloton, saying, "OK, how can we sort this out?" Leblanc was really good at trying to deal with it. He was always on the riders' side, saying, "let's try to find a solution",' Riis recalls. 'Of course, his interest was that the Tour should get to Paris, that's fair enough and I think it should have been for all of us. But it was a good dialogue.'

'Riis was of a certain age, he'd already won the Tour, he was somebody people would listen to,' Leblanc recalls. 'He had a certain authority and charisma and we knew each other a little. He knew I was no ruffian and we told each other the truth. That's what tipped the balance.' He was in any case much more straightforward to deal with than Jalabert, 'who was under the influence of Manolo Saiz'. But Leblanc is adamant that there was no payoff involved in the deal, saying when asked that he gave and offered Riis 'Nothing, *rien.*'

Riis calls his role at the time one of 'natural leadership, somebody taking responsibility'. But not everybody – including Jaksche – felt Riis was the right person for the unofficial mediator's job. 'I never talked to Riis about being the spokesman but nobody ever wanted him to be it, he self-proclaimed himself to be it,' Jaksche said. 'No one knew what kind of deal he really did. He probably saved the Tour de France and as a reward never got into trouble with the Tour.'

Jaksche doesn't answer when asked if there could be anybody else in that particular role. 'I'm sure that the Spanish argued that Riis sold the souls of the cyclists, by agreeing there would be no more raids on the riders.'

Nor was it clear, in fact, as Riis seems to make out now, that he was 'destined' to take that role. 'Bjarne came up to me and said, "you have to talk to these guys",' Bobby Julich now recalls, 'and I was like, "are you kidding me? You do it. Who am I?" I've seen photos of me that day and I'm sitting there with my head on my hands going, "let's just race, or not, let's not just sit here and do this." Then Bjarne came up to me, he speaks very calmly and I said, "Bjarne, there's no way I'm going to talk on behalf of anyone. I'm nobody." "You're up there, Pantani's up there, Leblanc is up there, you guys deal with it." I didn't really know the gravity of the situation because I elected not to speak French.'

Even Riis, now, has his doubts about whether he took the right course of action. 'Maybe,' he reflects, 'I was thinking I was afraid of what was going to happen to cycling if we had gone home. And who would have known what would have happened if we'd gone home. Maybe it would have been the best solution, maybe, who the hell knows?' However, at the time, Riis appeared to have no such doubts, putting one arm around Jean-Marie Leblanc as – for a second time – the riders stopped again. This time, though, it was much briefer and, to judge by the waving from a Telekom rider for the peloton to halt, not so spontaneous.

Riis briefly explained his deal with Leblanc, that even if the day's racing was over, the police would ease back a little, that the riders and teams would be treated with respect. But it went, at the time, no further than that. 'You're not going to sit on the side of a climb and resolve cycling's problems,' he reasons. 'What we agreed on was that they [cycling's underlying problems] had to be resolved in another way, which actually, afterwards, the UCI was not capable of doing.'

Circumstantial evidence suggests, from the way riders stayed standing in the road, straddling their bikes rather than sitting on the tarmac or in the shade, that the Tour's third stoppage that day – if you count the two-minute protest delay in starting – was more of an information break than the full-on strike that had immediately preceded it a few kilometres before. Only one rider appears to have taken up Jalabert's role as stand-out French rebel by that stage: Polti leader Luc Leblanc. His finger wagging furiously in Riis's direction as the Dane communicated the deal in the midst of the peloton, the former World Champion was clearly unhappy with it. 'We were no diplomats' is Riis's terse recollection of their angry face-off. The next morning Leblanc, who opted to quit regardless of what the rest of the Polti team did (they stayed), would explain to the media at the start that he had left the Tour because of the way riders had been treated – and the lack of support from the UCI.

The rest of the bunch, numberless and with no objective but merely to get the stage completed, meandered on. But their numbers were shrinking steadily. Two more squads, Spanish team Banesto and the three remaining riders from the small Italian Riso Scotti outfit, also opted for an early exit at the feed zone in Lescheraines. If Riso Scotti's exit was barely noticed, the departure of Banesto, a team which had won five Tours with Miguel Indurain, was another symbolic blow to the race's prestige. So, too, were the photos published in Spain next day of one rider, Txente García Acosta, in tears as he sat in the team car, using a race jacket to wipe them away. For the rest, another 90 km of meaningless riding to Aix-les-Bains continued, amid boos and jeers and not a few members of the public baring their buttocks as the Tour director's car passed by.

With a delay of two hours, evening shadows were growing longer when the peloton finally reached the outskirts of the venerable spa town at around 7.20 p.m. Then, just under four kilometres from the line, after Marco Pantani and Erik Zabel, as the green points jersey leader, had spent some time at the head of the pack in what looked like a first display of solidarity, the TVM riders moved to the front, with TVM's Steven de Jongh gesturing that the pack should slow down even further. Thus, with the four of the six TVM riders lined across the peloton, the Tour finally completed the most crisis-ridden day in its history. It turned out to be a seven hour day of racing for 149 km – an average speed of 22 kmh an hour, compared with the normal minimum of 36 kmh. TVM crossing the line first together was a bizarre image, but one which showed the world exactly who the Tour's most high-profile protagonists of the previous 24 hours had been – much to Jean-Marie Leblanc's chagrin. With the official clocks (sponsored by Festina) showing a black screen rather than their usual digits, too, it was clear that the stage had been cancelled, even before a single sheet, containing the overall classification from the previous day, was passed to journalists in the press room. And that, at least from an official point of view, was that.

For all riot police from the RDI were drafted in, the riders got a surprisingly warm reception from the finish crowd. Perhaps it was because they were now resigned to the fact they were going to be witnessing an unusual spectacle, although some of the media even claimed that fans' hostility to the media – widely blamed for worsening the situation – had meant the police had been drafted in to protect journalists from the public. Certainly the finish-line spectators were not as angry as those who had spent all day in blazing heat, some in fields or Alpine forests, for little reward other than a bunch of slow-pedalling, miserable looking riders and a few photographers and race officials to blame.

TVM's dour Russian national champion Sergei Ivanov technically 'won' the stage in that he was the first across the line, a fact that would have some bizarre echoes in later cycling history, both in terms of doping scandals and French geography. Excluded from the Tour in 2000 because of a high hematocrit value, in 2001 Ivanov was again a winner on the Tour's return to Aix-les-Bains, taking a transition stage. 'Last year I made some mistakes,' he was quoted as saying in 2001 in his stage winner's press conference, before adding a cryptic punchline worthy of Manolo Saiz in his prime: 'but they were not my mistakes.'

As for the 1998 strike, 'You could see it coming,' Rabobank's Australian rider Robbie McEwen told Channel 4's 30-minute programme on the Tour de France a few metres after crossing the finish line. 'The other day [on the first strike in the Pyrenees] it was almost like this when the whole thing blew up, but last night, they took the guys from TVM out of the hotel, they were there all night ... they were giving all sorts of samples, the guys haven't returned a positive test or something, it's five days to go in the Tour, you can't have the police taking the guys out of the hotel at night for no reason, it's not on.'

Asked by reporter Gary Imlach exactly how many riders had wanted to go on and how many wanted to stop, McEwen described the Spanish team's departure as 'their bad luck' but that they had 'done the right thing letting TVM cross the line first'. 'We've had to put our point across,' added Stuart O'Grady. 'It had to happen.' 'The Tour is no game,' added Pantani, 'at each stage, we take huge risks, even our lives on descents, and it's outrageous that the police can come into my room, looking for vitamin C or put me in jail for something in my suitcase, forbidden or not. It's unfair that a rider, a champion, be treated like a murderer.'

The Tour by this point was now down to 117 riders, lacking the world number one and the number one-ranked team (Jalabert and Festina respectively), the most consistently successful team of the 1990s (ONCE) as well as the team that had won the Tour for six of the last 10 years (Banesto). That it had been a brilliantly fought race up until that point was undeniable. But so, too, were the scandals that had laid open a sport rent asunder with doping, ridiculed in the general media. Such was the degradation of the Tour's image in just two weeks that an event Charles de Gaulle once said could only be stopped by world wars had only been prevented from collapsing altogether by one civil servant's throwaway line and a race director's ability to spin those words into something vaguely convincing, if not a little fictitious.

There is no doubt that the Tour could have come to a premature end somewhere on a back road outside Annecy. But *should* the 1998 edition have folded there and then? Curiously, for all their huge differences in the future, both Jaksche and Saiz agree that it would have been best for cycling if the Tour had stopped in Aix-les-Bains. 'If you're honest it would have been the strongest [best] thing to do. Just leave the Tour and see what happens,' Jaksche says.

'The Tour is the race I love the most,' Saiz says. 'It's the best race in the world. But at that point in time, we should have been talking about the dignity of the riders. And instead the race tried to put itself ahead of the riders. If it had stopped, cycling would have retained some sort of credibility. Instead, since 1998 it has been under suspicion. And thanks to the Tour we've created that status for cycling, because every government knows that while they can't have it in the football World Championships, in 1998 all we showed the world was that we were really weak. Really, really weak. And nobody listens to the weak.'

15

Early Exits

Thursday, 30 July. Stage 18:
Aix-les-Bains–Neuchâtel, 218 km

Friday, 31 July. Stage 19:
La Chaux-de-Fonds–Autun, 242 km

Anyone who thought the battle to save the Tour de France was 'won' when the TVM riders reached the line in Aix-les-Bains was sorely mistaken, as events a few minutes later would show.

The contradictions between Riis's assurances to the rest of the peloton that 'if the police go to the hotels tonight, we go home' immediately became clear. Even as Riis was repeating the promise to the world in general after he was invited on to the French post-race chat show *VeloClub*, and claiming that 'everybody wants to go on to Paris, everybody', the gendarmes were searching the hotels of Casino, ONCE and Française des Jeux. Two other teams would shortly quit. It was hardly, therefore, either a reassuring or credible message.

In ONCE's case the search had begun well before the peloton had actually reached the finish. Barely half an hour after the Spanish squad had turned up at their hotel for the night, the police turned up, too. 'We saw what they had taken and they took away our team doctor, Nicolás Terrados,' Saiz observes. 'We'd already been in touch with lawyers who then headed to France to fight our case. And we were' – he observes for the third time in the interview – 'the only people to walk clear.'

He confirms, as has been stated elsewhere, that the police were very thorough in their search, which lasted nearly 12 hours, leaving papers, suitcases and team material strewn across the floor. 'I don't mind, in fact it was good that they should check right down to the last mote of dust, and place them all in plastic bags for checking up on them. We didn't mind, because we were free by that point. A totalitarian group can be controlling you, but your freedom is yours. And in that moment we had a lot of freedom. Pablo [Anton, team manager] stayed behind as coordinator and I headed for Spain. I just wanted to get home.'

That night Vitalicio and Kelme, the other two Spanish squads of the original four, then also quit. Although Vitalicio, essentially a team built around breakaway specialists, had little left to play for, Kelme was another story, given their rider Fernando Escartín was lying, at the time, fourth overall.

Seventeen years on and Escartín still says he has no regrets about leaving the race, even though he says he was 'in the best shape of my life. I'd seen it coming, I'd done really well in 1997 [finishing fifth overall] and I did well again later on in the race. So I'd been able to fly under the radar a little, because the other top names were looking more at Olano and Jalabert in the Spanish teams, and although I'd done well in the Pyrenees, the time trials were always my problem.'

At the point of the strike, Escartín says that although winning was way out of the question, and even finishing second was difficult, he might – just – have moved into third had Julich run into difficulties. That, in any case, he felt would have been 'complicated'. He does not feel he would have been happier had he had the chance to try to do something, as he would have done in any normal race. Rather, Escartín prefers to put things in much broader perspective. 'What I most regret about ... the strike was that the union between all the different riders that day was terrible. It was the day that cycling changed. We weren't asking for anything out of the ordinary, but what we asked for ended up breaking what little union remained between us.' If he had to quit again, he says, 'I'd do it again, I would do, because it was a decision taken by all of us – ONCE, Banesto, all of us – and I was disappointed that the other teams didn't do the same.'

Barring Riso Scotti, the other Italian squads – Mercatone, Polti, Saeco, ASICS – did not pull out, after 'backtracking' on an unwritten agreement to do so, although Jaksche, for one, did not want to go and Traversoni says that, in an informal vote, Mercatone was too divided to end up quitting. 'The Italians had Pantani as their leader and so they didn't do it. But I still think that that was the day that changed things.' And not, Escartín would argue, for the better. 'If we had continued to Paris', he says, 'we would have been lessened as people.'

Kelme were not the only ones to leave. *MARCA* also opted to pull out its correspondents from the race, with the full, extraordinarily lengthy front-page headline on the next morning's paper reading, 'You're all getting dumped ... France, for being such a bad host; the [investigation's] police, for abusing your power, Jean-Marie Leblanc, for playing cheap politics with sportsmen, and Tour' – with the definite article removed for good measure – 'for sinking so low'.

'Our riders could not stand any more humiliation,' *MARCA* continued, 'so they're coming back to Spain feeling sad but with their heads held high. *MARCA*, with the permission of you, the readers, could not stand by when faced with such an outrage and our reporters are coming home too. Those who are interested, if there is still anybody who cares, can follow the race on the news agencies.' 'Let them race it,' wrote *MARCA*'s chief cycling reporter,

Josu Garai, in a front-page editorial, and reflecting the widespread anti-French sentiment in Spain concerning the police raids in the Tour, condemned by leading sports figures from the country, including the usually mild-mannered Miguel Indurain. 'Because it's the French who want to impose some new ethical standards, in cycling and by extension to world sport ... as if they were the only "clean" ones. So why didn't they do that in the football World Championships? everybody asks here. Why didn't they search through the rubbish bins in the hotel rooms belonging to the [teams named] team doctors and soigneurs? Because they weren't brave enough and FIFA wouldn't have let them.' Garai, like Saiz, attacked the media's 'excessive and forewarned' presence at police raids, rather than the raids themselves. He asks why TVM's 'affair' was 'revived' at the time of the Tour, 'taking them off for blood tests in order to find out if they failed to stop at a pedestrian crossing' and demanding to know if there were 'hidden powers' seeking to overturn the Tour de France.

At the press centre, as the searches went into overdrive so did the rumours. All that was known for certain, at this point, was that three teams – ONCE, Banesto and Riso Scotti – had left the race, that more were probably quitting, and that searches were proceeding at multiple team hotels. When the dust settled, which was not until next morning, although it was clear that the Spanish had gone, as well as Luc Leblanc, there was one other important exit: Rodolfo Massi, the first leader of a classification in the Tour de France to disappear from the running since Pascal Hervé, the King of the Mountains during the first week. But, unlike the Spanish, Massi had not left by choice.

Seventh overall at the time and the King of the Mountains with a massive lead on Christophe Rinero of 335 points to 197, as well as being a stage winner in the Pyrenees, Massi was detained by police after banned products, thought to be corticoids, were allegedly found in his hotel room that evening. He was then charged with trafficking banned drugs, media reports stated at the time. Surprisingly, given the number of riders who had passed through the hands of the police by this point in the Tour, and for all the confessions that had appeared in grisly detail, Massi was the first member of the Tour peloton actually to face charges since Voet had been detained.

The sudden police interest in the Italian veteran was – it was reported at the time – due to his being named by a former Festina rider within his new team, Gilles Bouvard, who had been questioned by police earlier in the week. Massi defended himself in *La Gazzetta dello Sport*, saying that he and Bouvard had fallen out earlier in the season and the products in his room were for treating his asthma.

Massi's case was eventually dropped by the police and no charges brought, but in just one day layers of suspicion and rumours had relentlessly wrapped themselves around a rider who had broken his femur and collarbone badly when he smashed into – of all things – a Roman arch in the first week of the 1988 Giro d'Italia. Subsequent surgery following a year on the sidelines left him with one leg shorter than the other, but Massi stubbornly raced on until, in 1993, he broke his collarbone again. Until 1998, the Italian had been an outstanding example of a rider who tenaciously raced on against overwhelming physical odds. Suddenly, he was nicknamed 'the Pharmacist' by newspapers, and, as Jeremy Whittle wrote, 'his supposedly frequent trips to Mexico weren't to enjoy the benefits of altitude training, but [supposedly] for more sinister purposes. Anonymous riders still racing in the Tour were said to be queuing up to reveal what and how much they'd bought from Massi in recent years … it was a hard fall for a long-suffering rider.' However, the way he was handled by the media is illustrative of how interest in the Tour had veered from the purely sporting stories with an occasional dash of scandal, to pure scandal stories with an occasional sliver of sport. All in the space of two weeks.

For the press, with one team after another facing arrests or raids, the state of uncertainty and rumours which had driven Saiz and ONCE to quit the race altogether reached fever pitch – then blurred, oddly, into silence. By the small hours of the evening of stage 17, as final rounds of drinks were ordered in hotel bars, the final edition of their papers went to press and mobile phones were switched off, the sense that events were finally and definitively out of control produced a kind of odd indifference. A million solutions might be found, but, for now, after three weeks of constant tension, there was an overwhelming collective desire for the race to end, one way or another.

Exactly when it would end – on the Thursday in Aix-les-Bains or the following Sunday in Paris – nobody could predict. Even if the Tour seemed set to have a start village for stage 18, nobody knew which squads would actually be present for the mid-morning race *départ* itself.

The first thing that seemed to help the Tour regain its sense of normality early on the morning of stage 18 and another hot, dry day, were the local freeloaders. With their *invité* passes flapping around their necks, they sturdily stocked up on the ample supplies of free food and coffee that never seemed to be lacking in the Tour's start village.

When Casino's team vehicles, despite the absence of their King of the Mountains leader, pulled up, another piece of the jigsaw fell unexpectedly into place. 'My riders don't know what to do, but I told them that it's better to die in a battle than on the sidelines,' said team manager Vincent Lavenu.

Another arrival was Rabobank, whose one, all but forgotten, moment of glory had come thanks to Léon van Bon at Pau.

Team-mate Patrick Jonker, after confirming to van Bon, sitting next to him in the start village, told me they were in a state of total panic. 'We have thrown away everything – glucose, amino acids, vitamins. We are shitting ourselves that the police will come through the door.

'It could be a salt drip, a glucose drip, that could be an anabolic steroid or a masking agent as far as they're concerned. In this weather you take lots of salts and magnesium, but we've thrown it all away. By the time the lab has found out what it is, you could have been in a police station for two days.'

The sense that the race was in a state of suspended animation, that the riders were no longer battling for a result, was all but universal. 'Physically it may be possible for me to get Paris, but mentally, for me, it's over,' Dane Bo Hamburger, later to be named as an EPO user by a Danish anti-doping investigation, told *Cycling Weekly*. 'The Danish police wouldn't strip me and look up my arse' – as was rumoured to have happened to some riders, although only Willy Voet has directly confirmed a rectal search took place in his arrest – 'as the French police have done to friends of mine.'

Telekom's presence at the start line was no surprise, and nor, once they were there, was Cofidis or Mercatone's. Finally, although the number of team vehicles had dropped by a quarter since stage 17, the race still seemed to have some kind of structure. 'If we start today, we'll make Paris,' Bobby Julich predicted.

However, Julich's next words seemed to contradict his own optimism: 'There will be no more doing this stuff in half-assed ways,' reported *Cycling Weekly*. 'Either we will start and finish in Paris with our heads high, or we won't do it. If the consensus of the riders is that we are still not being treated like human beings, we will have no choice.'

It was an indication of just how jittery everyone was, though, that when one of Pantani's team-mates got lost and rode away from the signing-on podium by mistake, it briefly caused a rumour that Mercatone were going to quit at the last minute. In fact, Pantani, despite being one of the very last to sign on was willing to comment on the tumultuous events of the previous 24 hours. While calling for a fresh start for the sport it also seemed clear that he was not willing, with Paris now just three days away, to sacrifice his yellow jersey. Instead, he opted for the middle road, saying, 'the sport has to change and the rules, too. But I don't think what has happened besmirches my victory.'

The sense that the Tour had broken into new terrain, however, was unescapable. Rather than asking riders whether they would be finishing the world's greatest bike race, the pinnacle of nearly every professional bike rider's dream, the question on everybody's lips that day was whether they would start, and if they wanted to start. Marco Pantani's epic victory at Les Deux Alpes was, incredibly, just over 48 hours old. It felt as if it had happened in another world.

But all the untimely exits, the resentment and the anger of the previous days, the actual abandons on stage 18 were limited to just two: Stéphane Barthe of the Casino squad, whose enthusiasm for dying in battle, as his manager had recommended, became clear, climbed off the bike shortly after the race had rolled out of Aix-les-Bains. Second to go was TVM's Jeroen Blijlevens, who quit the minute the race entered Switzerland on its brief excursion to Neuchâtel, not before – some said – making a few choice gestures back at France as he did so.

Bizarrely enough, even as TVM's sprinter was bidding farewell to the Tour at the French border, it was only when the race reached the neutrality of Switzerland and left its motherland that a sense of momentum returned to the racing. The chance of police raids, after all, was far less likely in Switzerland, and the change of country unexpectedly introduced a feeling of business as usual.

Four riders, including former 1998 race leader Laurent Desbiens and Cédric Vasseur, winner of a spectacular lone break to a spell in the *maillot jaune* across the plains of central France in the 1997 Tour, had made it away from the pack. But despite a stiff tailwind, Mapei and Telekom, with Bjarne Riis driving at the head of affairs in person, managed to reel the quartet in, with Tom Steels taking his third stage of the race.

Steels said his only regret was the absence of Cipollini, but with only 101 of 189 starters left in the race, the smallest Tour peloton in years, the race had shrunk severely in size. Survival, it seemed, had come at a very high price. There was one final reminder of the tense start that the Tour had left behind only that morning, as Cofidis' Christophe Rinero refused to put on the King of the Mountains jersey that he had only inherited from Massi by default.

Perhaps it was appropriate that the 1998 Tour's first fully calm stage in three days, stage 19, was one of pure transition, running for an almost interminable 242 km westwards to the nondescript town of Autun. Largely flat but for a chain of hills near the finish, this was a day for the GC riders to ease back, waiting for Saturday's final time trial – and on this occasion, to put memories of the Tour's near-demise behind them.

But it was not quite as easy to do that as the Tour organisation might have wished: the final realistic opportunity for a long-range attack in the Tour started with a breakaway of a different kind, for the five remaining members of TVM. Perhaps fearing for their *liberté* in the land of *égalité* and *fraternité*, Steven de Jongh, Servais Knaven, Bart Voskamp, Sergei Outschakov and Sergei Ivanov all opted to remain on neutral Swiss soil. That brought the number of riders in the Tour down to double digits – 96.

For Mercatone Uno, as Traversoni recalls, the day was unusually stressful, but more because of the structure of the team than because of any last-minute hitch. 'The problem was that Marco was adamant we did not negotiate with anybody. We never asked for help. That was his policy, and we followed it to the point that' – with no alliances to be forged, as would be standard practice on such a long day in the saddle – 'the stage we feared the most wasn't the mountainous one, it was that long, flat one. No climbs, it was like riding across a billiard table!'

Victory went, as might be expected, to a breakaway rider, Magnus Bäckstedt. Adopted by the Tour's English-speaking journalists, after the big Swede had taken his first – and only – Tour stage victory, the main peloton rolled across the line 15 minutes later. For all Mercatone's worries, Pantani had come through the Tour's last main road stage unscathed. That it had taken place at all, though, was no small matter.

16

Can I Still Be Second?

Saturday, 1 August. Stage 20:
Montceau-les-Mines–Le Creusot, 52 km

On the morning after Marco Pantani's victory at Les Deux Alpes, Bobby Julich, finally third overall in Paris, discussed with his girlfriend – later his wife – something which had long been on his mind: that he had used EPO. Sitting in the start village, surrounded by the usual melee of VIP guests, media and team staff, and as one of the greatest successes the rider would have in his career beckoned ever closer, Julich and his future wife held what must have been a difficult, painful, personal reality check on professional cycling and its doping hinterland. It was very probably not the only one in that year's Tour, but, given the deception involved, not just to the outside world but also to someone very close to him, it was surely one of the most traumatic.

'It was not an easy conversation to have,' Julich now says, with more than a hint of understatement. 'She found out right in the middle of the Tour and that's what made it … she goes, "listen, we're not going to talk about this now, but we are going to talk about this as soon as the Tour is over." And that next day [after the Tour had ended] she nailed me with it, and said, "listen, this had better be all over"', to which Julich says he replied, 'Oh it's over, it's over, it's a totally different sport, it's going to be so great.'

That was when Julich, unlike many in the peloton, confirmed he had called time on his doping. But after, Julich says, first learning of it from fellow American Frankie Andreu's wife, Betsy (later to become one of the earliest, most outspoken campaigners against Lance Armstrong's doping activities), Julich's future wife first knew for sure it was happening the morning after Les Deux Alpes.

'That stage 17, I almost missed the start because we stayed talking in the race village for a little bit too long,' says Julich. 'And that's when she asked me about it straight up. Of course at first I denied it – "you know, I don't know what you're talking about" – "But it's starting to make sense to me, those little things that were in your refrigerator". And I told her. Finally I told her. I said, "But it's all over now". That was not a good conversation to have, for sure. But she was serious. And at that moment, I was just so pissed at Betsy, because Frankie was doing the same thing, and like, "how dare you?"

'Finally,' he concludes that the discussion and its consequences 'really helped'. Because even if the sport did not move on after the 1998 Tour, Julich did – although in sporting terms, it took him over five years truly to reap the benefits.

For Julich, the way into doping was far more straightforward than its exit. As a professional in Europe since the mid-1990s, it came about almost as a matter of course.

'Back then, I knew about it, I knew I'd have to make a decision and I was on that fence for a long time and I made that decision to do the minimum of what I was told it took to be professional.

'It wasn't like, "oh, you're doping". You were "prepared", that was the word. "Oh, yeah, I've done some good preparation this week."' ('Prepared', in modern cycling argot, now has no automatic associations to taking banned drugs and is generally considered shorthand for 'training and only doing off-the-bike activities which will ensure good race condition is maintained'. But it's indicative of how enduring the effect of doping can be at a mental level, that Julich says that he still does a slight double-take when somebody uses the term, even in the most innocent of ways.)

Disconnecting himself from the world of banned drugs in the Tour de France 1998 was something Julich did out of necessity and also by default. Up until Les Deux Alpes, Julich had mostly been able to keep both the doping issue and doping raids at arm's length, even though he was one of the race's top protagonists. The reason was simple: during the Tour, the police did not investigate his team on the ground at least, none of the Cofidis staff were arrested or even questioned and their vehicles were not searched.

'Everyone had the same thermos [for transporting EPO], I guess, and you hear all these things about people throwing their stuff away and that happened,' he recalls. 'But [once the drugs had been trashed] it was like, OK, now we're all in the same situation. When we landed in France, the French guys were panicking, but we were like, "what's going to happen?" and nothing did happen. We weren't raided, although I'm sure there were undercover police there.'

As ever in a cycling team, though, there were worlds within worlds. Julich recognises that some riders, in order to maintain their supply, 'like [team-mate Philippe] Gaumont, got a little bit crafty, a little bit creative. But for us, it was like, "that's over, it's done, it's gone".' What had been in his own thermos 'had gone, to say the least', although not the receptacle. 'Why throw away a perfectly good thermos?' he asks in a comical, 'hicky' voice. Returning to his more serious recollections, Julich observes that 'Everyone was nervous about something, but I was like, "hey, I've nothing on me, what's going to happen?"' He is puzzled, though, even now, that he was labelled as 'questionable' in the French Senate findings for dope tests from the 1998 Tour, and questions the validity of their test, given that, prior to the Tour, 'we were all taking it. Somebody texted me and said, you were so stupid to admit to anything' – as he had done already – 'you were "came up as a non-negative" ... Well, too late now.'

Other drugs were still present in the Cofidis team, albeit the legal ones. 1998 was the first time that Julich heard of Stilnox, for example, a sleeping pill that he did not take and which 'scared the hell out of me' because of what he witnessed within the team during the Tour.

'Guys would have a Stilnox, and then waking up in the morning I remember one guy had 21 Kit-Kats, the mini ones, so that was his bonus at the end of every stage.

'Evidently on the fourth or fifth stage he had a Stilnox and [when he woke up] there was nothing but Kit-Kat wrappers, and he came down and he was so mad at us, and I was saying, "*je ne comprends pas*" and asking who came into his room to eat his Kit-Kats. Then his room-mate came down and said, "dude, it was you, you went off and ate every single one of them and stayed up until 2 a.m. in the morning eating Kit-Kats". But if that was as bad as it got, I could have lived with that, but then you heard of guys doing stuff out in the hallway they didn't even remember the next day.'

An article in the *Sydney Morning Herald* in 2008 confirms that although Stilnox has some strong defendants who say they have had no issues with it, 'Callers to a national hotline for Stilnox users have [also] reported incidents such as crashing cars, having sex, fighting and binge-eating while apparently asleep.' The after-effects of the medication for the team were not so simple to escape, either: as David Millar writes in his autobiography *Racing Through the Dark*, it continued to be heavily used as a recreational drug by some members of Cofidis long after the 1998 Tour.

Yet even as the Tour's hidden relationships with the world of banned drugs were surfacing, Stilnox incidents notwithstanding, Julich could, like so many of the riders, continue to try to bypass the consequences of the police raids and confessions. And by and large, up until Les Deux Alpes, he succeeded. 'It was a race, a beautiful race,' Julich insists, even now. 'It was a bizarre turn of events, but not talking French, it was easy to just kind of zone out, not listen to what was going on, or even care, really, and that was what saved me. I was rooming with Kevin Livingston, we'd go into our room, switch on MTV and just block it out and then in the morning we'd hear this, "did you hear what happened, did you hear what happened?" and we were like, "no, who cares?". It was just "ignorance is bliss" at that point.' He was, he says, 'Living on an island, oblivious to the political stuff. Nor, really, did I care.' Although he remembers the second strike well, he barely recollects the first, beyond wondering why Jalabert had first led the strike and then was racing so hard, admitting, 'I was totally out of touch with what happened.'

With only a ninth place in the 1996 Vuelta a España and a 17th in the 1997 Tour de France as his standout Grand Tour results, Julich, through all the tumult of the 1998 race, was actually having the ride of a lifetime. But he never expected it, he says, 'and that's maybe what helped me do so well. I wasn't stressing, all I thought I would do would be to work for [Cofidis leader] Casagrande.

'It was different, I felt like I was coming up in the [pre-Tour warm-up race] Route du Sud. But I hadn't won the Midi Libre or the Dauphiné. I did do a normal training ride with Kevin, a test up the [Col de la] Madone' – later used by Armstrong for his test climbs – 'and Kevin was maybe a minute faster. So then at Dublin, when I was fourth in the prologue, it was a major surprise.'

The surprise might, he believes, have been even better with just a little more decisiveness on his part. 'I think I would have won it, but with one kilometre to go, I felt pretty good and I heard the speaker saying "best time, best time" and I was thinking "best time of my team, of the entire race, what does he mean?"

'I had very little confidence in that, because in the French teams they had the habit of telling you you had the best time, but they would mean of the squad. So it was only with 500 metres to go that I suddenly thought, "it doesn't matter, just go!" And I lost four seconds there, and Boardman beat us all. But I felt good, I felt good, but I wasn't really sure I'd be able to pass these guys on the mountains. It wasn't until every day you passed the test, you got a little lighter, you were still up there and kept your morale high.'

Indirectly, though, the raids were providing a kind of assistance. 'Because it was nerve-wracking, people were always tense because of coming back to France, then they kicked the Festina riders out, then it was the mountains. There was always something. I was able to block it out. It was not a stressful situation for me at all. There were no decisions to be taken, just a realisation that the sport was going to be better. You always looked at it like, "that's the other guys' problem". I never was nervous.'

Julich recognises, too, that the absence of certain figures favoured him. 'I never expected to be where I was, and I don't think that I would have been where I was in the overall if all those guys hadn't left the race. I was beating all of them before they quit anyway, but Festina, ONCE, Kelme ...' The rider who caused him most concern, he said, was Escartín, fourth overall by Aix-les-Bains, but who had left by the end of the Alps. 'He would have fought me all the way through to the podium in Paris,' Julich says. 'Pantani and Ullrich were in a different league, but I felt that I had a couple of those guys pinned. Olano wasn't very good, he was overweight, Jalabert was good but inconsistent.' Although Italy's Leonardo Piepoli was an occasional concern – the Saeco rider was an attacker on the Madeleine and lying ninth as they went into the final Alpine stage when he finally blew badly in the last time trial and dropped to 14th by Paris – 'It was,' says Julich, 'Escartín I feared the most.'

It wasn't just the American who was on a roll. Cofidis concluded the 1998 Tour de France with the Best Teams prize, the

King of the Mountains prize, a spell in yellow for Desbiens and Julich's third place on the podium. They also placed Christophe Rinero in fourth overall, Roland Meier in seventh and Kevin Livingston in 17th.

This made Cofidis the best overall, all-round performers by a long shot, even though they had lost their nominal leader, Italian Francesco Casagrande, as early as the Pyrenees when he crashed out, not to mention Philip Gaumont through tendinitis. Yet if they would never have taken such exceptional results in a 'normal' Tour – Rinero's polka-dot jersey, for example, was only 'inherited' from Massi after the Italian had been arrested – that power vacuum created by the absence of Festina and the rest only partly explains one of the more curious success stories of the 1998 Tour de France. It is a reflection – one of many – of how the race simultaneously disintegrated and yet continued to function.

Team support, for example, did not crumble, as Julich points out. There was the case of Meier working his heart out for Julich on the Madeleine, but also of Christophe Rinero, 'who waited for me after the descent of the Galibier. I think the team management must have thought we were closer together because he was told to wait for me and pace me up the Deux Alpes, but he must have got fed up waiting, 'cos he finished ahead of me, and I smoked him in the final time trial anyway. But that decision of his to wait, maybe that could have been the difference between third for me and fourth for him in Paris, and it'd have been a totally different scenario. As it was, everything fell my way.'

After the Dublin prologue, Julich's third place in the Corrèze time trial in the first week moved him on to the provisional podium. After one day in the Pyrenees, where he finished in the Ullrich group, he was second overall. But the abandon of Casagrande, sixth in the 1997 race, did not create a power struggle to be protected rider, Julich says. Rather, it was the Italian, who had signed for

238

Cofidis that year, whom Julich sees as being 'responsible, he and he alone, for what we managed to achieve in 1998' by collectively pulling the team's racing and training practices up another level.

'From the first training camp in January, in Perpignan, he was amazingly switched on' – giving advice and instructions on everything from diet to resting strategies – 'and so strict about his training, did his training by the numbers; he was a great influence. He was the most professional guy I've ever been around.'

There was the issue that Casagrande was 'doing some extra-curricular stuff, as was everyone at that time'. But as one former 1990s pro put it, 'you could have a pool of EPO and without that other stuff – training properly, reconnaissance, diet – you wouldn't do shit', and thanks to the Italian's influence in other areas, according to Julich, Cofidis suddenly found themselves collectively punching above their weight.

But having had such a positive effect on his new team, just when it mattered the most for a French squad, at the Tour, the Italian then suddenly – and according to Julich, somewhat inexplicably – abandoned. That Casagrande crashed on the Aubisque on the mist-shrouded descent, like so many others, was unquestionable. But by his own admission Casagrande was able to start training again four days later – which does not make it sound like serious injuries – and indeed he then went on to win three races in eight days, including the World Cup's Clásica San Sebastián in early August. It later emerged that Casagrande had already tested positive in the Tour de Romandie, and that the result may well have been confirmed to Cofidis, off the record, before the Tour de France started. If so, Casagrande's exit from the Tour, given the circumstances surrounding the race, might well have been a logical move.

As a result Julich was soon to be cast into the role of team leader, but for a few moments, on the fog-covered Aubisque, he found himself at the head of the entire race.

'The Aubisque was crazy, you couldn't see anything. I remember they attacked for the King of the Mountains prize, and I stayed back and rode my tempo. And the next thing I know – you couldn't see off the side of the road, there were just people climbing over the guardrails – when I reach the foot of the descent, before the next climb [the Tourmalet], and there's me and Rolf Aldag, nobody behind us, nobody in front of us.

'All of a sudden we see the lead [Tour de France director's] car and we're like, "are we, are we in the lead?" And Rolf says "yes, I think so, shall we go?" And then we're like, "awww, I don't know if this is a good idea, you know,"' and then other guys start catching up and we formed a group.'

Appropriately enough, though, given he had just – albeit unwittingly – had a brief spell as joint leader of the race, it was at that point that Julich then discovered that the leader's role at Cofidis had fallen vacant, after Casagrande had abandoned. But his first impression was, almost, that he was hallucinating.

'I thought something was strange. When Casagrande stopped, I expected him to be shattered, in a hospital, his arm in a sling. I came down to breakfast the next day and I remember it very vividly, because we'd slept above what must have been the hotel boiler room and I was sweating the entire night.'

Having got downstairs for breakfast, Julich was surprised to find Casagrande seated there as the first rider down from the hotel rooms, calmly putting jam and butter on the single piece of toast the diet-conscious Italian only ever allowed himself for breakfast. 'Maybe the sleep-deprived dehydration made me think "is he actually in the race still, or out of it?"' Julich recalls. 'He seemed way too happy to quit the Tour de France. And I later discovered he already knew he was positive.

'This was a big objective, in theory, for him, he was our captain. And it had given us some security to know that, hey, we'll knock off whatever we can for ourselves before things get serious, and even if I was ahead of him on GC, he was like a safety blanket for me. I could say "I'm just here to work for him".'

Once Casagrande left, though, Julich was forced to step up to the plate – and, initially, not entirely willingly. 'That evening, Kevin said, "dude, you gotta, you gotta do something here, you gotta lead us. And I was like, "Kevin, come on, me?" It was a weird situation. But a power struggle? It never happened. We were all so young, and we never expected to be in that situation.'

'I remember how insecure I was because I had no idea I could have the ability to be with these guys,' Julich comments. 'The year before, try as I may, I think I was 17th overall and fought for some stage wins, but I always had that one bad day.'

Having stayed with the pre-race contenders on the Plateau de Beille stage, where he gained seven seconds on Ullrich in the final kilometre, Julich's thoughts began to turn towards how he could, at the very least, consolidate what would be a career-changing placing. The next crucial moment came in the stage over the Galibier to Les Deux Alpes, which – given how it changed the Tour – Julich has no problem recalling, even now. 'It was one of the few races that while I was in, a voice came on to me and said, "Bobby, remember this moment because it will go down in history as being one of the most epic races, ever."

'And I said that to myself at that moment, and very few times did I have that sort of revelation of, "Bobby, enjoy where you are. You're suffering like a pig, it's cold as hell, but just remember, people are going to be talking about this." It was the freeze-frame moment of that Tour.'

Given the heavy rain and the plummeting temperatures, freezing was a word that had other associations for Julich and the peloton that day. 'Right as we cleared the Télégraphe [prior to the Galibier], Hamilton attacked and I remember he had a rain jacket in his back pocket, and I saw it and thought "good idea", so I went back to Roland Meier and asked him if he could get my rain jacket. I didn't have space in my pockets so I put it under my race jersey – not a good idea,' he adds with a grin before the trainer in him briefly shines through and he adds, 'kids, take note'.

Following Pantani's attack and Julich's ride to the summit – which he recounts elsewhere in this book – the rain jacket was to feature again on the descent of the Galibier. 'I knew it was going to be cold on that descent and I was just thanking God I'd told my team-mate to get that jacket.

'What I felt like doing and what I should have done, with hindsight, was to stop on the crest, put it on, zip it up and then start the descent. But when I got there, I was a little bit caught up in the moment, I thought I can get it on [anyway].'

In what is a minor YouTube classic, the ensuing events show how Julich's Tour, which had gone so well, came within metres of a finale bordering on both the farcical and the potentially dangerous. 'I got one arm on and then immediately after the Galibier's summit there was that [downhill, right-hand] switchback, and right then and there I said, "don't crash into this camper van". However, even though he deliberately stopped, because he could see he was not going to make the turn, Julich all but wobbled into the van – I hadn't had time to brake to heat my wheels up so I would stop, because I was trying to put my jacket on – so I'm just two hands on the bike, "brake, brake, brake" and I come to a stop right at the camping car.

'So I said, OK nobody hurt, learned my lesson, never do that again, but the guy whose camper van it was, was pushing so hard I didn't have time to zip up my jacket. So I'm going down the first part of the climb in the same shit that I was when I started it. Then I spent another kilometre trying to put this jacket on and there was another voice saying, "if you don't put this jacket on, you're done".

'So I basically got dropped, and I was shaking so hard, I could barely turn. But I come back up the chase group and everybody's the same, Jan looks like he's frozen solid and I'm just like, "what's going on here?"'

What had happened was that Julich's foresight had allowed him – close encounters with camper vans and their owners notwithstanding – to remain in contention. One seemingly tiny decision, with much greater consequences, such as heat retention on a bitterly cold day, made all the difference, as Ullrich – for one – was to find out.

'Then when we got to the valley, and because of that jacket, I was suddenly warm again, and I was actually hot. The guy at the foot of the climb must have been made out, we were ripping off everything we had, rain jackets, helmets, gloves.

'Then I attacked and it was an eight-kilometre time trial. I thought I was alone and it was only when I got to the top I realised Boogerd had been behind me. But it was so cold, it was survival. And that's why even today when the weather is beautiful here on the Côte d'Azur, nine times out of ten I'll always bring a rain jacket in my pocket. Because of that day.'

On the stage to Les Deux Alpes, Julich finished fifth, 5′ 43″ down on Pantani, a point at which he realised he had reached his upper limits and that the Italian was in a class of his own. 'I thought I was going fast up that climb – but Pantani put three minutes into me just on the final climb. I was the best of the rest that day. Three minutes – unbelievable.'

But the 'bad day' that Julich had feared then came close to sinking him, as he reached near-meltdown on the Madeleine the following stage. 'I thought I was done: Escartín was attacking. Fortunately [Cofidis team-mate] Roland Meier, he pulled the entire Madeleine, till about two kilometres from the top and I was going cross-eyed by that point, but I knew if I could get to the top of the climb, I'd have a chance.'

Divine intervention, of sorts, played a part. 'I was on the rivet there, thinking, "this is it, I'm done", Piepoli was attacking, Axel Merckx, Boogerd, all attacking, and all of a sudden, I look to the side of the road and I see this "Angel"' – in fact, the fan who for a few years would stand on the side of the road dressed in white, celestial garb, topped off with a halo on a wire, urging on the riders – 'and see this bottle of Coke, with the top on it.

'And I'm like, "whoa, this is a sign", honestly of all the weird things that go through your head … I thought, "this was here for a reason" and I grabbed the Coke and I drank it.'

Spurred onwards and upwards and provided with some extra energy by his heavenly supporter, Julich was nonetheless cramping so badly that 'on the little bump that follows the Madeleine, I was pedalling but it felt like I was ripping my muscles'. He tried pedalling by putting his weight on his toes, but if it worked short-term, that evening, after the stage, 'that was what made me so sore the next day, trying to pedal through the cramp.

'If I could have just relaxed, breathed through it and let it release, and then pedalled, I wouldn't have had a problem the next day. But I told myself, "either I pedal here or I get dropped".'

He survived one day, but 'I started paying the price for all the cramps I'd had and I thought, OK, this is it, I'd had a good run at it. That'll be the end of me.'

Stage 17, then, was where Julich anticipated that he would crack completely. Instead, with the strike going on, he got to live to fight another day – in a surreal twist, the stage that could have sunk the Tour ended up being the one which guaranteed Julich a place on the podium. 'We wound up not doing the stage, and honestly, I think if we had done it … I'd done all the recon. on it,

I would have suffered that day, big time. It was just one of those things, just, gosh, how lucky could I get that the day that I was feeling bad was the one we turned into an eight-hour training ride.'

But by keeping himself out of the loop of the scandals, Julich was able to treat the Tour de France as the classic voyage of exploration of a young outsider in a three-week stage race. Yet it was a story – like so many in that race that were not immediately associated with doping – which failed to generate long-term media interest, particularly after a certain Texan won the Tour the following year and set the bar far higher for American riders. Briefly seen as the next Greg LeMond, Julich's star, until 2005, faded steadily, and what might have been a story of inspiration for future generations of American riders in other circumstances became blurred by the clouds of suspicion and Lance-worship.

Julich's performance is also testament to the fact that, with the exception of that Alpine day though, as Julich can testify, for all the Tour was disintegrating, it continued to work. 'The racing was always on, but' – and partly as a result of that disintegration – 'the characters were constantly changing.'

It may sound surprising that a rider could cut himself off to that point. But Jaksche says he did the same, and so, too, from what Traversoni tells us, did the Mercatone riders. Nor yet does Riis sound overly troubled by outside events. As Julich points out, even within a flat stage, when the riders are all largely part of a huge bunch, they remain atomised, aware of their goals and their team's goals, but beyond that only vaguely aware of the bigger picture. More than being egocentric – although that is a factor – it's more like an energy-saving strategy, a way of ensuring maximum effort is placed on obtaining the best possible performance. But it was also one which meant that understanding what was happening to the race in general – to cycling in general – was limited.

Julich gives an example of how each rider, and each team, was living in their own bubble. 'I remember when we had the yellow jersey with Desbiens' – stage 9, following the Corrèze time trial – 'Kevin was in charge of going back and getting bottles and policing and stuff and I'm just sitting on the wheels going, "oh man, this is boring, this is beautiful, five guys ahead of me".

'And Kevin comes up and says, "dude, it is absolute chaos back there. People are all over the road, sweat stains everywhere, everybody's on the limit. And I was just like, "that's their problem, not ours".' In fact, that day, riders like Hamilton suddenly lost colossal amounts of time, while Cipollini abandoned altogether.

But that Julich was operating on another level was clear, even to those not involved in the direct GC struggle. 'We've all lived through this, when you're all riding on the rivet, and another guy stops, has a piss, and then comes flying through the peloton. And Frankie goes "that was you". We were on the rivet, me and George [Hincapie, US Postal] and Tyler was out the back [dropped, on stage 9] just swinging. And you stopped for a pee, came by, and it was like you were on a motorcycle.'

That Andreu noted that Kevin Livingston was on equally strong form and able to maintain Julich's pace that day is in some ways testament to Julich's comment that Cofidis collectively were in good shape and with sky-high morale. But if Livingston had not built on a low but potentially promising 38th place in 1997, Julich on the other hand, was flying.

Whatever the situation, then, the Cofidis riders not only felt that they had to salvage what they could from the wreckage of the Tour, collectively they were a team performing more strongly as well.

'We were all just squirrels out there trying to get nuts,' Julich says. 'Desbiens took a big opportunity to get the yellow jersey which was something that eluded me my entire career. I thought that year I would get it for at least a day, and I kept trying, I kept trying. And Rinero got a "nut", too, with that King of the Mountains jersey.'

Given he was making his debut in the higher rankings, for a general classification rider such as Julich, '[I said to myself] this race could stop at any moment, but that yellow jersey, that would last forever. I was thinking on the day by day, there was no long term for me. I was not thinking about the podium in Paris, up to the last couple of days. It never crossed my mind that I would be able to win, that was reserved for Ullrich and Pantani, but I wanted to get as close as possible.'

Yet there was another reason that Julich might not have been able to hang on to his podium place. 'It was a drama bomb every single day, I remember after that first protest, when it looked like the race was going to stop, the only question I had was, "so does that mean I get second?" I didn't care if we kept racing or not, because to me, I was just waiting to have that one bad day. So to be honest, when they said they were going to stop the racing, I was like "fine, but do I keep second?"

'That just goes to show my immature mentality. I was only 26. And you wish you had known how serious it was and what an opportunity it was. But it's like me, now, as a 43 year-old man trying to give advice to the 25-year-old riders that I work with. It's so hard to get through that wall and it reminds me of something my dad would say to me: "Bobby, the older I get, the smarter I will become." And I didn't know what that meant, because talking to a 25-year-old, it's in one ear and out the other. I just wish I could go back to being that 25-year-old and listen to what I'm telling my riders now. But we're all like that, hindsight's 20-20.'

Similarly, for all the Tour was in no way a reflection of racing normality, Julich – like Jaksche – learned career-forming lessons there. 'It was something that I think saved me through the harder points of my career. Whereas Lance [Armstrong] would have a "win at all costs, second is the first loser" attitude.' Julich harks back to Bob Mionske, an American who placed fourth in the 1998 Olympics, and the cruel nickname, 'Almost-Bronze-Bob', that he ended up being landed with as a result. 'I would consider podium as a success; fourth place, no way, that was a waste. But I was satisfied, if I gave my best, with second or third.'

It's indicative of how much lower, in the pre-Armstrong years, across-the-board media scrutiny was for non-European riders, that for all Desbiens had already 'flown the flag' for Cofidis with his spell in the race lead, Julich says there was never any sense of stress from the team that he had to turn in a top Tour performance. 'Back then, there just wasn't that kind of pressure,' he explains. 'At Cofidis it was very much a mom-and-pop organisation, and by then [world -famous sports director Cyrille] Guimard' – previously running Cofidis in 1997 – 'was gone, so we didn't have the pressure of a big high-paid sports director there, either.'

Sadly, this was due to change shortly afterwards, when Cofidis introduced its notoriously stress-producing UCI-points-related salary system, criticised by riders as diverse as David Millar and Philip Gaumont for wrecking team solidarity, and by Gaumont for indirectly encouraging doping. It is also interesting to note that following its introduction, although Millar was, for many years, their top Tour rider and won the opening prologue in 2000, Cofidis never had such a successful GC performance as in 1998. But for Bobby Julich and his future wife, the 1998 Tour had very different connotations indeed.

The final time trial itself went more or less as expected, with Julich unable to prevent Ullrich, confirming his bounce back in the Alps, from taking the fourth time trial of his career and dropping to third overall. Julich lost 61 seconds to Ullrich, finishing second on the stage, but it was a result that left him deeply satisfied.

'There wasn't the sort of analysis course recon. we do now, from previous years. I'd drive the first part and ride the last part. I remember this one being quite long, it was an hour and 15 minutes effort, it was no walk in the park. I remember the end more than anything: I was coming to a very heavy, hilly section, the last real climb of the Tour, and I remember telling myself, this is where you've got to give it absolutely everything. I was going so hard I was actually out of my saddle and still on my aerobars, coming into the finish, I was like, "I have no idea where I am" [in reference to the other top favourites] at about two kilometres and you can see the finish line; I passed this guy in the side of the road and he says, "50 seconds to Ullrich". And I said, "well, that's 50 seconds up or 50 seconds down" and that's not going to change in the finish. And so I take it safer, cross the line, and my dad and my girlfriend are there and it turned out that I was third.'

But as he says, he already felt that third was good enough – and viewed from the outside, given how much Ullrich and Pantani had shaped the race, it was probably a just result, too. 'People were saying, oh, what a shame you made third not second, and I was like, "are you kidding me, there's no difference". Between first and second, for sure. And it was the same story six years later in the Olympics, when I got bronze [later silver after Hamilton's disqualification]. Fourth, though, would have been a different story.'

On a personal level, the time trial mattered to Julich, with hindsight, in a sadly unexpected way. 'My girlfriend and dad were at the finish there and he never really had seen me race since I was a junior. And I was so proud and he had this special nickname for me and he called me that and I know he was proud of me. It was quite special, because since then I haven't really had any relationship with my father. It's been pretty rocky, I probably haven't spoken to him for eight years. But I remember that day, that moment was something I'll always be really happy that I had with my dad, even though we've grown apart.

'He hasn't met my daughter who's eight years old, he's only met my son twice, but I had that moment with him there and he was my first coach and my best coach, so to share that moment with him was very special, not only to share with him but with my then girlfriend, who turned into wife and mother of my two kids. That was as good as the last day [in Paris] because on that day there's so much "what do I do and where do I do it?".

'With the overall classification now set in stone, the time trial was the moment you knew the Tour was over and that was the one night I broke my rule of eating exactly the same thing for 20 days. Literally, exactly the same, for breakfast, after the stage for dinner and then for dinner and my midnight snack. I just got skinnier and skinnier. But that night was the party.'

In terms of his career – which went on for another ten and a half seasons – the combination of the sense that he had crossed the red line of doping, as well as the difficulty of the race on a personal level, carries a weight for Julich. But it is not so simple to say that he feels he did 'wrong' and has struck it off the list.

'When you were doing something the wrong way, you always knew, I don't know if you could really enjoy it. I still think the best memories of my career weren't from the Tour de France, they were of the 2004 and 2005 seasons, where I wasn't doing what I was doing back then and I was still winning races and I got a medal in the Olympics. Getting third in the Tour is probably third or fourth on that list.'

There are those who will argue that given Julich's third place had its share of medical assistance, prior to the race if not during it, then it was worthless. But given the context, as well as the extraordinary difficulty of that Tour de France from a racing level, it is hard not to sympathise a little with his view that it should not be simply struck out. It's worth remembering that he places an asterisk next to it, and that he moved on to a different way of racing in the years to come.

For Pantani, meanwhile, this was as good as it got. Losing more than six minutes on Ullrich would have taken a catastrophe, but it was hard not to forget, with victory so close, that Pantani's career had already been filled with its fair share of cataclysmic bad luck. The heavy rain falling on the lengthy time trial course in central France that morning did not help lift anybody's spirits either.

Pantani took the logical option of taking some solid precautions. He avoided riding over the time trial course in the morning, preferring to see it from a team car, and instead opted for a quick 90-minute warm-up spin near the team hotel when the rain eased. Faithful to his image of an eccentric racing genius, he did his final 15-minute warm-up on the rollers, clad, as *Cycling Weekly* observed, 'in a wacky blue and green bobble hat'.

The course itself was long, but it was also a fairly flat, unspectacular affair. That Ullrich had reached the start line a little too close for comfort – just 15 seconds beforehand – after an overlong warm-up may have flustered the German slightly and as a result he could not wear his aerodynamic helmet, either, which could have cost him some time. (Pantani, as nonconformist as ever in his deliberate decision not to wear one, made one concession to getting a smoother airflow: he shaved his head a little closer than usual that morning.) Then, as the rain eased slightly, Pantani kept himself in third at each checkpoint. 'I told him not to take any risks,' said Mercatone Uno chief director Giuseppe Martinelli, 'and I think it was his best time trial ever.'

As it turned out, Pantani's time trial performance was more than respectable, finishing third in the time trial, just 2′ 35″ back on Ullrich. This effectively netted the Italian his country's first

Tour since 1965 and made him the first out and out climber to win the race since 1976, and the winner of a Giro–Tour double, too, the first since Indurain in 1993, and the first Italian since Fausto Coppi over half a century before. Just to round off the comparison with Coppi, Pantani used the same light blue Bianchi bikes as the *campionissimo* 50 years earlier.

What kind of a race had Pantani won? How much value could it truly be given? 'Tour winners – Pantani and the police' was *Cycling Weekly*'s headline the following week. The historical associations were there for all to see – Felice Gimondi, the previous Italian Tour winner, was present in the press room to give his successor a congratulatory hug as he entered the room. Yet Pantani's stream-of consciousness reflections – delivered in a brain-numbing, rambling, hour-long press conference that for once left journalists praying that the race would be over for reasons other than the doping scandals – were a bizarre and painfully tedious mixture of reflections. They somehow encapsulated the sporting schizophrenia produced by a great race and one which had seen its credibility go up in flames.

Sifting through them later, one of Pantani's points, that the Tour, already the hardest for him as a climber, had become even more difficult to race because of the scandals, seems a just one. Not everybody had the type of personality that could react in the same way as Julich and close themselves off, and as race leader, too, Pantani's sense of responsibility and pressure would have been far greater. There was a moving tribute to Luciano Pezzi, the mentor who had inspired Pantani to go for the Giro–Tour double, but whose death, in June, prevented him from seeing it. 'I wanted to do something for him, he would have been happy to see me win,' Pantani confirmed.

But these were lost in the fog of verbose and muddled comments, such as when he was asked if he had been playing games by claiming, as he had done early on in the race, that he had no interest in winning. 'Absolutely not ... you go through a lot of different moods in a Tour as long as this,' he explained. But then when he claimed that 'I'm maybe more honest than some of the others, because when I said those things, that was how I was thinking, even if deep down I still had thoughts of winning.' There was no sign that Pantani seemed aware he was contradicting himself in the space of a few sentences. Equally, given that he had expressed to team-mates and other sports directors that he was in favour of the strike and, indeed, of abandoning the Tour, as well as condemning the raids, it seems unusual that he should then, in his final press conference, declare that both the police actions were justified and that strikes benefited nobody.

In some ways Pantani's verbal smokescreens were an appropriate symbol of the predicaments facing the Tour de France. It had survived, there had been moments of glory and greatness, but the contradictions, deceptions and lies which lay beneath the surface had become so evident that its credibility had been almost completely wrecked and it had run within a hair's breadth of collapse not once, but twice. As Paris loomed – at last – into view, Bobby Julich was not the only part of the Tour standing at a crossroads: which direction would the Tour de France, and the international peloton, now take?

17

The Final Lap

Sunday, 2 August. Stage 21:
Melun–Champs-Elysées, Paris, 147.5 km

For an outsider, watching the Tour de France for the first time as the peloton hurtled by on the cobbles of the Champs-Elysées, it would have been hard to tell that, of all the Tours, this was the one that came the closest in its 95-year history to never making it to Paris.

Guiding the head of the pack were sprinters' teams, led by Tom Steels' Mapei squad and racing full tilt up and down what some consider the most beautiful boulevard in the world. There was a race leader, Marco Pantani, surrounded by a cloud of Mercatone Uno team-mates all with their hair dyed yellow to celebrate the Italian's triumph. There were the usual banners, and the long lines of barriers and the flag-waving spectators. If the crowds were not quite as large as usual, that might have had something to do with the steady summer drizzle.

For those spectators who had been there before, however, they would have immediately noticed that the size of the peloton was far smaller. True, this was nowhere close the Tour's historical low of ten finishers, in 1919, and a double-digit-sized bunch for the final stage was not unusual up to the late 1970s, when the Tour field began to swell past 100 starters.

But 96 finishers was – and has remained – the lowest since 1983, when 88 riders of 140 starters made it to Paris. In terms of a percentage of the starters, 96 finishers of 189 was the lowest since 1957, 41 years before.

Quite how alive the 1998 Tour was, though, was open to debate. 'A glassy-eyed impostor, clinging doggedly to a life-support machine' was Jeremy Whittle's memorable description of the state of the race in the latter half of the third week. And if everybody left on the Tour seemed keen to make it to the Champs-Elysées, it was more as a phase to be got through rather than because they were keen to celebrate.

There was one final hiccup for the Mercatone Uno squad, though, that felt very much in keeping with such a tortured event. Tradition has it that the overall classification is set in stone for the last stage of the race, but, on this occasion, 'Marco almost lost the race because he punctured and was a minute back when we were coming on to the Champs-Elysées,' says Traversoni.

'Fortunately he could get back on again, but I had been shouting and shouting [to his team-mates to come back and assist] and at first nobody stopped.' Traversoni still got a seventh place in the bunch sprint for the line, but was drained after working to bring Pantani back into contention to a peloton going flat out on the Champs-Elysées 'And it was the one damn day I could try for the sprint!' he concludes ruefully.

There were celebrations for the Mercatone Uno team, but they were limited. They, like many of the foreign riders present, were keen to get out of France once and for all and put such a tumultous race behind them. Bjarne Riis's recollection of the moment he raced up and down the Champs-Elysées hits the nail on the head: 'All I remember by that point is feeling like shit.'

'We couldn't believe we'd won. It was like a dream. I can't ever forget that we got a standing ovation on the Champs-Elysées. We were the only team that spectators in the stands would get on their feet to applaud,' Traversoni says. 'But' – as is usually the tradition for all Tour de France teams – 'there was no party [in Paris] afterwards, because after everybody had been treated so shoddily, Marco wanted the party at home in Italy.'

The Tour winner and his team were so keen to get out, they flew out of France that same evening, but Traversoni denies it was for fear of a last-minute visit from the gendarmes: 'it was just that we were pissed off with everything. Once that magic moment on the Champs was over, when we reached the Concorde Lafayette [the central hotel that for years was the Tour's operational headquarters for the stage] we each got a yellow jersey signed by Marco – I have it framed on the wall. That's my best memory of the Tour. But we all got out, not just our team. Only a few people stuck around. I just wanted to go and I wasn't the only one.'

After the damp squib of Paris, Mercatone made up for it with celebrations in Italy that lasted nearly a month, with the riders discovering that their dyed yellow hair made them an easy target for autograph hunters. 'I didn't stop signing photos, there was a bit of a break, and then a whole load of criteriums and a *mega-festa* in Cesenatico' – Pantani's home town – 'which managed to block up the whole of Emilia Romagna's road system. Not even Cristiano Ronaldo could have had such a good celebration.'

The man at the centre of it all, though, 'didn't talk about it much. He was already thinking about 1999, looking at the future.' That is, Traversoni says approvingly, 'the mark of a true champion.'

Traversoni says that inevitably, with so many top riders missing, there were mutterings that Pantani only won because of the absentees. But it is hard to disagree with him that nobody would have been able to match Pantani in the mountains and that Ullrich was unquestionably the second strongest. The tumultuous off-race events of the 1998 Tour, in any case, certainly added enough stress to compensate for the lack of competition. Furthermore, Pantani's final victory margin, of 3′ 21″ over the German and four minutes over

Julich, was not a narrow one, particularly for a climber on a course which was not very mountainous. It's a truism that you can only beat those you are up against. The most recent case of a Tour champion having his victory played down because of the lack of top contenders was, curiously enough, for the next Italian winner, Vincenzo Nibali, in the 2014 race, which he captured without having conclusively defeated two top pre-race contenders Alberto Contador or Chris Froome after both abandoned because of crashes. It got to the point where 2014 was dubbed by some journalists as 'the Tour of absences', a repeat of the same moniker given to the 1973 race, taken by Luis Ocaña when all-conquering Eddy Merckx was not present. But it is as unfair to accuse Pantani of 'not winning fairly' in 1998 (though perhaps not for other reasons), as it was Luis Ocaña in 1973 and would be for Nibali in 2014. It was hardly the Italian's fault that six teams of 1998's original 21 went missing, either.

Not everybody left Paris in a hurry, though. Bobby Julich, for one, was determined to celebrate in style. 'Everyone in the team busted out after the Champs-Elysées, we had drinks and finger sandwiches at the Concorde Lafayette and that was it,' Julich recalls. However, he stayed on. 'I deliberately went to the restaurant, a Mexican that I had read the 7-Eleven team had gone to every year, the Café Pacifico. Kevin was there with his girlfriend, I flew my mum and sister in, and my dad, so there was like eight of us.' Although a pleasant and memorable evening was had, as Julich admits, given all the tales of wild celebrations 'it was not how I envisioned the post-Tour party to be'. After three weeks on the road, the drop in adrenaline levels combined with even a small amount of alcohol tends to make most cyclists fail to remember more than hazy details of their Paris post-Tour evening. One anecdote, though, has stuck in Julich's mind.

'There was a guy at the bar and he keeps looking back at me, and I'm like, "wait a second, that's Dag Otto Lauritzen"' – winner on the ultra-difficult Luz Ardiden climb in the 1987 Tour, for the 7-Eleven team, which was why Julich had booked that particular restaurant in Paris, too. 'So I went up to him and said, "My God you were such an inspiration to me when I was growing up with the 7-Eleven team and that's why I'm here today." And he was blown away, [saying] like, "you know who I am, you just got third in the Tour de France".

'I think that really touched him and maybe one day that'll be me,' Julich reflects. 'I'll be sitting at a bar some day and a kid will come up and say the same to me. Who knows?'

***

In the summer of July 2015, when the Tour de France passed very close to a small northern French village of Fontaine-au-Bois on stage 4 of the race, one of the proudest individuals lining the route as the peloton roared through was – in no small part – responsible for its survival when it was at its weakest.

Jean-Marie Leblanc, deputy mayor of Fontaine-au-Bois, director of the Tour de France for nearly 20 years, leads a quiet life these days. The village in the countryside just a few kilometres from the Belgian border is emphatically rural: a mishmash of tractor repair shops, farmyards backing on to the few roads and just one bar. As Leblanc discusses the darkest days of the 1998 Tour, the most restless thing in the neighbourhood is probably a pilotless lawnmower, perpetually buzzing around and bumping against benches and trees as it cuts the grass, in the sunlit, windy garden outside his home. 'His name is Toto,' says Leblanc with a mischievous grin.

To find a darker side to humanity in Fontaine-au-Bois, though, you don't have to look far. There are two sizeable military cemeteries in the village. One is filled with long lines of graves of soldiers who died in some of the last battles of the war in late October and the first week of November 1918, when New Zealand forces took part in a dramatic assault on the German occupiers of the nearby fortress town of Le Quesnoy – and the inhabitants thanked the Kiwis by renaming several of their streets after New Zealand place-names. By that point in the Great War, even while the German fleet was mutinying in the Baltic and the Kaiser was packing his bags for his imminent exile in Holland, the British First, Third and Fourth Armies had combined with the French to drive the wavering German forces into southern Belgium and north-east France – and the killing went on.

It is perhaps appropriate that Leblanc should be surrounded by so much military history. One of the classic images of the Aix-les-Bains rebellion shows Leblanc standing alone in front of a melee of disgruntled riders, hands on his hips, for all the world like a general facing down his mutinous troops. Leblanc was certain that saving the Tour meant getting the race into Paris, and, like any commander, he was prepared to make the necessary sacrifices to ensure the race, and he, attained its objective.

Unlike some First World War commanders, it would be inaccurate to see Leblanc as some kind of authoritarian, overbearing figure with no understanding or knowledge of what the peloton was going through. He had been there with the Tour's 'poor bloody infantry', riding (and finishing) the Tour himself twice as an anonymous domestique in 1968 and 1970. Quite apart from Manolo Saiz's grudging tribute to one of his long-standing adversaries, there is other evidence of his huge empathy with all classes of rider in the peloton. One of Leblanc's first actions as the Tour's new director in 1988 was to move away from the rather patrician attitude of his predecessor – the pith-helmeted, khaki shorts-wearing Jacques Goddet, inspired by the British Indian army – and 'ensure that the riders were at the forefront of my priorities, when it came to good hotels, and better money. That meant that even if me and the rest of the management weren't sleeping in campsites so the riders got the best lodging available, we did have to put up with guesthouses.' At the same time 'because at the time riders weren't paid so well', prize money was increased substantially in the Tour. In the case of the winner – money which was traditionally divided between team-mates, as the Tour's official history testifies the first prize rose to 1.5 million French francs in 1989 and two million French francs in 1990. Two years before, in 1987, winner Stephen Roche (and his riders) had netted 300,000 French francs, 180,000 of which came in the form of a flat on a beach resort. Leblanc also resisted TV pressure to shift race finishes to 7 p.m., putting 5 p.m. to 5.30 p.m. as a time limit. There was also his sense of indirect responsibility for the death of Fabio Casartelli during the 1995 Tour, even if there was never any question of the organisers being at fault – the Italian skidded on a downhill in the Pyrenees. 'Yes, but I couldn't help feeling when I met his parents at a ceremony in his memory, that it was a little bit because of me that they had lost their child,' he says, even now, 'because it was on *my* race.'

At the same time, flashes of Leblanc's profound love of the sport, how deeply he lived for cycling, still shine through. He can still remember, for example, the exact gearing he used in a small, but personally significant triumph, a time trial stage of the 1971 Tour of Portugal. Then, when he recollects a chance meeting as a semi-professional racer in 1966, with one of cycling's great stars, Tommy Simpson, he says, 'I remember it as if it was yesterday. It was in May, my team were testing me out with some [low-key] professional stage races and Tom, having won the World's the summer before, had had an injury over the winter so he was getting some form back in the same events. In those days, there were no team vehicles, but it was sunny, so I was sitting on some kind of bench, fixing my shoes or something, when Tom came out, wearing his World Champion's jersey. *Monsieur Simpson*, someone I admired a lot, and he asked me,' – and he chuckles, still half amazed by the memory of his idol asking him for permission to do something – 'if he could sit down!

'Then he started to talk to me, in French, what I was doing, where I was from, and we talked for five minutes. He was so courteous! *Voilà*, that shows that he really liked talking to people, not at all stuck up, a really polite guy.'

Barely 12 months later, though, Simpson would be lying on the slopes of the Mont Ventoux, dying from a combination of heat exhaustion exacerbated by amphetamine use. Discussing his death, Leblanc recognises Simpson had 'too much pride, but in the good sense, he wanted to do too much, had too much self-esteem. It was one of the elements … but that is one of the elements that make a great champion, that they could drive themselves right to the end. There is always a drive to win in riders, but what goes with that, what precedes that, is self-esteem, pride, the desire to be the equal of their rivals. There are other parameters – money, women, and so on – whatever.'

Over three decades later, Leblanc was forced to tackle both sides of the coin of the consequences of those kinds of personal ambitions in the Tour de France 1998. His lengthy career as a journalist had deepened that knowledge of the murky places they could lead to, but it had not lessened his respect for his former colleagues, either. Leblanc had had some serious experiences of doping scandals and handling them. He inherited the position of Tour director immediately after the 1988 Tour de France winner Pedro Delgado had tested positive for a masking agent – not on the banned list. That was, Leblanc says, something which, 'poisoned cycling, and alas, by extension, it started to poison the Tour de France. That meant that the following year I was bombarded with questions about how we were going to tackle doping. If Jean Montois says that "the masks came off in 1998", then in 1988, they started to slip a little. We noticed, too, that the UCI were not capable of sorting things out. The riders, doctors and teams had "dropped"' – Leblanc uses the word *distancer*, meaning drop as in distance your opponents in a race, to outstrip – 'the rules'.

'I liked Delgado, I liked the way he had raced and he was not forcibly the most guilty. It obliged us to take precautions, as organisers. Before that year we said, "that's the UCI's responsibility". We had a "pi-pi" room [for doping control] and' – he makes a gesture of having completed their responsibility – 'that was it. Now, we started to push the UCI about it at our CCP meetings. I remember, I admired Verbruggen, but after that it was "doping, it's maybe just a few riders are involved". Perhaps he said that in good faith, but he denied that doping was generalised and the medical commissions and the laboratories didn't act quickly enough to stamp it out. We weren't in the front line, for sure, but we tried to mobilise and motivate the UCI to go quickly.' The media, Leblanc's old metier, he says, were 'pushing harder and harder on this question' and indeed, in 1990, *L'Equipe*'s Philippe Brunel, together with Dutch journalist Bennie Ceulen, published one of the earliest articles about EPO.

It is possible that Leblanc could have known the 1998 Tour was due to be a rocky one, had he been more superstitious. Jean Montois and Leblanc recall, curiously enough, their conversation in their 1998 pre-Tour meal, usually a breakfast, to discuss how they viewed the coming race. Playing a numbers game, Montois forecast that there would be some kind of major scandal, given that in 1978 race leader Michel Pollentier had been kicked out for doping at Alpe d'Huez and in 1988 the Delgado affair had again left the Tour with a serious image problem. (As it happens, 2008 was also a Tour fraught with doping problems.) But at the time the powers that be did not seem interested in Leblanc's increasing concerns. Regarding meeting Verbruggen in western Ireland just before the Tour began, although EPO (and the future test) was discussed, it was only done briefly and Leblanc says overall, 'we barely talked about doping ... "no, it's only one or two isolated cases, it's not as serious as all that"'. To this day Leblanc still wonders 'whether he really meant what he said.'

In Verbruggen's defence, Leblanc argues, is that as a Federation president 'you don't want to knock down the house that you're sitting in'. There were times, too, when the Tour was so close to Verbruggen that prior to Leblanc being chosen as Tour boss in late 1988, it was suggested that Verbruggen be given the job. (The Dutchman turned it down, arguing that he was not French, but it does lead one to wonder how cycling would have developed with Verbruggen in charge of the sport's biggest bike race.) 'But we were among those who said "watch out" [about doping] and Verbruggen, who was a little bit anti-French at the same time, thought that the French exaggerated the problem.' Leblanc cites the 1996 letter sent by the French cycling authorities to the Olympic Games president Juan Antonio Samaranch and other top authorities, expressing their fears concerning EPO. 'Samaranch sent back a three-line letter, saying, "we can't find EPO" right now; [former French Minister of Sport] Guy Drut replied in a page and a half saying that efforts to find EPO should be speeded up and Verbruggen never bothered to answer at all.'

However – and here he does coincide with Saiz – Leblanc felt that once the crisis blew open, excessive attention was paid by the media to the Tour's ills, overshadowing other doping problems in sport. 'At the time the disappointment of the journalists and their outrage about doping was concentrated on the Tour de France, it's like that saying *on ne prête qu'aux riche* [only the rich get lent money], because we were the number one race, so all the attacks, all the criticism, at the hands of the press was unloaded on to us. It was like if doping existed, it was the Tour's fault because "we didn't do the correct tests, we didn't write up the regulations correctly, we didn't apply the right sanctions." But, in terms of doping controls, actually we didn't have the legislative power, we didn't have the executive power, all we had was logistic power, as organisers.

'We could only provide the legislators and the commissaires what they needed to carry out [anti-doping] tests, and we had even less [operative] power when it came to the field of scientific investigation. No, no, we're blamed for everything and it doesn't matter what, but no, no – from my point of view, the Tour de France had no responsibility [for doing anything] when it came to the fight against doping. None at all.'

He confirms his previously stated belief that, 'If the Tour de France was a hair's breadth away from collapse, it was because of those elements of the media who carried out sensationalist, junk TV, investigations, forcing the riders into a corner.' Particularly guilty of that, he argues, were some television reports of the time, which were 'sensationalist, over-emotional, which never, *ever*, provided a solution or a real reflection on it [doping].

'As Tour director, I was on all the committees and commissions for professional racing at the UCI and we spent huge amounts of time trying to work out what we could do about it [doping]. I never saw the television [reports on the 1998 Tour] get interested in sorting out doping, never, rather than produce something sensationalist – they would be there for that all right. Their power was such that public opinion could be formed by them, and if they said it was like that, then everybody went along with it. That's what the powerful often get condemned for, people say, "oh but they must have known about it and they hid it." We weren't aware of anything at all. *Rien*.'

But ultimately, Leblanc feels that for all the events of that year nearly wrecked the Tour, they were a necessary evil, to try and turn the corner against doping. 1998 drew a line in the sand. 'If we hadn't had those scandals, the Festina affair and so on, we would have continued in the world of ignorance and supposition. This way, it [doping] was smashed right into our face ... it was clear that Virenque and others had cheated. Following their confessions, that was something that had a real impact.'

He has no regrets, either, about how he behaved in the Tour. 'On the contrary, I am very proud of how I got things done there, to have been able to save the Tour and bring it all the way to Paris. It was hanging by a wire, but we talked our way through it. We did it.'

The longer it went on, though, the longer the potential for the media, sensationalist or otherwise, to make the most of one of sport's greatest events already in tatters. Was it absolutely necessary that the Tour make it to Paris, rather than just ending it at some point earlier?

'There was an element of self-esteem in that goal, for sure. I was determined not to be the first ever director in the Tour's history who hadn't made it to Paris. But at the same time, I thought, if we didn't make it, if we hadn't done, would it really have gone on the next year?' A Tour that had ended in Aix-les-Bains, say, would have caused all parties to have lost faith in the race, everybody, everything. "Hey, what's this you've got here, is it broken, has it stopped?" There would have been a breach of confidence in the race, that confidence would have collapsed completely. There would have been all manner of press campaigns … *ooh lalalala*,' he concludes. 'This way, we saved' – *pffft*, he interjects, as if accepting the sacrifices – 'the core, the essential part.'

The Tour's status as a key part of the country's national heritage is well established in France. But in his bid to save the race there was never, he insists, 'one single contact with the Ministry of Sport, or with the Ministry of the Interior. That guy [on the Aix-les-Bains stage] was there by chance. And no orders ever came down from "above". What's more, they left us to disentangle it all.' Symbolising that abandonment, he says, is that 'when we finally made it to Paris, instead of the usual group of ministers who'd come out to see the race arrive, this time there was only one. They didn't want to show themselves.'

As has already been observed, Marie-George Buffet's failure to communicate with Leblanc at the Dublin start that she already knew about the Festina raid would seem to confirm that there was little or no information provided to the Tour organisation from official sources. (Her own conviction was that, as she told the French Senate committee in 2013, 'In the Tour "village", the day after the confiscations [of doping products] in the Festina team, everybody thought there would be no longer-term consequence. A member of the IOC even said, in front of witnesses, "you should have warned me about it earlier, I would have calmed the Minister down straight away".')

Rather than knowing one way or another, Leblanc lived through the same kind of day-to-day uncertainty which Manolo Saiz found so onerous, to the point where Leblanc believed that once Festina had been excluded, the police raids would be at an end. He says the only source of information 'was the radio and the TV, just like it was for the riders and the teams. Never with any direct official source.' As such, for the man in the eye of the storm, Leblanc felt curiously – and intensely – isolated.

Yet for all that, the attitude of the public was odd rather than, as it sounds, in any way intimidating, he says. 'The morning after I kicked Festina out, they threw stones at my car. Why? Because I'd taken away their idol and their best team, and they didn't like that. And it was the same again on the day of the strike in the Alps – stones and spit. It was always because of the same things. It was a disappointment. They [the riders] were late, there was no race, and on top of that we had broken their idols. *Oui, oui.*' Yet he feels he had no choice but to get rid of the French team. 'The doping masks were whipped away as a result of Festina. The strongest element were the confessions, and then later the trials. The sports director who says, "yes, there is an organised doping in my team". How can I let that team, if we don't know whether there is or is not organised doping in the other squads, continue? We have those who have confessed and those who can continue. For lack of proof.' Virenque's later, oft-repeated claim that they were scapegoats is brushed aside by Leblanc with a very Gallic harrumph.

'Could we have seen the signs that they were doping? With hindsight? When there were seven of the Festina riders on the front on one climb, the Madeleine, in the 1997 Tour and only one of them [from the start list] was missing? And even if you think, that's a bit odd, maybe one is injecting, how can you think it was organised like that? We had no idea, even if looking back, of course there are episodes that seem to be suspect.'

As for Marco Pantani, whom Leblanc publicly thanked on the Champs-Elysées, he argues slightly differently. 'Doped or not doped, and with hindsight we think he was, but I think the same goes for Ullrich and the others, I said *Merci, Marco Pantani* because he had such charisma, gave a sort of spectacle, he had glued together the bad parts of the Tour. His victory over the Galibier to the Deux Alpes, that was magnificent, that's why I said he saved the Tour, he set it on fire three or four times, just as well he was there. He was great, *chack, chack, chack*' – he makes a sound as if he was a bike pedalling – 'those legs. In my opinion,' he adds, just to make it clear this is not an official point of view.

Seventeen years later, the Tour was still racing onwards. It's perhaps appropriate that when the 2015 race finally passed close by Leblanc's village, it didn't do so en route to some dramatic mountain-top finish; rather, it would be heading westwards towards the French cycling heartlands of Normandy and Brittany. 'When that happens it will be quite a moment for me, coming back to my roots. *Le bouclé*' – the buckle, slang for the Tour, '*est bouclé*,' he says with a smile. Once so close to being broken, *le gran bouclé* is, at least in his eyes, once again intact.

18

Aftermath:
A Double-Edged Sword

'The fight against doping is a thankless one. You destroy beautiful jewels, moments of public celebrations, you disappoint ...' French Senate report on anti-doping, 2013

It is now nearly 20 years since Rolf Aldag poured his EPO down a Dublin hotel toilet; since Joerg Jaksche and his team-mates transferred their doping products, flask by flask and vial by vial, into a team bus vacuum cleaner; since Richard Virenque emerged sobbing from a tobacconist's shop in the depths of rural central France; and since after the welter of riders' strikes, expulsions, police raids and public protests, as well as one of the race's most epic days in the mountains, the Tour de France 1998 finally – somehow – crept into Paris.

The 1998 *grand boucle* might have been *bouclé*, as Jean-Marie Leblanc would put it, but in terms of prestige by the time it reached the French capital the Tour was a shadow of its former self. Yet it would be very wrong to think that the Tour abruptly stopped mattering to France after 1998. It still did, and hugely. That can be seen by the way the country's establishment reacted even *after* the wool had been pulled so brutally from the public's eyes by the 1998 doping scandals. In July 1999, during the Tour's build-up, *L'Equipe* compiled a weekend supplement by figures from the world of French sport and/or politics to try to tell the world why – even if some of the latter had shunned the race on the Champs Elysées – the Tour still mattered so much. Among their writers, perhaps surprisingly, was Sports Minister Marie-George Buffet.

'Simply, the Tour is something beautiful to live,' she wrote. 'I remember a childhood where we did not miss a single highlights show of each stage, each evening. Later, on family holidays, it was difficult to get my husband and children to move from the television in the afternoons.

'We all have a special rapport with the Tour. This feeling of a daily meeting. No need to buy a ticket or book a place. You decide at the last moment to turn up at the edge of the road, *et voilà* ... The Tour offers this opportunity: everybody has the sensation, a strange one, that all France has its eyes fixed on this single event.' It was for that reason, she wrote, that she suffered so badly in the 1998 Tour 'with the idea that it might be going to stop'.

Yet for all the outpouring of affection for the Tour by Marie-George Buffet and others, following the events of July 1998 it was all but impossible even for the most diehard fan to regard the Tour in the same unblemished light of before. As for the media, to say we were doubtful about the Tour's future is an understatement: I can recollect taking part in an unofficial sweepstake as we sat in the Tour's press rooms of July 1999, in which we betted on which stage the race would finally grind to a halt.

But we cynical hacks were proved wrong on that one, very major, count. The Tour has survived, it is still hugely popular and it remains both road cycling's flagship race and the biggest annual sporting event on the planet. The sponsors have not fled in droves – quite the contrary. Yet one crucial difference between prior and post-1998 endures: an outstanding performance by any rider still produces a knee-jerk reaction among certain sectors of the press and public of automatic suspicion. That suspicion was heightened, massively, by Lance Armstrong's years of doping and subsequent confessions, as well as by the many subsequent scandals cycling has lived through after 1998. But as a default setting, doubting achievements that we would have otherwise simply admired began somewhere early in that month of July 1998, as the scale of the fraud sank in. As Frankie Andreu says, 'all you needed was two riders to be going well for it to be "wow, look at that".'

It has been forgotten in the wake of the Armstrong confession and the CIRC investigation, but until 2012 and Armstrong's admissions, the 1998 Tour had the unenviable honour of being regularly described as one of the biggest doping scandals – if not *the* biggest – organised sport had ever known. There had been strong suspicions about how countries east of the Iron Curtain might have doped their athletes for decades at a national level, but for the first time in a major sport, systematic doping of a team of riders was clearly and unequivocally laid bare. For the first time, too, the unsettling possibility arose that doping might not lead to the expulsion of a rider or a team, but to the impromptu cancellation of an entire event.

Even after Armstrong, the 1998 Tour remains in a doping class of its own on one level: the scandal did not happen after the athlete in question had left the sport or somewhere away from the event. Rather than the centrepiece of the athlete's downfall taking place in a courtroom, an anti-doping lab or in the anaesthetised setting of a TV chat show, like Armstrong's confession, the consequences were lived out on the roads of the Tour de France themselves: as *Cycle Sport* observed less than a month later, 1998 was the Tour where the chickens truly came home to roost.

To understand the full impact of the 1998 Tour on cycling and its relationship with doping in the years that followed, it's worth remembering that if drugs scandals pre-1998 could be taken as early warning signs of Festina, some anti-doping measures prior to that Tour had already been taken – and their effect and importance were considerably magnified by the events of July. In France alone, the initiation of an early form of the biological passport, the *suivi médical longitudinal* and Marie-George Buffet's 1999 anti-doping law were developed from earlier projects far more quickly thanks to the 1998 Tour. Some were initially slated as toothless, but longer term they represented key steps in the right direction. The 1998 Tour both speeded up their growth and hugely raised their profile.

Outside cycling, the most high-profile international consequence of the Festina affair on the anti-doping front was the creation of the World Anti-Doping Agency (WADA). After the IOC convened the First World Conference on Doping in Sport in February 1999, WADA was formally created on 10 November the same year. In a 2009 interview with Reuters to celebrate its tenth anniversary, its first president, Richard Pound, attributed WADA's existence directly to the Festina scandals.

'The European-based international federations realised that there was now a problem when they had watched all these Festina (cycling team) folks arrested and taken to jail,' Pound said. 'They thought: "Wow, if this can happen to cycling, which is a really important sport in Europe, and in their blue-ribbon event, then this could happen to us." All of a sudden the question of doping got raised to a new high.'

It can therefore be argued that even if cycling took a hammering as a result of the Tour, on a broader front and in terms of a wake-up call, sport as a whole gained its key anti-doping reference point and organisation. But while WADA rightly states on its website, 'The Tour de France scandal highlighted the need for an independent international agency, which would set unified standards for anti-doping work and coordinate the efforts of sports organizations and public authorities', the actual working benefits of that agency arguably took far too much time to be noted as quickly as cycling needed.

Nobody can disagree, for example, that the total of WADA's anti-doping tests in cycling, for instance, which tripled from just over 5,000 in 2006 to just over 15,000 in 2009 was an advance. Equally, WADA's World Anti-Doping Code, 'the core document that harmonizes anti-doping policies, rules and regulations within sport organizations and among public authorities around the world', constituted a massive step forward for all sport. But if it cannot be criticised given the immenseness of the task involved, WADA's Anti-Doping Code took until 2004 to be drawn up and come into effect. For cycling – one of sport's walking wounded since 1998 – that was six years too long a wait: by 2006, the sport had gained fresh injuries, from Operación Puerto and numerous other scandals. By then, too, the roughest scandal of them all was already slouching towards Paris to be born: in 2004 Lance Armstrong won his fifth straight Tour.

If WADA was created and the French anti-doping legislation gained traction because of the Festina scandal, closer to the 'front line' of cycling and as the dust settled on the Tour it was harder to perceive if there would be any rapid gains on the ground in the battle against banned drugs. Four days after the Tour had ended an eight-hour meeting between the UCI, race organisers and teams in Paris reached an agreement that something had to be done about doping. What, though, was not so easy to put into practice. Hein Verbruggen, now back from his holiday, hardly oozed optimism. 'Doping is not just a cycling problem, we lack the resources to look deeper into the question,' he said. 'You cannot prevent the use of EPO.' Of the series of proposals that did emerge from the Paris meetings – new blood tests before the end of the year, the naming of a single figure in a team to be responsible for doping cases, a possible change in the UCI points system to incentivise riders to race (and therefore hopefully dope) less – none had any long-term effect. A full-scale riders' meeting with the UCI, the following Tuesday in Lausanne, was hardly more productive. Although numerous former and current top names were present – Miguel Indurain, Johan Bruyneel, Tony Rominger, Stéphane Heulot, Luc Leblanc, Maurizio Fondriest, Pascal Richard and Laurent Jalabert – and there were repeated calls for the season and races to be shortened, they failed to be implemented. 'Maybe we have to review the entire system to avoid inciting certain racers to use doping,' commented Jalabert, once again acting as an unofficial spokesman. Not for the last time, the idea of a general amnesty for prior doping offences failed to get off the ground.

A UCI communiqué issued on 13 August provided a summary of the various meetings and acted as the governing body's road map for the sport's future struggle against doping. However, perhaps 'map of a labyrinth with no clear exit' is a more accurate description of that plan. Certainly the communiqué's contents suggest that, despite all the encounters the UCI had organised, neither the full gravity of the problems highlighted by the Tour nor the strength of the riders' response had struck home in Lausanne. With a degree of understatement that would be amusing had it not been discussing the fact that cycling's flagship event had nearly collapsed, the UCI's one referral to the strikes in the Tour came when it claimed, 'It is understandable that the riders should feel somewhat annoyed about the methods used by the police.' However, they then solemnly warned that the 'primary responsibility falls upon the person who is in breach of the law'.

The UCI initially distanced itself from all possible blame for police action, stating, 'the UCI had no means of intervening in the actions of the French justice authorities either during or after the Tour'. But the summary then flatly contradicted itself by stating the UCI 'used certain appropriate channels to exhort the French authorities to show greater discretion, which seems to have been the case for the end of the Tour'. It would seem, then, that the UCI's 'influence' on the French authorities did exist, but not for the difficult moments, only when the UCI was attempting to take some of the credit for the drop in pressure. Given the degree of 'spinning' going on here, it almost goes without saying that Hein Verbruggen's failure to show up at the Tour for more than a few days is not even mentioned or explained.

Equally confusing, contradictory statements permeated the whole summary, most importantly when the UCI argued the purpose of the rider–organisers–UCI team meetings 'was not to change our "anti-doping" systems. Indeed, the UCI believes that it is difficult to do more than is already being done, particularly in terms of: 1. Wide-ranging anti-doping controls for detectable products 2. Blood tests, which have already been conducted for the last 18 months, *enabling us to control the EPO problem* [my italics], and to establish that the goal of protecting health, by limiting EPO abuse, has been achieved.

'Taking this into account,' the UCI cheerfully concluded, 'whatever criticisms may be levelled at cycling, we can never be accused of hiding our heads in the sand when it comes to anti-doping and health controls.'

However, given the events of the previous month, on reading the above perhaps the politest accusation that can be levelled at the UCI is precisely that – of near-wilful ignorance, even after the Tour had all but fallen apart. To insist that the EPO problem was being 'controlled' when the world's number one ranked team had been using it systematically for the previous five years and had just been thrown off the Tour for banned drug consumption borders on the delusional. That impression is further reinforced by another observation in the same press statement which then claimed that the Festina case did not represent the situation in the majority of the teams, and that 'the UCI is quite certain that the majority of teams do not have recourse to such practices'. Again, it all but beggars belief that the UCI could not be certain about this – unless they had their collective heads in the sand.

But the contradictions and a certain tone of realism within the press statement, as well as Verbruggen's forthright declaration after the same series of meetings that EPO use could not be prevented, counter this optimistic world view about EPO being vanquished. Indeed, a few lines later, the UCI says in its communiqué, 'We have never shied away from admitting that the 1% of positive cases found in anti-doping controls do not reflect the reality of the situation.' The statement continues 'and the UCI has on several occasions acknowledged that, taking the undetectable products into account, the percentage of positive cases should be much higher'. Just to make it even clearer they are fighting an anti-doping war in which victories are only fleetingly successful at best the statements helpfully add, 'We are perfectly well aware that, as soon as it is possible to detect EPO, those who cheat will find new ways of doing so.' The underlying echoes of Verbruggen's previous observations about the role health controls played, prior to the 1998 Tour – 'why not prescribe certain limits, check the blood and the urine and say that as long as you stay within determined limits where there is no risk to health, that's fine by us?' – are unmissable.

Had the UCI simply been burying its head in the sand, that would have been bad enough. But, if anything, the flagrant contradiction between the simultaneous recognition that the doping problem was far greater than anti-doping tests showed, and the sweeping assertion that the majority of the teams were clean, was even more worrying. There was no clear vision of what was going on or how best to deal with it – not even a wrong-headed vision. It was hardly the most reassuring of situations, and even less so in a sport that the month before had seemed hell-bent on self-destruction.

Arguably, the one point on which it was possible to sympathise with the UCI's predicament is where it stated that, 'it is unacceptable to see ourselves criticized by anyone who is then incapable of showing us at least one alternative approach or telling us what additional action we should take'. There had, as Jean-Marie Leblanc points out, been much mud-slinging, and precious few real courses of action suggested by the media. Furthermore, the battery of measures that the UCI also announced in the same press communiqué 'to continue reducing the use of banned substances' – stepping up blood tests, keeping a much closer eye on team doctors' medical training and treatment of their riders, re-examining the banned list, and creating an independent commission to oversee its rules, were perhaps the most important – was a sizeable one.

But when combined with such a firm refusal to accept the current state of play in the peloton in full, no matter what the statement promised it hardly inspired confidence that the UCI was really grasping the bull by the horns. Nor did the UCI's recognition that it would be prepared to bring in a new measure that they were already convinced was useless. 'Even though our physiologists see no need for out-of-competition tests for road cycling during the period from November to January,' it said, 'we would be prepared to introduce these, despite the fact that the problem of use of undetectable products would not be reduced in any way.' Its ringing conclusion, that from the ashes of the 1998 Tour a new world would arise, is therefore hardly convincing. 'The UCI is fully aware that its sport has been seriously affected by recent events. It also realizes that this attack on the credibility of the sport, which remains no less noble and historic, provides it with a unique opportunity to build new solutions for the future.' When they announced that they would be creating a special fund – coming from the UCI itself, national federations, organisers, teams and riders – to fight banned substance use in 1999, it sounded encouraging. But the actual sum available, 3.8 million Swiss francs (£1.72 million) turned out to be risibly small. The scope of the UCI's involvement was later summarised in a press release issued on Wednesday, 1 November 2000. This specified that, from 1998 to 2001, 8.45 per cent of its total budget (5.7 million Swiss francs out of 67 million) was spent on anti-doping controls and health checks as well as research, and that in 2000 the total expenditure of the cycling community in the fight against doping totalled 4.3 million Swiss francs (€2 million). In comparison, Festina's annual team budget until 1998 was estimated at some $6 million, roughly double that sum.

Despite the UCI's confidence about the EPO problem being under control – or perhaps because of it – it was obvious that the most important and urgent step forward was that of finding an EPO test. But progress in that quarter had suffered a setback after the Conconi fiasco and another after the Brisson test had been stillborn – and the scientist in question later accused the UCI of being partly responsible for that. In yet more meetings, organisers and anti-doping officials found themselves coming up against the same major stumbling block: 'In 1998 I was really pessimistic,' says Montois, 'because we had a meeting in Grenoble at the end of the year, different journalists and the anti-doping authorities, and somebody from Châtenay-Malabry said we'd need another 20 years to conquer EPO. I remember Jean-Marie Leblanc, who was also there, was completely destroyed by that, saying, "God what are we going to do, we can make them swear on the Bible, but there's nothing as dissuasive as an actual test".'

277

Boardman felt it was too easy to blame the authorities of the time for this particular problem. 'It got to a point where it is, where it was not easy to deal with, if you've got undetectable products, you take those measures to put in place but you are bound by the law, what the hell do you do? I felt for the UCI at the time, regardless of who it was, because what the hell were you supposed to do?'

If the lack of tests hamstrung the fight against EPO post-1998, there were nonetheless some indications of the potential for a sea change in the peloton – in that using banned drugs was not automatically accepted, at least at a social level, by parts of the bunch. The 1998 Tour drew a line in the sand beyond which riders would no longer discuss taking EPO, as Bobby Julich memorably puts it, like they were going to have a coffee or because, as another 1990s pro said, because 'it was part of their job'. And if that was the attitude among the dopers, for those like Julich looking for a way out there was another encouraging development. The unspoken *omertà* surrounding doping was, if still largely present, no longer so intimidating. Rather, it became something that could – albeit still at a high price – be negotiated a little more easily.

Paul Kimmage's book *Rough Ride* stands out as one of the very few pre-1998 books on doping in the peloton. But after Festina there was a substantial increase in 'tell-all' works as harrowing and graphic as, to mention only three from 1999, Willy Voet's *Massacre à la chaîne* (published in English as *Breaking the Chain*), Erwann Menthéour's *Secret défonce* (the secret addict) and Christophe Bassons' *Positif* (published in English as *A Clean Break*). Thereon, exposing the underbelly of doping became more and more frequent. A small but significant number of riders and other members of the cycling community who reneged publicly or privately on their doping past or present began to come forward. It would have to wait for another huge scandal, that of the 2006 Operación Puerto anti-doping probe, before that trickle became a steadier, although still narrow, stream of confessions and exposés. But post-1998, the figure of the anti-doping campaigner and in particular that of the *repenti* – the repentant doper – became a much more familiar one in cycling, and, albeit very patchily, a more acceptable one.

Christophe Bassons, who had always refused to dope, was a leading symbol of the first part of the teams' progressive change in attitude – some of it, it has to be said, simply because they realised that was the way the wind was blowing. 'In 1995, several team managers had been weighing up my sporting future,' he later wrote. 'By June 1998, I was no more than a guinea pig on which to test alternatives to doping. In early 1999, I was a brand of washing powder: Bassons, with outstanding cleanliness, washes whiter. Guaranteed without chemicals, it works only with *l'eau claire*.' He then compares his fortune to that of another, earlier, anti-doping crusader in the peloton, Gilles Delion. 'He had to quit for being too clean. I think I would have suffered the same fate if the revelatory events of 1998 hadn't happened.'

One of those who, as we have seen, opted out of the doping system regardless and as a result of 1998 was Bobby Julich. Prior to the Tour that year he says, 'Obviously there were guys who had a different level of program, but as far as the oxygen carrying capacity aid which is known as EPO, that was pretty much "fair game" with everyone.' But the 1998 Tour rammed home to Julich that the game was not worth the candle. 'It hit you for the first time when guys were going to gaol. It was like "wow", this is serious.'

As for the Tour de France itself, although it continued, the sense that it was living on a knife-edge was not going to go away so quickly. 'I won't be able to relax until I see the Tour on the Champs-Elysées,' Marie-George Buffet wrote for *L'Equipe* in early July 1999, just as the race – and Armstrong's reign in yellow – was about to begin in Puy du Fou.

Attitudes within the Tour organisation varied radically. Some, like Jean-Claude Killy, head of the Tour de France parent company ASO, made one patent attempt to 'share the blame' for the doping plague among all sports. 'We reached rock-bottom. First we thought it was a problem concerning one team, then cycling, then we realised that the whole of sport is dashing towards death,' he argued at the 1999 Tour de France presentation on 5 November 1998. 'The Tour lives on but it will never again be the symbol of doping, it will be the symbol of the fight against doping.' Jean-Marie Leblanc, on the other hand, dealt with more specific cycling questions and promised that both teams and individuals on the Tour would be vetted for their anti-doping credentials before being let on to the Tour. 'We'll start the Tour with 16 or 18 teams if we have to.'

Financially the effects, in any case, were comparatively minimal, both for the Tour and for Festina, which that winter announced an increase in sales in 1998. 'The following year, we lost some sponsors,' Leblanc says, 'others asked that it be specified in their contracts, that in the case of a repeat scandal blablabla ... but things were re-established very fast. The same went for the public, there was a drop in popularity, but it came back very fast and these days ...' Even during the Tour, the decline in the number of its fans was not perceptible, and although in France there have been several reports of an ageing fan base, it retains massive popularity further afield. The German TV channel ARD announced in one 1998 survey that, even during the final week, five million spectators watched per day, with peaks of seven million. Some 87 per cent of their spectators wanted the Tour to go on, although, confusingly, 77 per cent were in favour of the protests – which, if successful, would have meant it stopped.

Elsewhere, as in the 1998 Tour's start country of Ireland, the impact of the Festina scandals was more marked, with talk of the

World Championships in 2003 quietly dropped. 'It didn't leave much of a legacy, beyond a few cases like [Sky rider] Philip Deignan getting into the sport,' Barry Ryan adds. 'At the time, afterwards, it didn't feel that huge. Part of the blame was laid on the fact that the "Tour in Ireland" was also "the Festina Tour", it was very much associated with that. It also happened to take place in Ireland on the weekend when the French won the soccer World Cup and there was a feeling in the papers they'd given it to us to look after whilst they were doing that.'

However, in France, even if the Tour remained in relatively rude health, the rest of the racing calendar and interest in the sport withered in the early noughties – and is only now returning. The French's lack of success in the Tour was never going to help. But cycling's popularity as a sport, even if the Tour was still a major draw, dipped in the home nation – and it is hard not to see a connection between that and the perception of cycling as a 'doped' sport. Among top level races post-1998, the Midi Libre, Classique des Alpes and GP de Nations all disappeared while both the Dauphiné Libéré and Paris–Nice hit financial difficulties before being taken over by ASO. And that was just the top of the pyramid.

Pierre Ballester's *Fin de cycle* paints a view of the sport in France described by William Fotheringham as 'apocalyptic'. According to Ballester, mid-level races in France dropped by 36 per cent between 1998 and 2008. Post-Tour criteriums halved from 37 in 1997 to 18 in 2011. Road racing licences dropped by 11,000 between 1998 and 2011. In such circumstances, credit is due to ASO, a private business when all is said and done, for buying up a number of races with limited profitability and attempting to maintain the 'pyramid' of professional racing in France as best they could.

One consequence of the Festina expulsions for the Tour was that, given it had been an action taken by the Tour's organisers rather than the UCI, a template was created for the future of the race in its own role in the battle against banned drugs. After 1998, there was a widespread expectation that the organisers had some power to fight doping with direct action, rather than waiting for the authorities to do their job, not just in the present but also in the future.

In 1999 the Tour's gestures were rather on the level of two steps forward, two steps back. A series of 'suspect' riders and individuals, including Richard Virenque, Saiz and the entire TVM squad, as well as Vini Caldirola, an Italian team embroiled in a minor possible doping scandal that June, were excluded from the Tour that year. But then both Saiz and Virenque were re-admitted at the last minute, when the UCI ruled the Tour had no right to stop the Frenchman from racing. Perhaps more worryingly, Festina, albeit with a much less powerful line-up – of 1998, only Brochard, Rous and Moreau were present – also took part. Pre-1999, the organisers also gave team personnel a general warning about use of drugs, and a reminder of the rules that had allowed them to expel Festina. On top of that, every starter was blood-tested before the race got underway.

The trend of highlighting the battle against doping has continued, with serious anti-doping statements of intent included in subsequent speeches at the Tour de France presentations, and lists of measures sometimes produced to prove the race's renewed dedication to the anti-doping struggle. One of the most important came on 6 April 2001, when ASO produced a list of ten measures, including the Tour's Ethics Code, which included a written agreement by team staff to 'neither administer nor prescribe any substance subject to restriction'. Anti-doping check-ups were increased to ten riders a day, including the EPO test, and research partnerships to investigate doping, education sessions and prevention campaigns were all created. The Tour is still prepared to bar squads from its race, as it did Astana in 2008 after Vinokourov's blood doping positive during the year before.

The 1999 Tour itself survived with no police raids, no strikes, no arrests and – Armstrong's near-miss with the corticoids positive notwithstanding – no positive tests. Nor yet were any riders prevented from taking part because of the pre-Tour blood tests that had left Pantani out for the count in the middle of the Giro d'Italia. Only one rider, Ludo Diercksens of Belgium, quit in what was a confusing possible doping case where he won a transition stage but did not have the correct prescription for a banned substance which was permissible for riders to use for health reasons. But Virenque's presence on the final podium as King of the Mountains, taking the title for the fifth time in six years, was ample proof that the Tour's ghosts of the past had not been laid to rest. Neither was Alex Zülle's second place overall behind Armstrong and Laurent Dufaux's fourth, as well as Virenque's eighth, exactly indicative of rapid change. Essentially, only the man at the very top of the classification was, allegedly, different.

At the same time, the fact that the Tour did not go under in 1998 produced a different kind of momentum, the feeling that, come what may, it would continue. In July 1999, *L'Equipe* dedicated an entire section of its colour supplement to that idea, entitled *Tour de Toujours, et Pour Toujours* (Tour as always, and forever). In the background was an overhead shot from 1998 of a group of unidentifiable riders pounding through somewhere in south-west France in the blazing heat, hayfields on one side, ploughed field on the other. 'Like the day before yesterday, like tomorrow,' read the caption. In other words, stopping the Tour was not an option. The show had to go on, no matter the cost.

There are still those – like Jaksche and Saiz – who believe it should have ended, for very different reasons. Saiz, for one, believes that the Tour organisers were too narrow-minded about their own race to see what was at stake.

'The thing that annoyed me the most about the Tour directors was when you were talking to them [to explain why it should stop] and they would say, "Nooo, but this is the Tour." What do you mean, this is the Tour? Sorry, the Tour is a lot of different families, among whom are the reporters, the media, the public, the riders, the commissaires, the team, the TV cameraman who films the rider – he's the Tour, we're all the Tour's family. And they forget that. I'm the Tour, too. The Tour is the rider who's last overall and the rider who's first overall and the Tour is the guy who stands on the roadside, cheering them on.'

'If I had stopped the Tour in 1998, cycling would never have recovered,' Leblanc argued in 2000. But one consequence of it continuing was that, post-1998, cycling became a living laboratory of doping scandals, the extent of the damage they could cause and how both to deal with them and how not to deal with them. Armstrong is the most obvious case of the latter, but there are plenty more of both, ranging from individuals right up to countries. 'After the Festina affair, only France reacted,' Leblanc's successor, Christian Prudhomme, once observed. 'We had to wait another eight years after the Festina affair for Operación Puerto to take place and for Jan Ullrich to be removed from his pedestal as a hero in Germany! Festina wasn't their problem. Everybody had made the terrible mistake of saying that only Festina were cheating, whereas the gangrene was everywhere.'

Attempts to speed up the process of change at team level, Prudhomme argues, by limiting high-profile appearances of some familiar faces of cycling's dubious past, are not straightforward. 'One year, we didn't give Bjarne Riis his accreditation as a manager on the Tour'. Like Pantani, Riis was another 'saviour' from the 1998 Tour. 'But when he decided, as if by chance, to book a hotel on the race and to go there with his computer and mobile phone, what more could we do? The solution only comes through the arrival of new generations of managers.' But ultimately, the final decision had to be made by the riders – whether to stop, whether to continue, whether to dope or not to dope.

'I know there's guys that still today, think like I was thinking, "everybody else is doing something",' argues Julich. 'And I say to them "no, stop worrying about what other guys are doing, concentrate on what you can do, 'cos it's not going to help". Take it from me, I wasted three or four years of my career because I was too scared to make that step – and thank God I was – back to the dark side. But I was still too worried about it. I should have been, "I don't care". Because there were other guys – [former World Champion and Tour leader] Thor Hushovd, [multiple Tour stage winner and Vuelta King of the Mountains] David Moncoutie – guys that never touched stuff, that were winning races against these guys. And I was, too, in 2004 and 2005 but I wish I'd started a little bit earlier.'

It was clear that the 1998 Tour had created a template for how the race would react to the many cycling doping scandals that followed. Suspicions and accusations of doping, combined with a police raid or positive test that effectively confirmed them – as happened in week one of the 1998 Tour – would often be followed by furious denials of cheating and claims of victimisation, using all manner of possible explanations and justifications – as per week two of the 1998 Tour – and lastly by an admission of guilt – as per the 1998 Tour's third week and/or thereafter. After which, the same old arguments would be trotted out yet again by the powers that be – that this latest scandal proved the doping tests were working, that cycling's repeated tripping over the same stone was due to its greater assiduity when it came to rooting out drugs from the sport and that yet more would, of course, be done in the fight against banned drugs. With each scandal that broke, too, the holier than thou elements of the mainstream sports media that wrapped itself in the anti-doping flag whenever they deigned to deal with cycling would be heard once more, uttering their apocalyptic warnings with even more self-righteous fervour. After which proclamation, they'd go back to reporting on golf, tennis or football. Then the vicious and virtuous circles – the fresh suspicions of doping and finger-pointing and the claims of a renewed determination to beat it – would happen all over again.

Perhaps that is being too cynical. Occasionally fresh cases of riders with a genuine desire to set the sport straight, to work hard at it, and an honest regret at past errors would emerge. The UCI has, particularly since 2006, completely overhauled and improved its anti-doping policies with a degree of diligence that, at the time of the confused and contradictory stance it took in the immediate aftermath of the 1998 Tour, would have been very difficult to foresee. And by a long and tortuous trail ultimately the rider confessions, the anti-doping investigations and some exceptionally persistent components of the mainstream media were some of the key ingredients that contributed to the destruction of the myth of the rider once hailed as the Tour's greatest ever athlete, and to another watershed moment for cycling. No single one of these factors brought the Armstrong story to the point where the USADA could decide to strip the American of his seven Tour titles; rather, there was a wealth of circumstantial evidence put together by tenacious journalists, positive EPO tests uncovered in research by the Châtenay-Malabry laboratory in 2005 and detailed accounts by, among others, Armstrong's team-mates Hamilton and Floyd Landis of doping practices. But if the impact Armstrong had on the Tour would never have been so great and enduring without 1998, the original determination to root out the cheats in cycling and the research that did so would never have gained such traction without 1998, either. Bizarrely enough, the same seismic shift which produced the ideal conditions for the Armstrong myth to take such rapid root also contained the seeds of its destruction: a real double-edged sword.

It's appropriate then that the 2013 French Senate report on doping in sport and the anti-doping struggle is dedicated to a hardened cycling 'user' who was also a whistle-blower – Philippe Gaumont, author of *Prisonnier du dopage* and present in the 1998 Tour for ten stages. Gaumont collapsed from a heart condition on 23 April 2013, the day before he was due to testify to the Senate, and died three weeks later. 'He both witnessed and participated in doping,' the report says, before later adding, 'He helped advance the fight [against doping] with his words and commitment.' Perhaps that is the most important lesson from the 1998 Tour, that from that point onwards, these two activities – riders realising the errors of earlier doping and then joining the struggle to stamp it out – were no longer widely viewed as mutually exclusive. Active repentance, rather than just taking your anti-doping ban and then going straight back to cheating again the minute it was over, became an option as it never had done before. But that was one light in what remained, for many years post-1998, a depressingly dark tunnel.

Meanwhile, one of the most pernicious consequences of the 1998 Tour was that doping systems in cycling became more efficient, not less. There is a bitter irony that the biggest doping scandal in cycling convinced some riders that cheating was the only way forward, only in a more subtle format. Simultaneously it created a scenario of a need for redemption and renewal, a figurehead with whom media and fans could identify as a 'saviour' of the sport, somebody who would move cycling forward and restore its credibility. However, rather than redirecting the sport purely in a good way, this quest proved to be the most damaging of solutions. For it gave some riders who were willing to cheat a much firmer foothold inside cycling. The harder cycling tried to dig itself out of its hole in terms of credibility, in other words, the deeper it sank.

The inherent risks of such a quest for a 'saviour' became clear in the 1999 Giro d'Italia. Marco Pantani was already considered to have redeemed the 1998 Tour, to the point where Jean-Marie Leblanc had thanked him in Paris for his stunning mountain performance. And, in 1999, Pantani the cycling saviour was dominating the Giro d'Italia with almost insolent ease. But then two days before the finish, the Pantani myth all but collapsed: tests showed Pantani had a hematocrit level which was in excess of the permitted 50 per cent threshold. Not proof of banned drugs use, but a possible indicator. As a result, even though he was leading the Giro and had won the stage the day before, Pantani was suspended, his legend suddenly enveloped in an omnipresent suspicion of doping. His ten-month role as the figure who would guide cycling out of the wilderness in terms of its credibility came to an abrupt, brutal end. Rather, the last impression of Pantani in the 1999 Giro d'Italia was the most damaging, as he was escorted by a knot of carabinieri away from the race. Once again, just as in the 1998 Tour, images flashed worldwide of the police taking away a bike rider over a potential doping question. Hardly surprisingly, the disgraced Pantani opted out of racing the Tour de France that summer as well. What had felt like the start of a new era of gutsily challenging mountain climbers, rather than the relatively clinical time trialling success of earlier 1990s stars like Miguel Indurain, suddenly collapsed. And with it went the Tour's 'saviour' of 1998. The sport was back to square one.

Longer term, though, Pantani believed he still would have had some kind of compensation for his efforts to ensure the 1998 Tour reached Paris – not of the financial kind, but in terms of a warmer relationship with ASO. But from the Italian's point of view that was never the case, with the biggest slap in the face coming in 2001 when Mercatone Uno did not receive a wild-card invitation for the Tour. Despite last-minute rumours that Pantani would sign for a Spanish team that had been invited to the Tour, the Italian did not make it to the race.

'We know that he was disappointed that he didn't get into the Tour two or three years later, but we'd set up some guidelines that year and even if he was strong, his team wasn't,' Leblanc explains. 'There were better, well-rounded teams. The same went for that World Champion, the Italian sprinter who won in Belgium – Cipollini, when he switched to Domina Vacanze. He made a whole song and dance about it, but he could never finish the Tour. Never.'

Pantani believed, though, that he had a free pass after 'saving' the sport and the Tour against his better wishes in 1998. As Traversoni says Pantani told him, '"[He would say] I've done so much for cycling and they've betrayed me. They are all against me. I was prepared to throw away the Tour, I did something great for cycling, not just because I have won the Tour for the first time in 40 years, but because I brought home a Tour which nobody had wanted to finish."'

Pantani remains one of the sport's icons, although the doping revelations about him, of which there were many more in the years after his death from an overdose in 2004, have brutalised and deformed much of the original magic. For proof that his image as a cycling star still endures in some quarters, you need look no further than the graffiti scrawled on a rock wall on the Madonna di Campiglio pass – where his overly-high hematocrit level was revealed in the 1999 Giro, hours after one of his most spectacular triumphs on the same climb – in the 2015 Giro d'Italia. It reads simply: '15 years can't wipe out a legend'.

Back in 1999, though, Pantani's sudden discrediting made the Tour's continued quest for redemption even more urgent. Purely by chance, a seemingly ideal candidate was waiting in the wings: a young Texan, returning from a lengthy battle against cancer, who became the Tour's new champion, just when the race was once again up against the ropes.

Crucially, Armstrong had not raced the 1998 Tour de France and so was not as exposed to the sweeping generalisations concerning the peloton from that year. Equally crucially, he had returned to cycling after successfully combating a life-threatening illness. His return to health and a new beginning at the pinnacle of his sport was therefore a story which was easy to associate with a fresh start, a clean beginning, beating the disease – be it cancer or doping. As José Miguel Echavarri, Miguel Indurain's old manager put it, 'Armstrong is the best symbol of the struggle against the impossible.'

Others, better informed, were more realistic. 'He was doing the same stuff as he'd been doing in 1998, but the story was that he was the clean guy,' Andreu comments, 'and people latched on to that. You could almost say he was the new generation.'

In terms of an absence of rivals, there was certainly a gap to fill, given the three previous Tour winners Pantani, Ullrich and Riis (the latter two because of injuries) were all missing from the 1999 Tour. Armstrong also had the UCI's blessing, if not its direct support. As the CIRC report into doping in cycling put it, 'The UCI saw Armstrong as the perfect choice to lead the sport's renaissance after the Festina scandal: the fact he was American opened up a new continent for the sport, he had beaten cancer and the media made him a global star.'

The long-term effects of Armstrong on the Tour are still to become completely clear. But in the short-to-medium term, Armstrong broadened, strengthened and embodied several key issues which had their roots in the 1998 Tour de France. The tendency for doping to go underground and become much more efficient, if not more sophisticated, was one key area. So, too, was the perpetual, and partly self-perpetuating, media suspicion of any outstanding performance, and so was the increasing distance between the media and the cycling stars to whom they had once been so close. The curtained-off team bus doors, the refusal in hotels to put phone calls through to bike riders, the shirking from all bar the most anodyne of comments and the general absence of access were all part and parcel of the 1998 Tour. They would all become standard features of the Armstrong era, when press officers, barriers round buses at starts and media training and in Armstrong's case, bodyguards, became a common sight. Regrettably, this sometimes deliberate distancing between riders and media largely endures today and it does nothing to help the sport when it runs into its umpteenth doping scandal, or suspicions of them. The worst effect is to create a vacuum of knowledge, to be filled by far more damaging speculation, the bugbear of any team, and in particular, one imagines, of those press officers who over-obsess with 'controlling the narrative' and deliberately reduce access. Those strategies just help foster doubt and overly large egos among riders, both of which cycling – a sport with foundations built on its democratic, accessible, everyman nature – can ill afford.

Armstrong's first brush with generalised suspicion was not long in coming, ranging from *L'Equipe*'s double entendre headline of 'The Extra-Terrestrial' when he won in Sestrieres in 1999, a victory that effectively netted him the Tour, to the questions about a backdated medical form to cover a banned drug in the third week. But if those areas of Armstrong's rise to fame have been relatively well documented, one has not.

The incarnation of Pantani in the 1998 Tour as a redeeming figure meant it was a role that Armstrong inherited rather than invented, and the Texan certainly played it brilliantly. But it is surely no coincidence that if both Pantani and Armstrong could be seen as 'saviours', it was because part of that role was to be viewed as nonconformists, swimming against the tide of a dope-fuelled peloton. Ullrich was always cast as the squeaky-clean, ultra-dull but reliable boy next door without a subversive thought in his head, but Pantani – *Il Pirata*, swashbuckling on cycling's high seas, Dumbo the friendless Elephant, or the *artista*, as Armstrong called him – fostered the role of the rejected outsider. Armstrong in turn was an American in an American team, therefore automatically a different entity in a European-oriented sport, and, as one who had survived cancer, something new and unusual and, for many at the time, inspirational. But Armstrong also brought with him other anti-establishment credentials in what seemed to be an increasingly professional and pioneering attitude to the sport, in terms of heavily emphasising specific training techniques, team-building, race reconnaissances, and the like, which Pantani never had. That near-revolution in technology and methodology effectively provided Armstrong with a new layer of credibility to Pantani's 1998 role as a saviour, and (importantly) separated Armstrong from the Italian, making him an inspired and different-sounding voice in the wilderness which triumphed over the conventional, doping plagued approaches of the past. As such, Armstrong the dramatically successful innovator-cum-redeemer was – at least initially although with disastrous long-term consequences – viewed as the sport's fastest way out of its drug-ridden problems.

The figure of cycling's saviour, then, continued and was strengthened by Armstrong after the 1998 Tour. But the pattern of high-profile police actions against or because of doping in cycling established by the 1998 Tour did anything but disappear, either in France or from 1999 onwards in the Giro, too. Professional cycling's constant entanglement with the law courts, a sprawling mass of cases that stretched across western

Europe and which continue to surface, albeit much less frequently, first became truly familiar in the police investigations of the 1998 Tour. To name but a few of the highest profile events, the Giro d'Italia raids of 2001 in San Remo were followed by the scandal surrounding 2002 Tour podium finisher Raimondas Rumšas and the 37 different medical products discovered in his wife Edita's car, which in turn was followed by the Cofidis arrests of 2004 and the fallout from Spain's own mass anti-doping probe, Operación Puerto, in 2006. The one figure who seemed unbreakable in these constantly evolving scandals was, during those bleak years for the sport, Armstrong himself – just as Pantani had appeared to be all the way through the 1998 Tour – with his mantra he had never doped and never tested positive.

It was only in 2006 with Puerto and the positive dope test for Floyd Landis as the Tour de France winner, that the damage to the sport became so extensive that cycling's anti-doping struggle regained the traction that it so badly needed. The UCI, too, has distanced itself hugely from the role it played up to the Armstrong era, and its anti-doping stance is far tougher – another key development. But there is a strong case for arguing that, had the 1998 Tour not happened and without the safeguards already in place, the post-2006 impetus in the fight against banned drugs would have drained away much more quickly, too.

The lack of a definitive EPO test gnawed at cycling's credibility during that era, with the first only coming into effect at the Sydney Olympics in 2000, two years after the events of 1998. Although there are obvious scientific reasons concerning research to explain that delay, for directors of races, it was as Leblanc says, 'a very long time'. Nor, regrettably, was the initial test so straightforward that it immediately began to show clearly who was taking EPO and who was not. As an article published in the *New York Times* in 2005 made clear, after Armstrong's tests for EPO in the 1999

Tour were published, 'The test for EPO, unlike, say, a test for cocaine use, requires skilled interpretation; it is more like reading an X-ray.' It quoted Dr Martial Saugy, head of the anti-doping lab in Lausanne, as saying, 'you are looking at numbers and signals, but in the end what is most important here is the experience of the eyes of an expert. It's the "now we see it, this looks like someone who has injected EPO".' Room for reasonable doubt, therefore, existed and so, too, did the questions, rarely dealt with during this era, of where the line between 'victim' and 'offender' in cycling's battle against banned drugs could or should be drawn.

Leblanc is equally adamant that the Tour was never able to be certain of Armstrong's doping until it was too late. 'Everybody says we should have known. But we trusted the regulations and in accordance with the regulations we made him piss out a sample 50 times and he was 50 times negative, what else was there for us to do or say? You can say "Yes, but he was pedalling like this or like that" ...' – a reference to Armstrong's ability to do stretching exercises on the bike on downhill sections of mountains, a display of physical power taken by some observers to indirectly show something suspicious, 'but give me direct proof. There never was, right up until those posterior tests, ten years afterwards.'

Certainly at the most extreme edges of the fight against doping – such as the tragedies of those who died as a result of banned drug use, or the cynicism of those who willingly used substances to improve performance for purely maximum financial benefit – it is easy to pin labels on riders. But the collateral damage from such a struggle also endured, particularly with weapons that were blunt instruments at best. Even in 2005, WADA was recommending that a second opinion from other laboratories was always in place before announcing a result for the EPO test. Once again, the 1998 Tour de France had already provided a key indicator of how high the cost of that anti-doping war for everybody in the sport, not just the cheats, could be. It's all too often forgotten that alongside the unmasked cheaters were cycling teams, riders and staff that would also lose their livelihoods and their reputations, not to mention see their personal lives potentially wrecked. Some riders from Armstrong's Discovery Channel, for example, were as guilty as the American of doping. But others had their careers tarnished purely by association with that team, when it was conceivable they had never taken banned drugs. From the 1998 Tour onwards, each sweeping generalisation about 'cycling, the tainted sport' saw the innocent, or partially innocent, not to mention their achievements, risk being mown down by the court of public opinion as quickly as the obviously guilty.

This tendency to generalise about cycling did nothing to resolve one of the most urgent questions arising from the 1998 Tour de France, either, which was how the sport would treat those who had been unmasked as cheats. It produced anything but a unified answer. The most obvious split was between Spain's attitude to the expelled racers and the teams that had abandoned the Tour and the way they were considered north of the Pyrenees. It so happened that the first major race to be held after the Tour was the Clásica San Sebastián in Spain on the following Saturday. Laurent Jalabert and the Festina squad were given massive support by local crowds, who mobbed their teams' hotels amidst chants of 'Long live Festina' and 'Now it's time to win'.

'This was a weird race,' Max Sciandri, the one British participant, told *Cycling Weekly* – who ran an editorial that week brightly announcing that, 'Basically, the cycling world has gone mad'. 'Everybody's fed up to the back teeth with everything after what happened in the Tour. They're all sick to death of the season. It was like people were there in body, but their minds were elsewhere.'

Spain was not the only country in which the disgraced Festina riders were treated like all-conquering heroes in a surreal setting where everything looked the same as before the Tour but which had in fact suffered radical, imperceptible changes beneath the surface. In Switzerland, two days after the Tour had ended Alex Zülle, Armin Meier and Laurent Dufaux, Festina's three locally-born components, signed on for their first race, A Travers Lausanne, the town that was home to both the headquarters of the UCI and the IOC, to a warm reception from the crowds. As the *Guardian* pointed out, 'If the trio had wanted to underline the apparent lack of interest on the part of the governing body in punishing them, they could not have chosen a better location.' The UCI regulations stated that the punishment for confessing to banned drug use – considered equal to a positive test in their own rule books – involved up to 12 months' suspension for a first-time offender. But when it was indicated to the UCI that three such riders who had confessed were racing within a stone's throw of their own headquarters, the UCI's anti-doping committee pointed out that any suspension had to be meted out by national federations. The Swiss national federation, meanwhile, said that was unacceptable. So with the buck duly passed, the Festina riders raced on, much to the delight of the local public, some bearing banners proclaiming 'Everybody with Festina' and 'We will always support Dufaux'.

Two other 1998 Tour Festina riders, World Champion Laurent Brochard and Pascal Hervé, had already raced by then, at a criterium in Lisieux, where organisers of the exhibition race presumably thought that, regardless of Brochard's confession, a rider wearing a World Champion's jersey would pull in the crowds. They were right – the crowds were huge. Meanwhile, Virenque received a warm welcome in Germany the following day at the start of the Regio Tour, and the Tour of Portugal, which started eight days after the Tour de France with Festina in their line-up, promised there would be 'no police raids' and just the normal anti-doping tests.

But it was Spain where pro-Festina support really endured. Resentment and anger over the police raids had been whipped up by an influential sector of the Spanish media determined to see the 1998 Tour as an assault on workers' rights, regardless of any doping issues, and the returning teams were subsequently treated as heroic victims. Support committees, most of them short-lived, sprang up across the country to 'defend riders' rights', with organisers of local races, local town councillors and even – ironically enough – the director of one Athletes High Performance Centre signing up. Anti-Tour de France feelings briefly threatened to tip into generalised resentment against French cycling, with one newspaper asking the Crédit Agricole team if they were worried about racing in the Vuelta in September. Fortunately that was as far as it went: a team spokesman said they had 'no reason to doubt the sportsmanship of the organisation or of the Spanish public' and he seemed to be proved right when Casagrande won the Clásica San Sebastián for Cofidis and there were no complaints that he was racing in a French squad.

Even so, for the Spanish a self-imposed boycott on racing on French soil became the short-term norm. The Vuelta, which had a segment of one stage in France that September, promptly altered that day's route to avoid crossing the border and the Spanish Cycling Federation withdrew its team from the Tour de France Féminin, which started on 11 August, too. ONCE, perhaps less surprisingly, withdrew their team from the Tour de l'Avenir, the Tour de Limousin and Paris–Tours, announcing that they would not race again in France that season.

As for ONCE's leader, Jalabert was no less vocal than he had been when he quit the Tour, saying he would 'do the same again,' and rejecting claims that ONCE had quit because they had nothing left to win there. 'At the time of the first strike I could have made it on to the podium,' he pointed out, 'and the day we left the race [the Aix-les-Bains stage] was the ideal one to attack from the gun. But I felt my dignity was more important than the overall classification.'

Whatever the rights and wrongs of Jalabert's arguments, if attitudes towards drugs in cycling in Spain had never been the most aggressive of the anti-doping war, they now softened further. The defence of 'the workers' and a camouflaged defence of doping in some quarters became almost impossible to distinguish. This same attitude endured in Spain right the way through to Operación Puerto in 2006, when riders went on strike – again – at the Spanish National Championships in 'defence of workers' rights', as they put it, when a list of 50 suspects from Operación Puerto was published in the media.

The effect of this blend of self-justification and justified anger was to make Spain a country notorious for its alleged high tolerance towards doping. 'The peninsula remained a sanctuary,' Bassons wrote. 'In Italy, France and Belgium, the authorities were hovering over the cycling scene like vultures. But in Spain the Guardia Civil maintained a respectable distance. Having arrived [at the 1998 Vuelta] in a manic depressive state, the peloton rebuilt its morale in the Andalusian sun. Ultimately, what had been cast as the end of the world was no more than a passing episode. They had been silly to get so worried, and they returned to their old habits. The Vuelta beat all speed records, with one stage run at average of more than 51 kilometres per hour.'

Two decades on it is still not clear how determined the Spanish peloton is when it comes to rooting out doping. As recently as June 2015, Spain's head of what is effectively its anti-doping agency, the AEPSAD, and the former head of the Operación Puerto investigation, Enrique Gómez Bastida, pointed out that since that time cyclists' collaboration with the authorities in anti-doping operations had been minimal, and with no confessions.

'Here the most that has happened is that riders will say, "it happens, but it's nothing to do with me".' Within that context, he called Puerto 'a failure, because [nationally], it's not had the same effect that, on an international level, the Armstrong affair has managed to achieve'. But it's definitely possible to trace a line of thought between Puerto's failure to shake the riders' collective consciousness and the way the Spanish media and the riders had treated the 1998 Tour and its consequences, principally in terms of the riders' tendency to see themselves as victims.

Over the border in France the attitude and lessons learned from the Tour could not have been more different. Contrasts such as these, inspired by events in the Tour de France, were to shape doping, and anti-doping – and, by extension, a significant percentage of results within the sport – from 1998 to 2009. That was the golden age of 'two-speed cycling' – those who presumably doped and those who (allegedly) didn't. 'From 1999, a big part of French cycling changed its philosophy and stopped doping,' Montois says. 'Just look at the results, and with the Française des Jeux team as one of those spearheads of that change, attitudes changed completely. That's not always been the case, look at Italian repeat doper Danilo Di Luca who says he had changed, but in fact didn't. But Française des Jeux and others really did. There was a change of mentality, across the board, and it has to be said it was more due to the sponsors and from inside the team than to the journalists.'

In France there was one new anti-doping weapon, too: longitudinal testing. 'This threw a new stick in the wheel of the dopers. The cycling fraternity regarded this medical oddity with disbelief,' Christophe Bassons wrote. 'The initiative was studied from every possible angle in order to detect a weakness in it, in the way a cat burglar examines a safe before breaking into it.'

Consisting of four detailed medical examinations of a rider every year, any abnormality in their physiological values would lead to a temporary withdrawal of their licence. It would not produce a positive or negative test in the conventional anti-doping manner, rather a preventative measure.

'Initially it sounded great. In reality it meant nothing' is David Millar's blunt analysis in his autobiography. 'There were no sanctions attached to an anomalous longitudinal test and even if a rider's profile suggested doping, there was no way to target them with specific anti-doping controls.' 'Only the gendarmes produce fear,' one French rider of that period, Carlos Da Cruz, said. That was perhaps so in the short term. The *suivi longitudinal*'s importance was ultimately that it contained some key elements of the biological passport, which has widely been seen as a major advance against doping.

Quite apart from the embryonic form of the biological passport, the creation of the *Conseil de Prévention et de Lutte contre le Dopage* (CPLD) – a Council for the Prevention and Fighting Against Doping – added another important layer of legal authority, investigation and anti-doping testing in France. It was also, arguably, the most important feature of the so-called *Loi Buffet*, already grinding its way through French parliament at the time of the 1998 Tour but given fresh impetus and support thanks to the events of July. The CPLD was an independently created nine-person commission that coordinated anti-doping testing and penalties outside the remit of any federation and on any athlete on French soil, be they training or racing. France's one accredited laboratory, at Châtenay-Malabry, remained outside its control, however, and would do so until 2006 when both the CPLD and the laboratory merged under one new organisation, the *Agence Française de Lutte contre le Dopage* (ALFD). Although trafficking for doping was already illegal in France – the investigation into the Festina riders and the other enquiries had taken place under the auspices of the 1989 anti-doping law, the so-called *Loi Bambuck* – the terms were broadened by the *Loi Buffet* to include '*cession et d'offre de produits dopants* [delivery and offering of doping products]'. Significantly, the athletes themselves were not considered criminals.

Indirect evidence that French cycling was taking the anti-doping struggle more seriously than in, say, Spain can be found, too. In 1999, for example, there were no French winners of Tour stages, a first since 1926. Furthermore, as William Fotheringham suggests in his biography of Bernard Hinault, *Bernard Hinault and the Fall and Rise of French Cycling*, following Festina the proportion of French riders or French teams either involved in new police enquiries for haemoglobin boosters such as EPO or testing positive for these drugs is minimal compared to figures at an international level. With the exception of 2004, when the Cofidis drugs investigation erupted, from 1999 to 2012, just one French rider or team out of a total of eight internationally was implicated in a doping affair or positive, and in 2006, the year of the Operación Puerto anti-doping investigation, it was just one in 35. In terms of actual bans for blood-boosting related offences between 1999 and 2010, of 150 only six went to French riders or teams.

Among the French public, it's fair to say that views on doping were deeply divided. In her *L'Equipe* article, Marie-George Buffet claimed that opinion polls in France were in favour of ongoing doping investigations. But others, like David Millar, for example, argued in *Racing Through the Dark* that 'the elderly in France, who'd grown up with the Tour, understood that it was a preposterous sporting challenge. In their pragmatic manner, they didn't see it as being humanly possible, and considered it part and parcel of the job to do what one had to do in order to survive and perform.

'This didn't mean they believed doping was right' – Ms Buffet's opinion polls were correct on that count – 'but for them professional cycling was a brutal sport that only desperate or crazy men would become part of – a "peasant sport" … this was a far cry from the romantic and ultimately naive perspective held by the modern generation of Tour fans. There's no doubt that the older generation's view, no matter how preposterous, was wrong, but was it better to be naive and believe in what was essentially a corporate-funded fraud?'

Yet as Millar now points out, he nonetheless began his 1999 season with hope that there had, in fact, been a sea change in the system. 'I was really happy in 1999, because post-Festina everybody thought the sport was going to clean itself up,' he recalls, 'and in fact when I started there was a sense it already had because I don't think people started on the gear till much later.' For proof, he felt he had the results to show that. 'I killed it, in March or April I was number three in the world, I did really well in the Etoile de Bessèges, got fourth there, third in the GP Chiasso, the Tour of Valencia I got fourth and the KOM [King of the Mountains title], the Critérium International I was second. I was in the final at Milan–San Remo and there was a real sense of hope. Then I saw what was going on with [Cofidis team-mates and notorious dopers Frank] Vandenbroucke and Gaumont and it was, fucking hell, no it hasn't changed.'

When did that fleeting hope of change kick in for Millar? 'For the guys of my generation, we were at training camp in Alsace in July that year [1998], I think, and when we found out that, we were so happy watching the Tour, we were like, "fuck, yeah, it's going to stop, this does mean that we're going to get our opportunity." Because otherwise there was always a certainty, even if you didn't admit it, if you were going to make any progress in the sport, that you were going to have to make a decision [about doping] at some point, whenever it was, because there was no way you were going to win the big races clean. And although you were adamant you were never going to do it, at the back of your mind was always, "how long do you want to stay in this sport?"'

'At that moment, we erased that thought, it was suddenly like, "we're never going to have to think about it". But then the public would be shouting *dopé* when we were training and suddenly we were getting labelled as doped cyclists and we were so pissed off about that, me and David Moncoutie at training camp and Laurent Lefèvre' – like Bassons, and Patrice Halgand, named as one of three clean riders at Festina. 'So 1998 was a glimmer of hope, but then it was extinguished; we realised quickly nobody gave a fuck. It was so fundamentally embedded in the culture, one affair wasn't going to change it.'

Changes, then, were only going to come from the grassroots, as a result of managers or riders changing their policies and attitudes and in particular, in France, that change did come about. But – and this was crucial – it only happened in certain squads. 'Française des Jeux and [Marc] Madiot [sports director] made for a real clean slate, he was the real pioneer,' Millar recounts. 'My team, Cofidis, though, wasn't in the slightest. That's what happened with Vandenbroucke, he saw it as an opportunity and Lance [Armstrong] did, too. It was like, these guys are backing off, let's do this.' Tyler Hamilton describes the post-1998 doping practices very simply. It was, he said, in his autobiography, 'a new era'.

One example of that professionalisation of doping in the 'new era' could be how one of Philippe Gaumont's 'brainwaves' for getting supplies into the Tour in 1998 after the Festina expulsions was repeated in more elaborate form by Hamilton's Postal team in 1999. 'One of the [1998 Tour] riders was a very close friend with one of the motorbike drivers,' Gaumont wrote. 'Against a sum of 10,000 francs ... this motorbike driver accepted to take our cumbersome baggage. One by one we wrote our initials on the ampoules of EPO that belonged to us, then put them all in three or four Thermoses. When we needed some, it was enough to call our motorbike driver.' In 1999, the US Postal 'system' with Motoman, the motorbike driver used privately by Armstrong to bring in fresh supplies of doping material for three weeks – as opposed to three days for Gaumont before he quit – suggests the same supply system, whether or not Armstrong knew of Gaumont's method, had taken on a far more sophisticated form.

***

While the French peloton largely remained cleaner, another sector viewed the 1998 Tour as a lesson learned in a radically different way: to avoid detection, doping had to become more efficient, less high-profile. 'Nobody would have imagined that the worst was to come after 1998, not in terms of quantity, because that was in the 1970s, but in terms of "quality",' Montois says. 'In 1995, everybody was on it, or almost everybody, but in the 2000s there were those riders who took absolutely nothing and those who were chocked up to their eyeballs on EPO. That, to my mind, was the worst; fortunately in 1998 we didn't know that.'

There were those, like Julich, who opted out, but he believes cycling's non-stop calendar of racing made it hard for others to establish a different kind of momentum, and break with old habits. 'I don't think there's a doubt that at least 50 per cent of the peloton realised that "it's over". And that's where the cycling at two speeds came up, and if at the time you thought, "oh, he's just bitching", he was right … You really thought it was going to get better and then in 1999, you realised it just went deeper underground. And then you had a bigger discrepancy.'

The division into *cyclisme à deux vitesses* hardened and broadened as the years went by. 'In 1997 they introduced the 50 per cent hematocrit level because the UCI knew there was an EPO problem, but it was haphazard, people were mostly doing it by themselves, it was almost doping DIY,' Millar says. 'It was always a cynical world, but whereas before 1998 it was part of the culture – but hush-hush, everyone knows but we don't want to know, all eyes wide shut – then suddenly [the attitude changes to] people still know that it's happening, we know it's bad, but we're going to do it anyway and much more professionally. Before it was "get it off your mate" – which still happened, that was how I did it, I got it off a mate. But in other teams it became much more systematic. It was like organised crime.'

'The UCI's "no needle policy" should have been done in 1998. Maybe we should have saved a lot of shit years,' Riis argues, although his own contribution to those blacker years of doping use was apparently not a small one, with his own alleged tolerance of doping inside teams he directed in the early noughties. He does recognise, in any case, that some members of the peloton got scared and therefore eased off their doping in 1998. 'Definitely.'

As Gaumont himself put it in *Prisonnier du dopage*, 'I continued to dope. The only difference was that it wasn't talked about like before. Doping became a question of little clans, groups of riders. Instead of confronting the demons, cycling just bowed its head.'

As a consequence of banned drugs use heading underground, ultimately 1998 represented another step for Jaksche in his learning curve in cycling's nether-world of doping: 'After 1998 I knew I never wanted ever again to be on a team where you had to carry your drugs yourself.' So he joined Telekom. Rather than stamp drugs out, long term the police action had simply reshaped the way he carried out his doping and probably rendered it less detectable.

On the other side of the fence, for Julich, ironically enough the realisation that others would not be sharing in his rejection of doping came when Cofidis riders travelled together for the first *suivi longitudinal* tests. 'That January of 1999 when we started doing the blood tests, I remember we were all bussed from Amiens, where we had our presentation, up to this lab and we all had our blood tests. I remember there were some guys that said, "oh, so you guys have taken everything?" "[I answered] what are you talking about?" and they're like "well, you can't start at 40"' – a reference to the hematocrit threshold established by the UCI, and the only widely known physiological parameter known at the time – 'and then in the season be at 50. But if you start at 50 and every health test is a 50 then you can't say you did anything wrong.' Julich names drugs they highlighted as suffering from this risk as '"cortisone, growth hormone and all this other stuff". And I thought they were kidding, but if you look at the guys who were talking and what has happened to them since, they were serious. They were preparing for that test.'

'The biggest shock was how scared everybody was,' Andreu says. 'There were certainly stories in 1999 that maybe half the peloton would be cleaner, so that would give some people [who doped] more of an advantage.' But he says of the average speed in 1998, 1999, 2000, 'nothing changed at all. It was warp speed. Guys would go for it at the bottom of a climb and just keeping going all the way over the climb and keep going. Now you see a difference, guys wait and wait, they go and go a kilometre and a half, they blow. That is a big difference. For me from 1992 till I stopped it was hanging on for dear life.'

For Andreu, there was a brief period where he felt certain that, 'this was really going to clear things up, wipe the slate clean because it was so shocking. Something that no one expected, a big wake-up call. But it didn't happen.' He went on doping, forming part of Lance Armstrong's Tour-winning team in 1999. 'I saw things hadn't changed that much' was his reasoning at the time, 'because after the [1998] Tour, I didn't take stuff – I didn't need to, you could get through the end of the season. Thing weren't changing, so you just revert to your old habits.'

But whatever option a rider took after 1998, continuing in the sport came at a painfully high price. 'I felt and still feel an immense bitterness, because I thought about what an expensive price so many people have paid for cycling over the last 20 years,' Erwann Menthéour told cycling writer Daniel Friebe. 'I thought of how, when the Festina affair happened, overnight a group of young men who were just doing what they had to do to earn a living suddenly lost all responsibility, all dignity. These were guys riding 35,000 kilometres a year, people were in awe of them and then all of a sudden they were treated like shits. And somewhere, even if they knew that they were only doing what everyone else did, those guys also had to look themselves in the mirror and feel shame, guilt, because that was what everyone was telling them that they should feel.'

Post-1998, those who came off worst, though, were the riders who opted to stay or turn clean, as the realisation sank in that cycling had only partly changed – and that they were set to be on the losing side for the foreseeable future. Riders like Boardman, although in his case, he had been enduring a long defeat since the start of his career.

'I dealt with it [the prevalence of doping] for years,' Boardman argues. 'I was really fortunate that I had one thing I could do that had a value, which was win time trials, albeit short ones, because we [Boardman and his support staff] understood demands of that event about a decade before anybody else.'

As the 1990s dragged on and systematic doping kicked in harder and harder to cycling, Boardman says, 'Racing became really unpredictable. For years even though you suspect things yourself, see things yourself that just look wrong, there's no evidence, it's not like people are going to talk about it over a beer, so you're scrabbling for ways to find why it is your fault, "what can I do different, can I get super-lean?" and so on.

'Really it was all out of my control, but I had my one space [the prologues] that belonged to me, that I could control, but by the end of the 1990s, I didn't even have that ... What was I, eighth in the the last Tour prologue I rode? Even that wasn't possible. So everything was just miserable. I never have been one to look back, you just get bitter and twisted, so you focus on what you can do. So that's what I did, focus on what I could do in that environment.'

'Before, everyone was doing it, when it was out in the open, it was fair,' Julich now argues in his account of how, as a non-doper, he lived through what Montois describes as cycling's darkest period post-1998.

'But you were still thinking, "they're going to get caught" and then a year went by and two years went by and the same things were happening, it just became either you suck it up and deal with getting dropped, which is what I did, or you go back over to the dark side and have to live that life of smoke and mirrors and lies again.'

There were points, Julich says, when he almost went back on his decision not to dope again – a situation numerous riders must have found themselves in during that era, what he calls 'foggy days'. 'It was hard to take, because I was left, forgotten about. You guys never called me or interviewed me but for good reason.

'I remember having this conversation with Floyd after a Tour of Georgia stage (in 2005) where he got into a big fight with Lance, it was ridiculous, like two little kids, and afterwards I'm in the food room and Dave Zabriskie's on the table getting a rub [massage], and Floyd walks in to see Dave cos he was friends with Dave. And Floyd says, "I can't believe Lance is saying this about me, and yelling at me because"' – and Julich emphasises the words – '"*we're all doing the same thing*".'

The barrier, the gap between the dopers and the non-dopers, could not have been more obvious for Julich at that point. 'I looked at him and I said, "that's where you guys are fucked up because, no, Floyd, we're not all doing the same thing." So that was the thing that was frustrating, specially with the Americans, we all thought that everyone was doing something that maybe they weren't. Or if I'm not doing it, I'd better do it because of him.' He compares the scenario among the American riders as 'like high school girls in a locker room', a situation aggravated personally by a team-mate based in Girona giving him updates on the banned drugs 'situation' such as '"they're hiding 'it' in the cereal box" and all this stuff ...' Julich's career spiralled steadily downwards, in what was a mirror image of fellow American and former team-mate Armstrong's succession of Tour wins at the time, and in what is effectively a painful reflection of the underlying reality of a sport that in theory had been 'saved' by the Texan.

A revival of the career of the rider once tipped as the next Greg LeMond came when he had reached a dead end, and Armstrong had taken five Tours. 'When I basically had no job, Bjarne Riis [in 2004, with CSC] offered me the same money, €25,000, as back when I signed up as a neo pro with Motorola in 1995.' Julich describes the day he signed for CSC as an 'epiphany moment' but points out that 'It took for me to have nothing to say "what am I doing this sport for?" And I wasn't finished, people were telling me that I was this once good guy and I'm not good any more because I had made these decisions [doped until 1998], but I knew it was more in my head than anything.'

Aside from tumultuous personal odysseys like Julich's – who would win Paris–Nice in 2005, the year of Armstrong's seventh Tour, before retiring – *cyclisme à deux vitesses* had other effects. As part of the increasingly efficient use of doping, Gaumont also commented that this was the start of media training in Cofidis. The new party line to be trotted out at interviews, he said, was, 'Festina has opened up our eyes, thanks to it we've changed, cycling is changing.'

Rolf Aldag echoes that, pointing out that 'Up until 1998 you wouldn't have had that pressure, the situation between riders and journalists was friendly, they'd all hang out, you talk. But from 1998 onwards, there was an understanding that it was part of the job [asking questions about doping] but there was still an attitude among journalists of, 'then OK, we have to do this question about doping, I come back in the interview to the sport in a minute. But will they be super-hard on us? No.

'There are three periods. In the Tour 1998 they would still be like, "there was still no evidence against us, everybody in Germany liked to believe that in Ullrich we have a national hero. But they don't expect a correct answer, I'm a journalist, I'm just doing this to make me, the journalist, sound more credible.' After the race there were signs of increasing doubt, but only up to a limit. 'From then to 2006, I ask the anti-doping question and it's done.' But after Operación Puerto, Aldag says, the attitude moved to a much more hardline, arbitrary attitude among the German press of, 'the sport is not clean anyway, I already know the answer to my question and it's all bullshit'.

Overall, though, it was perhaps inevitable that for many riders and team staff, 1998 marked an end of an era where being a bike rider was something of which you could automatically feel proud. Bassons recalls, that July, the other guests' embarrassed silence in his hotel dining room, because they knew he was a Festina rider. And it was not just the peloton itself: '1998 went from being a year in which you were proud to be driving a team car, to being one in which you knew you'd have an 80 per cent possibility of being stopped by the police,' Saiz says. The effects stretched into Saiz's personal life, too. 'It's true that up to then I'd been a person who slept little but well and after that [1998] I slept little but badly. But I don't have to say I love the Tour. That's inside me and I don't care what the rest say. I know what my feelings are.'

As for the legally charged 'villains' of the 1998 Tour, France's police enquiries continued unabated. A week after the race had finished TVM soigneur Jan Moors became the third member of the team's management to face drugs charges, along with Cees

Priem, the team manager, and Andrei Mikhailov, the team doctor. All six riders who pulled out of the Tour, meanwhile, visited Reims court to declare in the case.

The Festina riders and team staff found themselves with cases to answer to both the sporting and legal authorities. Regarding the former, the three Swiss riders faced risibly small sanctions for their confessions: Alex Zülle, Armin Meier and Laurent Dufaux were each given an eight-month suspension, later reduced to seven months, and were fined 3,000 Swiss francs (£1,360) apiece. Roussel was banned from directing for five years, although that suspension was later rescinded. Brochard, Moreau and Rous all received six-month bans in November 1998, after their confessions to the French police. Voet, in a suspension that was widely viewed as overly severe in comparison, was barred from working as a soigneur for three years. (He has since quit the sport, and has gone back to bus driving.)

Police questioning of top figures in the sport in March 1999, including Jean-Marie Leblanc and French Federation president Daniel Baal, proved totally inconsequential in the mid-to-long-term, but nonetheless helped maintain the impression that cycling was under severe scrutiny.

The crunch moment came when Richard Virenque finally confessed in the Festina trial in October 2000 that he had used banned drugs. 'It was like a train going away from me, and if I didn't get on it, I would be left behind,' he said at the time. 'It was not cheating. I wanted to remain in the family.' Pascal Hervé, too, also used the trial to confess his guilt, saying – and echoing Virenque's line that they were scapegoats – 'I would have done it earlier if it had not been just us nine idiots who had been caught.'

Virenque had maintained his innocence up to the last moment, even denying his guilt in the court's opening session. But his repeated denials were left exposed by both Voet and Roussel's confirmations that this could not be the case. Matters were not helped by a fresh doping scandal in May that entangled his lawyer, Bernard Lavelot. Police said at the time that Virenque had cracked and confessed, although he later apparently backtracked, and went on to take a stage win in the Giro d'Italia.

By this point, for many Virenque had become a caricature. 'He saw himself as the victim because everybody laughed at him, but they weren't laughing at him, they were laughing at how the myth had fallen apart and, for two years, Virenque was unable to admit that he had doped,' argues Montois. 'His sense of injustice is understandable – others got off scot-free – but to call himself a victim, I think that's excessive.' Furthermore, had Virenque merely admitted to doping and moved on, he would have been able to put it behind him much more quickly: it was the denial that kept him in the news, where, coincidentally or not, he liked to be.

Following his confession, as the only rider charged by the court Virenque was cleared of actively organising doping. But he did not get off so lightly from his sports federation, being banned for nine months and fined £2,000, and did not ride his bike for four months. By March 2001 he was overweight, and after a drastic diet he finally secured a contract for the last quarter of the season for the minimum wage of €1,000 a month. He continued to ride until 2004, winning more stages in the Tour as well as wearing the yellow jersey for one last time.

The trial – shortly after which the UCI insisted yet again that they had 'no reason to believe that the model of behaviour followed by and discovered in the Festina team in 1998 is widespread' – also saw the legal punishments meted out. Voet was given a suspended ten-month jail sentence and fined 30,000 French francs (£2,390), Jef D'Hont received a nine-month suspended sentence for encouraging doping, Roussel received a one-year suspended sentence and a fine of 50,000 French francs (£4,880),

Christine Paranier and her husband Eric, the couple running the chemist's in Veynes where Voet would buy products for Festina, were fined €4,000 and €1,500, while Jean Dalibot, a Festina soigneur, and Joel Chabiron, the logistics manager, received a five-month suspended sentence. The case against Rijckaert was dropped completely on account of his ill health and he died of cancer a month later. 'The facts would have been enough to justify jail terms,' the court ruling said. 'But the court took other factors into account, especially the widespread recourse to doping and the failings of the fight against doping.' The only other individual facing prosecution, ONCE medic Nicolás Terrados, charged with importing four banned medical products without French customs authorisation, was initially given a €4,573 fine. Terrados fought on to clear his name completely and, in March 2002, a court in Douai absolved him of all charges.

Far from folding at the end of the 1998 season, Festina the team continued apace, albeit with a vastly reduced budget, slashed by 60 per cent. While Virenque moved on to an Italian squad, Polti, three of the Festina riders, Pascal Hervé, Christophe Moreau and Didier Rous remained. Festina finally called it a day in 2001, but not before winning their first ever Grand Tour that year, the Vuelta a España, with Spain's Ángel Luis Casero. As for TVM, in July 2001 – the same day that Lance Armstrong took a race-winning triumph in stage 10 of the Tour de France – Cees Priem was given an 18-month suspended sentence and fine of 80,000 French francs, doctor Andrei Mikhailov was given a 12-month suspended sentence and 60,000 franc fine, while Jan Moors, the team soigneur, was given a six-month suspended sentence and 40,000 franc fine. The three were also fined a total of 50,000 francs for customs violations. None of the riders from the Tour were charged. TVM-Farm Frites continued as a squad, only without the transport company's backing from the end of 1999 and relying on the support of its former secondary sponsor, Farm Frites, until 2001. It then merged with an Italo-Belgian team, Mapei, the following year.

With the exception of Voet, the penalties, compared with the damage the cases had done to the sport, seemed risibly small – until it is remembered that they were the tip of a very large iceberg, which remained at least partly invisible. The real individual price, though, was largely in terms of reputations, while for the sport the immense cost was to its credibility.

'Festina, though, what happened with them, they took one on the chin for the entire peloton,' Julich says. 'That could so easily have happened to any team. Virenque doing that drama and crying, that could have been any of us. You heard tales, though, of guys like Zülle, keeping the lights on and cavity searches and being alone in a foreign jail and it was like – OK, it's over. Those guys indirectly helped change the sport, particularly for the French peloton at that time.'

During the 2014 Tour de France, I went to see Richard Virenque. One of my two reasons for doing so was to ask him for an interview about the Festina affair. It would be the first time I had talked to him since 2002, but I was hopeful.

With about two hours left to race on a Pyrenean stage, he emerged, bronzed and smiling, from the commentary box where he was working and waved me across. The rain began to fall as we stood there. But despite the shower the former Festina leader was initially happy to talk about the French renaissance in cycling in the 2014 Tour. (Thibaut Pinot and Jean-Christophe Péraud were both battling for the podium for the first time, raising the possibility of a first French top-three position since Virenque had finished second in 1997.)

After Virenque had delivered some fairly anodyne insights on the current situation in French cycling, when I proposed to him that we could – after the Tour – do an interview about Festina, his face hardened noticeably and he half turned away.

'There's been too much talk about that,' he said. 'We were scapegoats, the rest continued doing what they wanted.' He continued in the same vein for a further two minutes. Could I call him for an interview, then? 'No,' he said and walked away.

Not everybody is so uncommunicative about their past involvement in Festina. Last year Laurent Brochard described his feelings.

'You're not a drug addict, but it's an illogical situation,' he told the magazine *Pédale*. 'You're taking products you don't need, you're hiding away to do it, you're obliged to lie about what you do. It's hard to live that sort of scenario.'

Asked specifically about 1998 and the year of the Festina scandal, he was, he said, 'still ashamed of that history. It comes back all the time. I'm not at all proud of it. I burned all my jerseys. In a fire outside. It was symbolic. The clothes, the extra bits of race kit, everything. I burned the lot.'

The smoke from the burning embers of the 1998 Tour de France continues to billow through the sport. Ask Servais Knaven, part of the TVM team in 1998, a director with Sky and whose physiological data during the race, collected by the Reims investigation, were alleged by one newspaper as recently as March 2015 'to have raised fresh doubts about alleged historic doping'. (For the record, Sky insisted that, in the view of three independent anti-doping experts who reviewed the case, 'on the basis of what has been presented to us … there is no proof of doping and Servais continues to maintain his innocence'). Equally there can be no doubt that much of the questioning of Sky's dominance in the Tour partly has its roots in the credibility gap established by the Armstrong era. But the overarching philosophy behind the remorseless lines of questioning, the 'why should we believe in you?' question asked by the same American reporter to almost every standout Tour performer of the last five years, the original point at which the tentacles of doubt first showed themselves – that all stretches back to 1998.

It is impossible to establish exactly where the total sum of the suspicion, the credibility gaps, the damaged prestige from 1998 ends, and where the fallout and damage caused by later scandals, particularly (but not only) that of Armstrong, begins. Does it matter? As Andreu put it in 2014, 'it's the same predicament [post-1998] as they have right now. A new positive case completely tarnishes everything. I'm not naive enough to think that everybody's clean but when somebody from the younger generation does, then you think "man, this is screwing up again". The sport still has a black cloud over it.'

'It's been ten years since the Festina scandal but ten years is simply not long enough to change a system which is so deep-rooted,' said the French anti-doping campaigner Jean-Pierre de Mondenard in 2008. 'It will take at least 25 years for attitudes towards doping to radically change.'

Yet, as Julich sees it, there had to be a starting point where those changes began, and that was when the police stopped a carload of drugs on the Franco–Belgian border, just days before the Tour de France began. 'For these generations, we have to look back at the 1998 Tour de France and say, "OK, things weren't handled perfectly, but it was where the rose-coloured glasses came off for a lot of people". And if we hadn't had the Willy Voet and the Festina affair, where would we be right now? As uncomfortable as it is, talking about that period, it was a very important race, maybe not for our generation, because our generation was tainted, but for this future generation that we can only hope to keep away from those decisions that we all had to make at that time. That's when you have to look the guys in the face and say, "I'm so glad you don't have to make those decisions. And you'd better stay on the line and not screw things up because we were very much on the limit there for a very long time."'

'I think it [the 1998 Tour] needed to happen,' reflects Boardman. 'At the risk of getting overly philosophical, in the 1980s money starts coming into the sport, LeMond is the first person to get a million dollar contract, and cycling starts to get more and more value. When money comes along, people take risks, and then how do you get back [to a sport's original values]?'

Boardman calls the 1998 Tour 'the start of something' – and if it represented a dramatic change compared with the past – 'everybody has to go through the same process.' He likens the process of cycling's coming to terms with its doping past to the emotions that follow a traumatic death of a close relative or friend.

'Ask anyone who counsels somebody through grief: stage one' – as it was so often in a doping scandal – 'is denial, stage two is anger, stage three is blame someone else, stage four is blame yourself, stage five is accept and look for solutions. You can't break the cycle of that process.' Each scandal may have repeated the cycle. But each step towards recovery has to be taken.

Even with the impact and media attention on the Armstrong years, the 1998 Tour therefore remains a live issue, the point where the balls that gathered pace in the US Postal-Tour era – from the doping scandals through to the saviour figures and the mistrust around the sport – began truly to roll. It is certain that the confessions and discoveries about banned drug use now reach back to previous seasons and previous Tours. But the fact that the 1998 Tour itself came so seriously under threat during the actual race allows it to mark a psychological borderline between the years where cycling could tap into seemingly instant credibility and the years where it knew any top performer – right up to Chris Froome in 2015 – would face a degree of instant doubt. The 1998 Tour was the first year that images of police raiding team hotels, standing guard over vehicles and leading away riders and management became a sadly familiar feature of bike races. No further revelations of doping will change that.

Rather than excessively centring on one individual or even one squad – for all Virenque may think otherwise – in fact the 1998 scandal's near-universal nature, the way it reached out and affected team after team, is what makes it so important. Later accounts of scandals have tended to zoom in on Armstrong with his rivals treated almost as film extras. But the 1998 Tour shows that the decisions Armstrong was taking over doping were more general, although that does not automatically mean, as he says, that those decisions only had one answer.

There were other answers for those brave enough to look for them, and, indeed, for those who cheated as well. Doping is a question of shades of grey. The rider in a top-ranked team who told me and another journalist in 1996 on the Tour's rest day that he was taking EPO in small doses was not a high-flyer. He never won a stage of a Grand Tour or a major Classic. Could he have done so if he took as much EPO and other drugs as Armstrong? Probably not, but we shall never know for sure, and that is what the 1998 Tour established once and for all. Professional cycling was anything but a level playing field. Once we knew that, we started to appreciate what the players – clean, doped or somewhere in a murky grey area in between – were capable of doing on that distorted field from a radically different perspective. It is sometimes an unpleasant perspective, sometimes one that can be seen as negative, but it is one that should not be pushed aside too quickly, either – if only to ensure races like the 1998 Tour de France do not happen again.

Where are They Now?

Rolf Aldag: Retired from racing in 2005. Working as a cycling team manager.

Frankie Andreu: Retired from racing in 2000. Working as a TV commentator and team director.

Christophe Bassons: Retired from racing in 2001. Working as a coach and writer near Bordeaux.

Laurent Jalabert: Retired from racing in 2002. Working as a TV commentator.

Joerg Jaksche: Retired from racing in 2007. Returned to university, working in business and economics in Australia.

Bobby Julich: Retired from racing 2008. Working as a cycling coach.

Jean-Marie Leblanc: Retired in 2006 from directing the Tour de France.

David Millar: Retired from racing in 2014. Working as a writer, designer and commentator.

Jean Montois: Continues to report on the Tour de France and cycling for AFP.

Marco Pantani: Retired from racing in 2003. Died of a cocaine overdose in February 2004.

Bjarne Riis: Retired from racing in 2000, now a team director.

Erik Rijckaert: Festina doctor, died 2001.

Bruno Roussel: Trainer with the National Mexican track squad.

Manolo Saiz: Lost his job as director in the fallout from Operación Puerto's anti-doping probe in 2006. Cleared of all charges. Now running a small Spanish team.

Hein Verbruggen: Ended his presidency of the UCI in 2005. Remains an honorary president.

Richard Virenque: Retired from racing in 2004. Now a TV cycling commentator and still advertising watches for Festina.

Willy Voet: Last heard of working as a bus driver in southern France.

1998 Tour de France: Start List

DNS = did not start that day's stage. DNF = did not finish that day's stage. DSQ = disqualified. HD = outside time limit.

TEAM DEUTSCHE TELEKOM
1 ULLRICH Jan (Ger)
2 ALDAG Rolf (Ger)
3 BÖLTS Udo (Ger)
4 FRATTINI Francesco (Ita)
5 HENN Christian (Ger)
6 HEPPNER Jens (Ger)
7 RIIS Bjarne (Den)
8 TOTSCHNIG Georg (Aut)
9 ZABEL Erik (Ger)

FESTINA
11 VIRENQUE Richard (Fra) excluded stage 7
12 BROCHARD Laurent (Fra) excluded stage 7
13 DUFAUX Laurent (Swi) excluded stage 7
14 HERVÉ Pascal (Fra) excluded stage 7
15 MEIER Armin (Swi) excluded stage 7
16 MOREAU Christophe (Fra) excluded stage 7
17 ROUS Didier (Fra) excluded stage 7

18 STEPHENS Neil (Aus) excluded stage 7
19 ZÜLLE Alex (Swi) excluded stage 7
(The entire team is excluded from the Tour for organised doping on stage 7)

MERCATONE UNO-BIANCHI
21 PANTANI Marco (Ita)
22 BARBERO Sergio (Ita) DNF stage 15
23 BORGHERESI Simone (Ita)
24 CONTI Roberto (Ita)
25 FONTANELLI Fabiano (Ita)
26 FORCONI Riccardo (Ita)
27 KONYSHEV Dimitri (Rus) DNF stage 10
28 PODENZANA Massimo (Ita)
29 TRAVERSONI Mario (Ita)

MAPEI-BRICOBI
31 BALLERINI Franco (Ita) DNF stage 16
32 DI GRANDE Giuseppe (Ita)
33 LEYSEN Bart (Bel)
34 NARDELLO Daniele (Ita)
35 PEETERS Wilfried (Bel)
36 STEELS Tom (Bel)
37 SVORADA Ján (Cze) DNF stage 16
38 TAFI Andrea (Ita)
39 ZANINI Stefano (Ita)

ONCE-DEUTSCHE BANK
41 JALABERT Laurent (Fra) DNF stage 17
42 BRUYNEEL Johan (Bel) DNF stage 10
43 DIAZ JUSTO Rafael (Spa) DNF stage 17
44 DIAZ ZABALA Herminio (Spa) DNF stage 17
45 GARCÍA Marcelino (Spa) DNF stage 17
46 MAULEÓN Francisco Javier (Spa) DNF stage 17
47 MAURI Melcior (Spa) DNF stage 17

48 PÉREZ RODRÍGUEZ Luis (Spa) DNF stage 17
49 SIERRA Roberto (Spa) DNF stage 17
(The entire team abandons on stage 17)

RABOBANK

51 BOOGERD Michael (Hol)
52 DEKKER Erik (Hol) DNF stage 2
53 DEN BAKKER Maarten (Hol)
54 JONKER Patrick (Hol)
55 MOERENHOUT Koos (Hol)
56 VAN BON Léon (Hol)
57 McEWEN Robbie (Aus)
58 VIERHOUTEN Aart (Hol)
59 ZBERG Beat (Swi)

CASINO

61 HAMBURGER Bo (Den)
62 AGNOLUTTO Christophe (Fra)
63 BARTHE Stéphane (Fra) DNF stage 18
64 CHANTEUR Pascal (Fra)
65 DURAND Jacky (Fra)
66 ELLI Alberto (Ita)
67 KIRSIPUU Jaan (Est) DNF stage 10
68 MASSI Rodolfo (Ita) DNS stage 18
69 SALMON Benoît (Fra)
Following his arrest, Massi fails to start stage 18.

BANESTO

71 OLANO Abraham (Spa) DNF stage 11
72 ALONSO Marino (Spa) DNF stage 17
73 ARRIETA José Luis (Spa) DNF stage 15
74 BELTRÁN Manuel (Spa) DNF stage 17
75 GARCÍA ACOSTA José Vicente (Spa) DNF stage 17
76 JIMÉNEZ José María (Spa) DNF stage 16

77 PEÑA Miguel Ángel (Spa) DNF stage 17

78 RODRIGUES Orlando Sergio (Por) DNF stage 17

79 SOLAUN César (Spa) DNF stage 17

The entire team quits on stage 17

GAN

81 BOARDMAN Christopher (GBR) DNF stage 2

82 BÄCKSTEDT Magnus (Swe)

83 MONCASSIN Frédéric (Fra) DNF stage 10

84 O'GRADY Stuart (Aus)

85 POLI Eros (Ita)

86 SEIGNEUR Eddy (Fra) HD stage 15

87 SIMON François (Fra)

88 VASSEUR Cédric (Fra)

89 VOIGT Jens (Ger)

LOTTO-MOBISTAR

91 MADOUAS Laurent (Fra)

92 FARAZJIN Peter (Bel)

93 LAUKKA Joona (Fin) DNS stage 13

94 TCHMIL Andrei (Bel) DNS stage 16

95 TETERIOUK Andrei (Kaz)

96 VAN DE WOUWER Kurt (Bel)

97 VAN HYFTE Paul (Bel)

98 VERBRUGGHE Rik (Bel)

99 VERHEYEN Geert (Bel)

TVM-FARM FRITES

101 ROUX Laurent (Fra) DNF stage 10

102 BLIJLEVENS Jeroen (Hol) DNF stage 18

103 DE JONGH Steven (Hol) DNS stage 19

104 IVANOV Sergei (Rus) DNS stage 19

105 KNAVEN Servais (Hol) DNS stage 19

106 MICHAELSEN Lars (Den) DSQ stage 11

107 OUTSCHAKOV Sergei (Ukr) DNS stage 19
108 VAN PETEGEM Peter (Bel) DNF stage 15
109 VOSKAMP Bart (Hol) DNS stage 19
The team did not start stage 19

SAECO-CANNONDALE
111 CIPOLLINI Mario (Ita) DNF stage 9
112 CALCATERRA Giuseppe (Ita) DNF stage 16
113 DONATI Massimo (Ita)
114 FAGNINI Gianmatteo (Ita) DNF stage 10
115 FORNACIARI Paolo (Ita)
116 MAZZOLENI Eddy (Ita)
117 MORI Massimiliano (Ita)
118 PIEPOLI Leonardo (Ita)
119 SCIREA Mario (Ita) DNF stage 10

LA FRANÇAISE DES JEUX
121 BERZIN Evgeni (Rus)
122 BOUYER Franck (Fra)
123 GUESDON Frédéric (Fra)
124 HEULOT Stéphane (Fra)
125 JAN Xavier (Fra)
126 MAGNIEN Emmanuel (Fra) DNF stage 10
127 MENGIN Christophe (Fra)
128 NAZON Damien (Fra)
129 SCIANDRI Maximilian (GBR) DNS stage 18

COFIDIS
131 CASAGRANDE Francesco (Ita) DNF stage 10
132 DESBIENS Laurent (Fra)
133 GAUMONT Philippe (Fra) DNF stage 10
134 JALABERT Nicolas (Fra)
135 JULICH Bobby (USA)
136 LELLI Massimiliano (Ita)

137 LIVINGSTON Kevin (USA)
138 MEIER Roland (Swi)
139 RINERO Christophe (Fra)

TEAM POLTI
141 LEBLANC Luc (Fra) DNF stage 18
142 BRASI Rossano (Ita)
143 CREPALDI Mirko (Ita)
144 GUIDI Fabrizio (Ita) DNF stage 6
145 GUIDI Leonardo (Ita) DNF stage 15
146 JAKSCHE Joerg (Ger)
147 MARTINELLO Silvio (Ita) DNF stage 6
148 MERCKX Axel (Bel)
149 SACCHI Fabio (Ita)

ASICS-CGA
151 BIANCHI Carlo-Marino (Ita) DNF stage 10
152 BONGIONI Alessio (Ita) DNF stage 9
153 FERRARI Diego (Ita)
154 POZZI Oscar (Ita)
155 ROSCIOLI Fabio (Ita)
156 SCHIAVINA Samuele (Ita) DNF stage 4
157 SHEFER Alexandr (Kaz) DNF stage 10
158 SIMEONI Filippo (Ita)
159 TURICCHIA Alain (Ita)

VITALICIO SEGUROS
161 BLANCO Santiago (Spa) DNS stage 18
162 BENITEZ Francisco (Spa) DNS stage 18
163 BUENAHORA Hernan (Col) DNF stage 10
164 CASERO Luis Ángel (Spa) DNS stage 18
165 FERRIGATO Andrea (Ita) DNS stage 18
166 GARCÍA David (Spa) DNF stage 10
167 GARCIA Francisco Tomás (Spa) DNF stage 5

168 INDURAIN Prudencio (Spa) DNS stage 18
169 RINCÓN Oliverio (Col) HD stage 8
The entire team quits after stage 17

KELME-COSTA BLANCA

171 ESCARTÍN Fernando (Spa) DNS stage 18
172 CABELLO Francisco (Spa) DNS stage 18
173 CONTRERAS Carlos Alberto (Col) DNF stage 10
174 DE LOS ÁNGELES Juan José (Spa) DNF stage 15
175 GÓMEZ José Javier (Spa) DNS stage 18
176 GONZALEZ Santos (Spa) DNS stage 18
177 RODRIGUEZ José Luis (Spa) DNF stage 16
178 SERRANO Marcos Antonio (Spa) DNS stage 18
179 VIDAL José Ángel (Spa) DNS stage 18
The entire team did not start stage 18

US POSTAL SERVICE

181 ROBIN Jean-Cyril (Fra)
182 ANDREU Frankie (USA)
183 BARANOWSKI Dariusz (Pol)
184 DERAMÉ Pascal (Fra)
185 EKIMOV Viatcheslav (Rus)
186 HAMILTON Tyler (USA)
187 HINCAPIE George (USA)
188 JEMISON Marty (USA)
189 MEINERT-NIELSEN Peter (Den)

RISO SCOTTI-MG MAGLIFICIO

191 BALDATO Fabio (Ita) DNF stage 15
192 BOBRIK Vladislav (Rus) DNF stage 11
193 BRIGNOLI Ermanno (Ita) DNF stage 17
194 CARUSO Roberto (Ita) DNF stage 10
195 CASAGRANDA Stefano (Ita) DNF stage 10
196 DE BENI Federico (Ita) DNF stage 4

197   MINALI Nicola (Ita) DNF stage 17
198   PISTORE Roberto (Ita) HD stage 8
199   SPEZIALETTI Alessandro (Ita) DNF stage 17
The entire team abandons on stage 17

BIG MAT-AUBER 93

201   LINO Pascal (Fra)
202   AUGER Ludovic (Fra) DNS stage 2
203   BORDENAVE Philippe (Fra)
204   BOURGUIGNON Thierry (Fra)
205   DJAVANIAN Viatcheslav (Rus)
206   GOUVENOU Thierry (Fra)
207   LEBRETON Lylian (Fra)
208   LEPROUX Denis (Fra)
209   SIVAKOV Alexei (Rus)

The 1998 Tour de France Stage Winners and Final Classification

Saturday, 11 July. Prologue: Dublin: 5.6 km (individual time trial) – Chris Boardman (GB) GAN

Sunday, 12 July. Stage 1: Dublin–Dublin: 180.5 km – Tom Steels (Bel) Mapei

Monday, 13 July. Stage 2: Enniscorthy–Cork: 205.5 km – Ján Svorada (Cze) Mapei

Tuesday, 14 July. Stage 3: Roscoff–Lorient: 169 km – Jens Heppner (Ger) Telekom

Wednesday, 15 July. Stage 4: Plouay–Cholet: 252 km – Jeroen Blijlevens (Ned) TVM

Thursday, 16 July. Stage 5: Cholet–Châteauroux: 228.5 km – Mario Cipollini (Ita) Saeco

Friday, 17 July. Stage 6: La Châtre–Brive-la-Gaillarde: 204.5 km – Mario Cipollini (Ita) Saeco

Saturday, 18 July. Stage 7: Meyrignac l'Eglise–Corrèze: 58 km (individual time trial) – Jan Ullrich (Ger) Telekom

Sunday, 19 July. Stage 8: Brive-la-Gaillarde–Montauban: 190.5 km – Jacky Durand (Fra) Casino

Monday, 20 July. Stage 9: Montauban–Pau: 210 km – Léon van Bon (Ned) Rabobank

Tuesday, 21 July. Stage 10: Pau–Luchon: 196.5 km – Rodolfo Massi (Ita) Casino

Wednesday, 22 July. Stage 11: Luchon–Plateau de Beille: 170 km – Marco Pantani (Ita) Mercatone Uno

Thursday, 23 July: Rest Day

Friday, 24 July. Stage 12: Tarascon-sur-Ariège–Le Cap d'Agde: 222 km – Tom Steels (Bel) Mapei

Saturday, 25 July. Stage 13: Frontignan-la-Peyrade–Carpentras: 196 km – Daniele Nardello (Ita) Mapei

Sunday, 26 July. Stage 14: Valréas–Grenoble: 186.5 km – Stuart O'Grady (Aus) GAN

Monday, 27 July. Stage 15: Grenoble–Les Deux Alpes: 189 km – Marco Pantani (Ita) Mercatone Uno

Tuesday, 28 July. Stage 16: Vizille–Albertville: 204 km – Jan Ullrich (Ger) Telekom

Wednesday, 29 July. Stage 17: Albertville–Aix-les-Bains: 149 km – cancelled

Thursday, 30 July. Stage 18: Aix-les-Bains–Neuchâtel: 218 km – Tom Steels (Bel) Mapei

Friday, 31 July. Stage 19: La Chaux-de-Fonds–Autun: 242 km – Magnus Bäckstedt (Swe) GAN

Saturday, 1 August. Stage 20: Montceau-les-Mines–Le Creusot: 52 km (individual time trial) – Jan Ullrich (Ger) Telekom

Sunday, 2 August. Stage 21: Melun–Paris: 147.5 km – Tom Steels (Bel) Mapei

Final GC

1 Marco Pantani (Ita) Mercatone Uno 92h 49' 46"
2 Jan Ullrich (Ger) Telekom at 3' 21"
3 Bobby Julich (USA) Cofidis at 4' 08"
4 Christophe Rinero (Fra) Cofidis at 9' 16"
5 Michael Boogerd (Ned) Rabobank at 11' 26"
6 Jean-Cyril Robin (Fra) US Postal at 14' 57"
7 Roland Meier (Swi) Cofidis at 15' 13"

8   Daniele Nardello (Ita) Mapei at 16′ 07″

9   Giuseppe Di Grande (Ita) Mapei at 17′ 35″

10   Axel Merckx (Bel) Polti at 17′ 39″

11   Bjarne Riis (Den) Telekom at 19′ 10″

12   Dariusz Baranowski (Pol) US Postal at 19′ 58″

13   Stéphane Heulot (Fra) La Française des Jeux at 20′ 57″

14   Leonardo Piepoli (Ita) Saeco at 22′ 45″

15   Bo Hamburger (Den) Casino at 26′ 39″

16   Kurt Van de Wouwer (Bel) Lotto at 27′ 20″

17   Kevin Livingston (USA) Cofidis at 34′ 03″

18   Joerg Jaksche (Ger) Polti at 35′ 41″

19   Peter Farazijn (Bel) Lotto at 36′ 10″

20   Andrei Teteriouk (Kaz) Lotto at 37′ 03″

21   Udo Bölts (Ger) Telekom at 37-25″

22   Laurent Madouas (Fra) Lotto at 39′ 54″

23   Geert Verheyen (Bel) Lotto at 41′ 23″

24   Cédric Vasseur (Fra) GAN at 42′ 14″

25   Evgeni Berzin (Rus) La Française des Jeux at 42′ 51″

26   Thierry Bourguignon (Fra) Big Mat at 43′ 53″

27   Georg Totschnig (Aut) Telekom at 50′ 13″

28   Benoît Salmon (Fra) Casino at 51′ 18″

29   Alberto Elli (Ita) Casino at 1h 00′ 13″

30   Philippe Bordenave (Fra) Big Mat at 1h 05′ 55″

31   Christophe Agnolutto (Fra) Casino at 1h 11′ 03″

32   Oscar Pozzi (Ita) Asics at 1h 14′ 54″

33   Maarten Den Bakker (Ned) Rabobank at 1h 16′ 21″

34   Patrick Jonker (Aus) Rabobank at 1h 16′ 49″

35   Pascal Chanteur (Fra) Casino at 1h 19′ 32″

36   Massimiliano Lelli (Ita) Cofidis at 1h 20′ 15″

37   Massimo Podenzana (Ita) Mercatone Uno at 1h 20′ 47″

38   Viatcheslav Ekimov (Rus) US Postal at 1h 22′ 40″

39   Denis Leproux (Fra) Big Mat at 1h 25′ 05″

40   Beat Zberg (Swi) Rabobank at 1h 26′ 08″

41   Lylian Lebreton (Fra) Big Mat at 1h 28′ 19″

42 Andrea Tafi (Ita) Mapei at 1h 29′ 22″

43 Rolf Aldag (Ger) Telekom at 1h 29′ 27″

44 Koos Moerenhout (Ned) Rabobank at 1h 29′ 37″

45 Peter Meinert (Den) US Postal at 1h 29′ 52″

46 Riccardo Forconi (Ita) Mercatone Uno at 1h 30′ 33″

47 Fabio Sacchi (Ita) Polti at 1h 31′ 53″

48 Marty Jemison (USA) US Postal at 1h 34′ 27″

49 Nicolas Jalabert (Fra) Cofidis at 1h 38′ 45″

50 Massimo Donati (Ita) Saeco at 1h 38′ 59″

51 Tyler Hamilton (USA) US Postal at 1h 39′ 53″

52 Simone Borgheresi (Ita) Mercatone Uno at 1h 40′ 04″

53 George Hincapie (USA) US Postal at 1h 40′ 39″

54 Stuart O'Grady (Aus) GAN at 1h 46′ 04″

55 Filippo Simeoni (Ita) Asics at 1h 47′ 19″

56 Jens Heppner (Ger) Telekom at 1h 50′ 43″

57 François Simon (Fra) GAN at 1h 52′ 41″

58 Frankie Andreu (USA) US Postal at 1h 53′ 44″

59 Thierry Gouvenou (Fra) Big Mat at 1h 55′ 20″

60 Roberto Conti (Ita) Mercatone Uno at 1h 55′ 33″

61 Laurent Desbiens (Fra) Cofidis at 1h 56′ 28″

62 Erik Zabel (Ger) Telekom at 1h 56′ 57″

63 Léon van Bon (Ned) Rabobank at 1h 57′ 30″

64 Paul Van Hyfte (Bel) Lotto at 1h 58′ 02″

65 Jacky Durand (Fra) Casino at 1h 59′ 42″

66 Christophe Mengin (Fra) La Française des Jeux at 2h 00′ 35″

67 Frédéric Guesdon (Fra) La Française des Jeux at 2h 05′ 08″

68 Wilfried Peeters (Bel) Mapei at 2h 06′ 16″

69 Rik Verbrugghe (Bel) Lotto at 2h 06′ 17″

70 Magnus Bäckstedt (Swe) GAN at 2h 08′ 30″

71 Eddy Mazzoleni (Ita) Saeco at 2h 10′ 19″

72 Fabiano Fontanelli (Ita) Mercatone Uno at 2h 11′ 37″

73 Stefano Zanini (Ita) Mapei at 2h 12′ 11″

74 Alain Turicchia (Ita) Asics at 2h 14′ 12″

75 Mirco Crepaldi (Ita) Polti at 2h 15′ 05″

76 Diego Ferrari (Ita) Asics at 2h 15′ 46″
77 Xavier Jan (Fra) La Française des Jeux at 2h 15′ 51″
78 Pascal Lino (Fra) Big Mat at 2h 16′ 13″
79 Fabio Roscioli (Ita) Asics at 2h 17′ 53″
80 Christian Henn (Ger) Telekom at 2h 19′ 52″
81 Viatcheslav Djavanian (Rus) Big Mat at 2h 21′ 31″
82 Rossano Brasi (Ita) Polti at 2h 22′ 10″
83 Jens Voigt (Ger) GAN at 2h 25′ 14″
84 Pascal Derame (Fra) US Postal at 2h 26′ 25″
85 Tom Steels (Bel) Mapei at 2h 26′ 30″
86 Eros Poli (Ita) GAN at 2h 31′ 56″
87 Alexei Sivakov (Rus) Big Mat at 2h 33′ 19″
88 Aart Vierhouten (Ned) Rabobank at 2h 35′ 06″
89 Robbie McEwen (Aus) Rabobank at 2h 36′ 32″
90 Paolo Fornaciari (Ita) Saeco at 2h 37′ 50″
91 Massimiliano Mori (Ita) Saeco at 2h 38′ 12″
92 Bart Leysen (Bel) Mapei at 2h 39′ 43″
93 Francesco Frattini (Ita) Telekom at 2h 43′ 16″
94 Franck Bouyer (Fra) La Française des Jeux at 2h 43′ 45″
95 Mario Traversoni (Ita) Mercatone Uno at 2h 44′ 42″
96 Damien Nazon (Fra) La Française des Jeux at 3h 12′ 15″

Starters: 189
Finishers: 96
Distance: 3,712.1 km
Average speed: 39.988 kmh

Bibliography

Interviews

The 1998 Tour was not a straightforward race to live through for anybody, and some of the key individuals involved refused pointblank to discuss it with me, on or off the record. On this occasion, therefore, I am even more grateful to the following, in alphabetical order, for their interviews, valuable insights and willingness to give up their time.

Rolf Aldag: 4 June 2014
Frankie Andreu: 5 July 2014
Ian Austen: 19 January 2015
Chris Boardman: 19 November 2015
Fernando Escartín: 3 April 2015
Joerg Jaksche: 5 June 2014
Bobby Julich: 6 May 2015
Jean Marie Leblanc: 17 April 2015
David Millar: 10 September 2014
Jean Montois: 23 September 2014
Bjarne Riis: 2 December 2014
Manolo Saiz: 25 June 2014
Mario Traversoni: 22 January 2015

Books
(Published in English)
Albergotti, Reed, and O'Connell, Vanessa, *Wheelmen*, Headline 2013

Bassons, Christophe, *A Clean Break,* Bloomsbury 2014

Fotheringham, William, *Racing Hard,* Faber & Faber, 2013

Fotheringham, William, *Bernard Hinault and the Fall and Rise of French Cycling,* Yellow Jersey Press, 2015

Hamilton, Tyler, *The Secret Race,* Bantam, 2012

Kimmage, Paul, *A Rough Ride,* Random House, 2009

Millar, David, *Racing Through The Dark,* Orion 2011

O'Reilly, Emma, *The Race to Truth,* Bantam, 2014

Parisotto, Robin, *Blood Sports,* Hardie Grand, 2006

Rendell, Matt, *The Death of Marco Pantani,* Phoenix, 2007

Riis, Bjarne, *Stages of Light and Dark,* Vision Sports, 2012

Voet, Willy, *Breaking the Chain,* Yellow Jersey Press, 2002

Whittle, Jeremy, *Yellow Fever,* Headline, 1999

(Published in French)

Ballester, Pierre, *Fin de Cycle,* La Martinière, 2013

Brochard, Laurent, w. Lambert, Matthieu, *S'ils Savaient,* Idoines, 2013

Gaumont, Philippe, *Prisonnier du Dopage,* Grasette & Fasquelle, 2005

Guillon, Nicolas and Quénet, Jean-François, *Un Cyclone Nommé Dopage,* Solar, 2009

Keil, Patrick, *Du barreau aux barreaux,* Jean-Claude Gawsewitch, 2009

Leblanc, Jean-Marie, *Le Tour de ma vie,* Solar, 2007

Lhomme, Fabrice, *Le Procès du Tour,* Denoel, 2000

Menthéour, Erwann, *Secret Défonce,* Jean-Claude Lattès, 1999

Penot, Christophe and Leblanc, Jean-Marie, *Jean-Marie Leblanc, gardien du Tour de France,* Cristel 1999

Roussel, Bruno, *Tour de Vices,* Hachette, 2001

Virenque, Richard, *Ma Vérité,* Rocher, 1999

Vespini, Jean-Paul and Virenque, Richard, *Plus fort qu'avant,* Robert Laffont, 2002

Newspapers, websites, news agencies, TV channels and magazines
(Published in English)
Cycling Weekly, *Cycle Sport*, *ProCycling*, Velonews, cyclingnews.com, the *Guardian*, *New York Times*, AFP, AP, *The Times*, the *Independent*, Reuters, the *Daily Telegraph*, the *Observer*, Channel 4.

(Published in French)
memoire-du-cyclisme.eu, *L'Equipe*, AFP, *Ouest-France*, *Le Soir*, *Le Monde*, *Le Dauphiné Libéré*, *Le Figaro*, *Le Journal du Dimanche*

(Published in Spanish)
MARCA, As, *El País*, *El Mundo*, *El Mundo Deportivo*, *El Diario Vasco*, *El Correo*, *La Vanguardia*, RTVE

(Published in Italian)
La Gazzetta dello Sport

Acknowledgements

Thanks first and foremost to Naomi, for her patience, thoughts and support. And to Mar, for the drawings, the advice and the hugs. And to both of them, for being there.

In terms of the book itself, my deepest thanks go to my brother William Fotheringham, a hugely valuable source of advice, memories, reflections, contacts, books, magazines and newspapers from start to finish, not to mention his own writings on the race.

After six years, 1998 was our last Tour de France working directly together, too, and sharing a car throughout – mainly writing for *Cycling Weekly* and *Cycle Sport* and in William's case, the *Guardian* and the *Observer* as well. It proved to be a stressful swansong. As the scandals expanded, there were constant requests for extra copy, incessant calls from various editors and an endless stream of British radio interviews to handle – the copy being written on clapped out office-issue computers, the phone calls handled on a brick-sized, brick-minded early-generation mobile phone. We found ourselves praying for weekends, the only time when it seemed that French police would stop dropping in on Tour team hotels ... But if I got through the 1998 Tour and to Paris in one piece, it was in no small part due to William.

Many thanks to Stephen Farrand for taking considerable time out to track down and help interview former Italian bike riders for me. Also, for a memorable evening in Aix-les-Bains during the 1998 Tour where we put the cycling world (or at least our respective shares of it) to rights.

And to Jacinto Vidarte, then a *MARCA* correspondent, for his recollections about the Tour and not a few phone numbers, as well.

Thanks to Barry Ryan, for his comments, recollections, knowledge and support as well as being a willing interviewee about his personal recollections of the 1998 Tour de France stages in Ireland. Thanks to Barry, *The End of the Road* was both more enjoyable to write and is surely better as an end result. Thanks also to Jean-François Quénet, for his assistance and whose book on the Tour de France, *Un Cyclone Nommé Dopage*, co-written with Nicolas Guillon, was a hugely valuable source of reference. Last but not least, thanks to Ian Austen for sharing his considerable knowledge and insights about the state of anti-doping in the mid-1990s onwards.

On the book production front, thanks to Charlotte Atyeo of Bloomsbury Publishing for yet more sound advice, enthusiasm and hard work, to Richard Collins for his thorough, thoughtful copyediting work and to my agent, Mark Stanton of Jenny Brown Associates for helping get the book from vague concept to concrete reality.

Also (in alphabetical order) to Sam Abt, Daniel Benson, Javier Bodegas, Pierre Carrey, Sam Dansie, Marc Ghyselinck, Ed Pickering, Dave Prichard of Metro Books, Granada, Julien Pretot and José Luis Benito Urraburu. Also to François Thomazeau, for serious amounts of advice and warm interest.

And last but very much not least, to my mother, the author Alison Harding, for the same reasons as ever.

Index